THE
IMMUNE
ADVANTAGE

THE
IMMUNE
ADVANTAGE

How to Boost Your Immune System:
The Single Most Important Thing You Can
Do for Your Health

ELLEN MAZO and the authors of **PREVENTION** Health Books
with **DR KEITH BERNDTSON**

RODALE

This edition first published in the UK in 2003 by
Rodale Ltd
7–10 Chandos Street
London W1G 9AD
www.rodale.co.uk

Prevention and *Prevention* Health Books are registered trademarks of Rodale Inc.
Printed and bound in the UK by The Bath Press using acid-free paper from sustainable sources
1 3 5 7 9 8 6 4 2

A CIP record for this book is available from the British Library
ISBN 1–4050–3339-8

This paperback edition distributed to the book trade by Pan Macmillan Ltd

The quiz 'How connected are you?' on page 146 is from *Connect* by Edward M Hallowell, © 1999 by Edward M Hallowell, MD. Used by permission of Pantheon Books, a division of Random House.

Editor's Note

This book is intended as a reference volume only, not as a medical manual. The information given here is designed to help you make informed decisions about your health. It is not intended as a substitute for any treatment that may have been prescribed by your doctor. If you suspect that you have a medical problem, always consult a conventional medical practitioner before following any complementary therapies.

Beginning on page 446, you will find safe use guidelines for supplements, essential oils and herbs recommended in this book that will help you use these remedies safely and wisely.

Mention of specific companies, organisations or authorities in this book does not imply endorsement by the publisher, nor does mention of specific companies, organisations or authorities in the book imply that they endorse the book.

Internet addresses and telephone numbers given in this book were accurate at the time this book went to press.

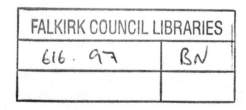
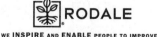

RODALE
WE INSPIRE AND ENABLE PEOPLE TO IMPROVE
THEIR LIVES AND THE WORLD AROUND THEM

About Prevention *Health Books*

The editors of *Prevention* Health Books are dedicated to providing you with authoritative, trustworthy and innovative advice for a healthy, active lifestyle. In all of our books, our goal is to keep you thoroughly informed about the latest breakthroughs in natural healing, medical research, alternative health, herbs, nutrition, fitness and weight loss. We cut through the confusion of today's conflicting health reports to deliver clear, concise and definitive health information that you can trust. We also explain in practical terms what each new breakthrough means to you, so you can take immediate, practical steps to improve your health and well-being.

Every recommendation in *Prevention* Health Books is based upon reliable sources, including interviews with qualified health professionals. In addition, we retain top-level health practitioners who serve on our board of advisors. *Prevention* Health Books are thoroughly fact-checked for accuracy, and we make every effort to verify recommendations, dosages and precautions.

The advice in this book will help keep you well informed about your personal choices in health care – to help you lead a happier, healthier and longer life.

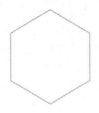

CONTENTS

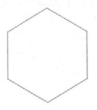

PREFACE

The Editors of *Prevention* Health Books are proud to present *The Immune Advantage*, one of the most valuable guides to optimum health we have ever produced.

Our mission was to bring you the newest, most effective, scientifically accurate information on how to harness our inborn, natural powers of wellness – to enhance and release the potential energy of the immune system. In order to accomplish this goal, our researchers and writers consulted with more than 95 doctors and health professionals – conventional doctors, herbalists, nutritionists, alternative practitioners and specialists in holistic medicine, Ayurvedic medicine, Chinese medicine and more. We spoke to psychologists, psychiatrists and family therapists. We also consulted hundreds of scientific papers and articles in professional journals. Then, our team of fact checkers verified the accuracy of every statement and every quote, so we are sure that we are bringing you the best available information on enhancing your immune system that exists anywhere.

We then went one step further. We consulted with Dr Keith Berndtson, medical director at Integrative Care Centers in Chicago and Glenview, Illinois, who specialises in bringing the best of conventional and alternative medicine together to treat his patients. We drew on his years of hands-on experience treating hundreds of patients and asked him to help us develop a simple, practical and effective programme for enhancing the immune system. The result of this unique collaboration is the Max-Immunity Plan featuring the Six-Facet Vitality Diamond.

We are convinced that the information we have gathered here will not be found in any other single source. If you follow the guidelines we offer, pay attention to our Immune Busters and Boosters and actively participate in our MaxImmunity Plan, you will reap the rewards of a healthy, vigorous life.

The Editors of *Prevention* Health Books

PART
1

The Immune
System:
What You
Should Know

Chapter

1

THE MOST IMPORTANT THING YOU CAN DO FOR YOUR HEALTH

Why is it that some people seem to have an endless supply of energy and others can hardly drag themselves out of bed in the morning? Or that some people seem to have one cold after another all winter long, while others are out there skiing and snowboarding without even a sniffle? Is it all just a matter of luck? The right genes?

Genes certainly are a part of the answer. But even genes no longer mean that we must be passive victims of fate. Today, we can measure our risk of getting various diseases that may run in our families and take practical steps to avoid them or lessen their effect. Some of these steps are as simple as avoiding certain foods and environmental toxins, and taking regular screening tests.

In addition to using knowledge of our genetic risk factors to safeguard our health, there are many other aspects of health that are in our own hands. In fact, there is nothing more powerful than the potential weapons of wellness that lie within us all. We are all born with an extraordinary system of immunity that serves as a natural defence against bacteria, viruses and other invaders. Your family tree may tell you a lot, but scientists now say that the strength of your immune system depends on your lifestyle choices: eating well, exercising, reducing stress and even taking a moment, perhaps, to say a prayer or simply think about the good things in life. It is that basic. That is why we believe that boosting your immune system is the most important thing you can do for your health.

If you take away nothing else from reading this book, remember this: you can take charge of your health and make simple lifestyle changes that might have a crucial effect on the quality – and perhaps even the length – of your life. Researchers say that it is never too late to boost your immune system. Scientists have proved that people who take steps to eat healthily show huge improvements in their daily lives, and that exercise is a kind of elixir of youth – a dramatic means of rejuvenating muscles and overall strength. As you adjust your lifestyle to reduce your risk of getting life-shortening diseases such as cancer and heart disease, you will increase your odds of living to a ripe old age. You may not have been able to select your genes, but you certainly can make lifestyle choices that will put your health in your own hands.

Learn How to Take Command of Your Health

To understand how your immune system works, think of it as an army. Imagine your cells as the soldiers gearing up for battle to defend against and attack invading germs and viruses. At all times, your immune system operates as a powerful defence, shielding you from the most common cold and the most deadly cancer. It is a magnificent machine that works with military timing and precision, with trillions of cells throughout your body moving in harmony through cooperation and communication.

Yet despite the awe-inspiring efficiency with which our immune systems work, they can also benefit from our help. This book will show you how to increase your defences with the Top 20 Immune Boosters, and what to avoid with the Top 10 Immune Busters. It will demonstrate how easy it will be to display a rainbow of fruits and vegetables on your dinner plate – a delicious way of making sure that you and your family consume the rich combination of phytochemicals that your immune system craves to protect it from the assault of free radicals. You will find out why it is so critical to wash your hands frequently, yet avoid common antibacterial products. We will show you how to protect yourself from environmental hazards that can weaken your immune system – including steps as simple as washing your new clothes before wearing them. You will also find out why parking your car at the far end of the carpark and taking the stairs to the office lavatory on another floor will add years to your life.

In fact, we will supply you with dozens of simple strategies that will help you live longer, including the most important supplements to take, the most promising stress-relieving techniques and some top exercises to boost your overall health and immunity. If you should experience health problems – perhaps you come down with the flu or pneumonia, get a sexually transmitted disease or experience chronic fatigue – we will show you how to work *with* your immune system so that your body best uses its innate healing ability to make you well once again.

Sometimes, your immune system can become confused and attack itself. In this book, you will learn how to care for yourself and your family when dealing with autoimmune disorders such as insulin-dependent diabetes, rheumatoid arthritis, lupus and multiple sclerosis.

The Vitality Diamond

Even when you are faced with immune-related diseases, you will discover the amazing power you have to enhance your immune system. You will learn how you can make your immune system shine – like the facets of a diamond. Rather than bore you with a regimented plan, we instead will give you health elements that you can easily incorporate into your life to ultimately create, for yourself and your family, a Vitality Diamond. With the guidance of Dr Keith Berndtson, medical director at Integrative Care Centers in Chicago and Glenview, Illinois, you will learn about all the ways in which you can boost your immune system for a long and healthy life.

SUCCESS STORIES

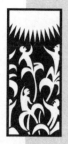

Together, They're Winning

Twelve years after his heart bypass surgery, John McCormick felt his pulse quicken. But a cardiologist's check showed that his arteries were clear – probably because of a major change in lifestyle that has left him full of energy and vitality.

If John hadn't taken such good care of himself, his quick pulse might have meant atrial fibrillation – an indication that his arteries could once again be blocked. But since his open-heart surgery at age 63, he's taken major steps to improve his eating and exercise habits – very specific immune-enhancing achievements – and he has a clean bill of health to prove it.

What's more, today, at 75 years old, he feels so much better than he did 12 years ago. He's also taken his wife, Connie, 74, along for the ride.

'I don't weigh any more than when I was first married,' says Connie.

'And I'm the same weight today that I was when I was drafted in 1944: 165 pounds,' John notes.

Granted, the parents of six children and 11 grandchildren do have a background in health. John worked in health education and research for more than 30 years, and Connie was a public health nurse for almost as long. They used to take their children ice-skating near their home in Dormont, Pennsylvania, and belonged to a local swimming club. They kept

Our Hidden Weapon

Would you ever have put peanut butter at the top of your immune-enhancing list? For years, diet books advised us to avoid peanut butter because of its high fat content. In fact, nuts and seeds are loaded with good fats, such as essential fatty acids, that actually *help* your cells to do their jobs. (Of course, if you have an allergy to peanuts, peanut butter is not suitable for you.) In this book, we give you the reasons why you should incorporate essential fatty acids and lots of other tasty nutrients sugary drinks out of the house and never served fried foods.

'I love to cook out (barbecue), though, and I used to grill hamburgers and steaks,' says John. He also enjoyed the occasional cigar and wine with dinner.

After his open-heart surgery, however, John took to heart his surgeon's recommendations. 'John has done what he was supposed to do,' says Connie. 'He exercises. He eats right. We follow a low-fat, low-salt diet with fish, chicken, turkey and lots of fruits and vegetables.' He also stopped drinking and smoking.

In the years since the surgery, the couple moved from their large home in Dormont to a townhouse in Bethel Park, Pennsylvania, which is close to a park, a golf course, a swimming pool, their church, shopping and three of their grandchildren.

'We looked at some places that would have required us to drive everywhere. They were much more isolated,' says John. 'Now, I can walk to church. I can walk to the post office, to the shopping centre. I can walk to the park. And that's what I do. Plus, I can take my bike out of the garage, ride about 1,000 yards on the berm (path) to the park, and then get on a path in the park.' John also plays golf every Wednesday during the summer in his church's golf league.

Arthritis plus a possible hip replacement have slowed Connie down somewhat. But they both enjoy swimming laps year-round in two local swimming pools.

Furthermore, both Connie and John are volunteers. They helped create and are active in a new health ministry at their church.

'We're staying busy and we enjoy it,' says John. Connie has another way of looking at it. She believes that an active, healthy lifestyle, at any age, leads to a better quality of life. By all accounts, it's working for this couple.

into your eating plan to keep your immune system strong.

It is no wonder that, for too long, we have been unable to stick to diets. Most diets are boring: not this one. Here, you will be able to refer to the MaxImmunity Diet to find a cornucopia of fruits, vegetables, nuts and seeds for a delicious, variety-filled diet to boost your immune system. As a special bonus, we will provide you with 50 tasty, healthy recipes to kick-start your immunity-boosting programme, such as Asian Green Beans with Beef (see page 427) and Citrus Chicken Breast with Mint and

Toasted Almonds (see page 404).

In addition, you will learn which vitamin and mineral supplements will boost your immune powers. After all, even the most healthy of diets cannot always provide all the essential vitamins and minerals that your body needs. (Refer to the Safe Use Guidelines on page 446 for specific dosage information as well as any other precautions and warnings associated with supplements mentioned in this book.)

The Emotional Connection

Finally, you will learn that your immune system is more than what you consume. A relatively new scientific field, psychoneuroimmunology, explains how your mind and body are inextricably linked. Your thoughts and emotions and your immune system are intertwined. What this means is that when you are tired, stressed, or depressed, you tax your immune system. Hormones are secreted that block your immune cells so that they cannot fight off bacteria and viruses. You become ill.

As Dr Berndtson will tell you, your immune system responds to *you*, to your choices. Caring for yourself is the most important thing you can do for your health. The best part is that you can take charge of your health, and we will be here to guide you every step of the way.

Chapter 2

THE BODY'S BEST NATURAL DEFENCE AGAINST DISEASE: YOUR IMMUNE SYSTEM

Have you ever known a family that has one member who catches everything that is going around, while her siblings seldom have even a cold? This occurs despite the fact that they share bedrooms, eat the same food and go to the same school. Long after she's become an adult, this person still has many more illnesses than her brothers and sisters – or anyone else. Why is it that some people are more susceptible to the germs that assault us every day? We all cut our hands on sharp objects, kiss people who are harbouring a flu virus, touch surfaces that are covered with microbes. Yet only some of us will develop an infection, come down with the flu, or be devastated by a bout of whatever is going around.

To guard us against these hazards, our body has a complex and sophisticated defence organisation: the immune system. Like any defence force, it is organised into different parts (like battalions) that stimulate each other and work together, although each one has its own special field of activity.

If they are functioning as they should, these defences protect us against the daily bombardment of infectious microorganisms, attacks that we usually do not even notice because our immune systems are so automatic and effective.

Our Defence Systems

The body's first line of defence is the *innate system*, which is the protections we are born with. They include our skin, mucous membranes, inflammatory response and secretions that contain toxic chemicals to destroy invading microorganisms. Bacteria and viruses are the most common invaders.

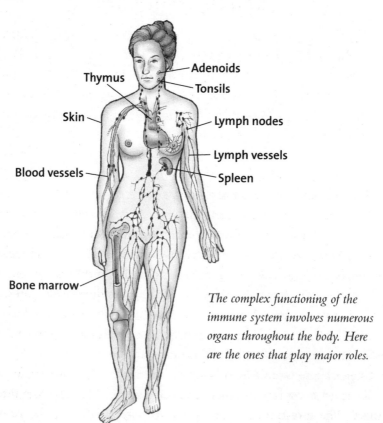

The complex functioning of the immune system involves numerous organs throughout the body. Here are the ones that play major roles.

The *adaptive immune system* is the body's second line of defence. It responds to an invasion of microbes by transforming whole classes of white blood cells into fighting cells, armed to attack specific invading microorganisms. This part of the immune system adapts its response to a particular invader. The process is complex, so adaptive immunity usually takes more time – days or weeks – to get under way.

The third defensive system is the *lymphatic system*. This is constantly at work filtering bacteria, abnormal cells and other foreign bodies from the lymph fluid.

Now that we have been introduced to the basic defence systems of our bodies, let us take a closer look at the individual parts that make up each of these general systems, beginning with the innate system.

Innate Immunity

The physical and chemical barriers we are born with provide a form of built-in, always present protection.

Skin. If it is whole – without cracks and scrapes – the skin is probably our most effective barrier against foreign microorganisms. The skin's protectiveness is enhanced by its secretions, which contain chemicals toxic to bacteria.

Eyes. The physical action of tears washes away any microbes. In addition, tears contain an enzyme that destroys bacteria.

Mouth. Saliva can also kill bacteria.

Nose. The mucus-coated hairs in the nose help trap organisms that ride in on dust particles. When we sneeze, we blow these organisms back out.

Respiratory tract. The cells that line the airways to the lungs secrete sticky mucus that snares invading microbes. Then, the movement of tiny hairs, called cilia, that line these airways carries the invading germs upwards out of the lungs and into the throat. Coughing then forces them out. This prevents germs from getting into the lungs, where the warm, moist environment would encourage their growth.

Stomach and intestines. Among the properties of stomach acid and enzymes is an ability to kill most microorganisms that enter the intestinal system. The intestines also are home to permanent colonies of helpful bacteria that destroy invading germs.

Reproductive and urinary tracts. These also contain helpful bacteria that compete with and reduce the numbers of dangerous bacteria. In addition, vaginal secretions are highly acidic much of the time, which protects the reproductive tract from microorganisms.

Natural killer cells. These are a type of white blood cell (or lymphocyte) which can destroy infected body cells and cancer cells before the adaptive immune system is alerted.

Dispersed throughout the body, they can act against any suspicious cell because they are able to recognise certain foreign substances on the surfaces of non-normal cells.

The inflammatory response. Inflammation is a defensive action that is usually limited to a local injury. It becomes activated when the body has been damaged – a muscle is torn or stressed, a joint overused, the skin cut or burned. It stops the spread of microbes from the site of an injury and removes cell debris and microbes so that repair processes can start.

Signs of inflammation are familiar: redness, warmth, swelling and pain. Blood vessels around the injury widen, causing redness, and more fluid than usual leaks from them into the surrounding tissue, which swells. These actions permit other troops of the defence system, such as white blood cells and certain blood proteins, to move in to fight the germs causing the infection.

Injured tissue releases inflammatory chemicals that attract armed white blood cells known as phagocytes to the area. Within an hour, phagocytes will be at the site of the injury, gobbling up dead tissue cells, bacteria and toxins, so that healing can begin.

Pus. If the injury is severely infected, creamy-looking pus may accumulate. This is a mixture of dead and living phagocytes, dead and living bacteria and bits of dead tissue cells. If the inflammatory process fails to clean up the site, the sac of pus may develop into an abscess and need to be drained before healing can take place.

Complement. This group of proteins circulates constantly in the bloodstream. When aroused by the presence of bacteria or fungi, they generate chemicals that augment or 'complement' the inflammatory response, hence the name.

CHILDHOOD IMMUNITY

A newborn is protected by the innate barriers we are all born with, plus antibodies and other protective proteins passed from the mother's blood supply before birth and in her breast milk afterward. These provide some immunity until the infant can develop her own antibodies to specific microorganisms. This is why modern research favours breastfeeding over bottle feeding.

Unfortunately, these early defences don't always stop every germ. As a child grows, she comes into contact with organisms that get past her body's basic defences and make her ill.

While her adaptive immune system is in the process of being activated to fight these pathogens, a child (or an adult) can become very sick and even die. In the past, in fact, many children died of common infectious diseases.

Today, the chances of a youngster avoiding serious illness are much better. Good nutrition strengthens young (as well as older) immune systems, and a clean water supply and better sanitation eliminate the sources of many serious diseases, such as cholera and typhoid fever.

Furthermore, timely vaccinations against common childhood diseases give most youngsters long-term protection against illnesses that once were devastating, such as measles, whooping cough, polio, diphtheria and mumps.

Adaptive Immunity

The various components of our innate immune systems are ready to function soon after they become aware of the presence of an invader. The adaptive immune system, however, takes longer to swing into action, largely because it is somewhat complicated. It must be triggered by contact with a foreign substance called an antigen before it can mount an attack. For this reason, the impact of adaptive immunity may not be felt for days, or even weeks, after we have been invaded by microbes.

Once it swings into action, adaptive immunity intensifies the inflammatory response. Most important, however, is the fact that this system mobilises an army of antibodies and killer white cells to destroy the invaders, whether they are floating in the blood and lymph or hiding in tissue cells.

The white blood cells then transform into warriors bent on finding and killing the identified invader. There are two types of fighting white cells, with the first letters of their names indicating their origins.

B-lymphocytes. These cells mature in the bone marrow and comprise about 10 per cent of the white cells that circulate in the blood.

T-lymphocytes. These cells mature in the thymus, a small gland that lies beneath the breastbone and is part of the immune system. T-cells make up 80 per cent of our circulating lymphocytes.

When attacking invading microorganisms, B-cells and T-cells have separate, but sometimes overlapping, tasks. The T-cells go after pathogens that hide inside cells. B-cells produce masses of antibodies to eliminate pathogens that are circulating in the blood or lymph.

B-cells: Armed with Antibodies

B-cell action is directed at many types of bacteria, some viruses and some parasites. Though it takes a while for the B-cells to recognise invading microbes as foreign, when they do, they manufacture antibodies

ALL ABOUT ANTIGENS

An antigen is anything recognised as foreign by – and that elicits an immune response from – its host. The word is derived from the phrase 'antibody generating'. Most antigens are large, complicated molecules.

The larger it is, the greater the number of *antigenic determinants* a molecule is likely to have. An antigenic determinant is a chemical on the antigen that arouses an immune reaction.

Because different antigenic determinants are recognised by different lymphocytes, a molecule that has a lot of them on its surface may provoke the development of many different antibodies against it.

Big, complex molecules, such as 'good' and 'bad' bacteria, can have hundreds of chemically different antigenic determinants, and so they evoke a big immune response. Simple molecules, such as those that make up hormones, produce little or no immune reaction. That's why certain plastics can be used for artificial body parts: they don't arouse a reaction from the recipient's immune system, so the replacement part is not rejected.

that flood into the blood and lymph (more about the lymphatic system later) and go hunting for the invading microorganisms. Antibodies operate by inactivating the enemy or marking it for destruction by other types of white cells.

Vaccines take advantage of the action of these B-cells. They arouse the B-cells to produce antibodies, which furnish a long-standing immunity to the particular germs – such as the polio virus – from which the vaccine is made.

Most vaccines are prepared from a whole microorganism or a part of a microorganism. To prevent vaccines from causing disease, however, the microorganisms are used in a weakened or killed form. They are still recognized as foreign by B-cells, however, which manufacture antibodies against them. When we are naturally exposed to germs or are vaccinated, we develop what is called acquired immunity. We develop this long-lived immunity because some of the B-cells that have been sensitised to the disease become 'memory' cells. If we are exposed to the

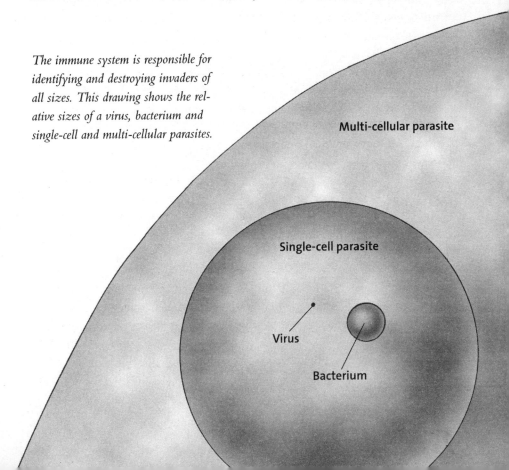

The immune system is responsible for identifying and destroying invaders of all sizes. This drawing shows the relative sizes of a virus, bacterium and single-cell and multi-cellular parasites.

Multi-cellular parasite

Single-cell parasite

Virus

Bacterium

OUR GENES DETERMINE
WHAT OUR IMMUNE SYSTEMS WILL RESIST

Although a lot of the features of white cell development are unknown, scientists do know that lymphocytes are changed into a disease-fighting form before encountering any antigens. They seem to be genetically programmed to recognise many different antigens as foreign. If the antigen makes an appearance, its presence mobilises the already primed white cells to act against it.

Our genes control our reactions to particular antigens. If we possess immune response genes, we're able to respond to a particular antigen; if genes are missing, we're unable to react. Our genes also can control how much of an immune response we're able to produce.

One of the most common immune problems is a deficiency of the immune system genes responsible for producing antibodies against upper respiratory ailments. People with this deficiency have more colds, flu and similar illnesses.

A much severer but rare genetic flaw that cripples both the innate and adaptive immune defences is severe combined immunodeficiency disease, commonly known as SCID. Babies born with SCID usually die of infections in their first year because they have no immunity against disease. In one well-publicised case, a boy with this deficiency survived because he lived in a huge plastic bubble, which protected him from contact with the ordinary germs of the real world. When he left the bubble aged 12, in the hope that his immune system might have improved, he became ill and died within 15 days.

same disease later, the memory cells will quickly generate antibodies to fight it off. Whether acquired naturally through contact with microbes themselves or artificially from vaccines, acquired immunity lasts a long time, often for a lifetime.

The secondary immune response aroused by memory cells actually is faster, more effective and longer lasting than the original response, because our immune systems already have been trained to attack those microbes.

Although the capacity of B-cells to produce antibodies and memory cells is an important function of immunity, B-cells have one major shortcoming. They are limited to the destruction of microbes that are not hidden within cells but are circulating freely, in the blood and lymph. Antibodies do not enter solid tissue unless the tissue has an opening, like a cut. This means that they are not very effective against those germs, such as tuberculosis bacteria, that hide in body cells in order to make thousands of copies of themselves.

Helper and Killer T-cells: Trained to Attack

Helper T-cells are the commanders of adaptive immunity. They are responsible for giving orders to all other white cells, which is why this is sometimes also called the cell-mediated branch of the immune system.

Helper T-cells stimulate B-cells to divide faster and form antibodies. They also use chemical messengers called cytokines to arouse other, more general immune defences. Without helper T-cells, our bodies cannot mount an effective immune response.

IMMUNODEFICIENCY

When a person's immune system fails to fight infections and tumours, that person is considered to be immunodeficient. Immunodeficiency can arise from an inherited problem that hampers the usual development of the immune system, or it can arise from a disease or a physical condition that injures the immune system.

Severe malnutrition, particularly protein starvation, and many types of cancer can lead to immunodeficiency. The best-known disease that causes this condition is infection with HIV, which precedes AIDS.

When a person's immune system is not working, she is susceptible to unusual problems. Infections by microbes that don't ordinarily cause trouble occur over and over again. Or she cannot recover from an illness despite getting treatment that is usually successful. She is often vulnerable to cancer. Such effects are often seen in seriously ill AIDS patients.

Autoimmune disorders are at the opposite end of the spectrum from immunodeficiency problems. With these disorders, a person's immune system is overreactive – mistaking cells that it should protect (body cells) for invaders that it should attack (for example, bacteria or virus microbes). When you have an autoimmune (literally, 'self-immune') disorder, your immune system directs its powerful defensive abilities against your own tissues.

Helper T-cells do not do it all, however. Another class of T-cells – the killer T-cells – shares in the heavy work of the immune response. Known as CD8-cells, these are the only lymphocytes that can directly kill other cells.

Killer T-cells circulate in the blood and cruise through the lymphatic organs looking for enemies they have been trained to kill. Some of these enemies appear on the surfaces of cells they have taken over. Their presence alerts roving killer T-cells, which then kill the germ-sheltering cells – a big step toward eliminating the disease.

'Their main targets are virus-infected cells, but they also attack tissue cells infected by certain intracellular bacteria (such as the bacillus of tuberculosis) or parasites, cancer cells and foreign cells introduced into the body by blood transfusions or organ transplants,' notes Elaine Marieb, R N, PhD, member of the Human Anatomy and Physiology Society, and textbook author.

Once an infection or disease has been eliminated, a group of lymphocytes called suppressor T-cells slows down or stops the action of B- and T-cells.

The Lymphatic System

Think of the lymphatic system as the body's own filtering system, sifting out or destroying bacteria, abnormal cells and other foreign bodies. The two major parts of this complex and efficient system are the lymph and the lymph nodes.

Lymph. Our bodies' tissues are constantly awash in fluid (lymph) that seeps from the blood vessels into the tissues. As it does, it collects cell debris and small, unwanted particles such as bacteria. Much of this fluid re-enters the blood system through the walls of the capillaries in order to maintain proper blood volume. The rest soaks into the even more porous lymphatic capillaries and is circulated back toward the heart via lymphatic ducts.

Lymph nodes. The lymph fluid slowly moves through the lymph nodes (also called lymph glands), which are strung along the pathways of the lymph ducts like pearls on a string. The lymph nodes are home to macrophages, T-cells and B-cells.

Lymph nodes function as filters, collecting microbes and other foreign material that the lymph has washed from our tissues. As a rule, lymph must flow through several nodes before being fully cleansed.

Also gathered in the nodes are many macrophages, large cells that ingest tissue debris, germs and anything else not wanted by the body. By cleaning this matter from the lymph, macrophages keep it out of the bloodstream.

Because lymph nodes are everywhere in our bodies, B-cells and T-cells are also widespread, ready to be mobilised against microbes.

Cleaning lymph is an important immune function of the nodes. Lymphatic capillaries are normally porous so that protein material can enter. When the tissues are inflamed, however, capillaries become even more porous, allowing larger particles, such as bacteria, viruses and cancer cells, to enter the lymph ducts. Although it is possible that infectious organisms could flow to other parts of the body via the lymph system, this danger is alleviated considerably by the filtering action of the lymph nodes.

When lymph nodes are fighting to contain an infection from spreading to the rest of the body, they become noticeably swollen and tender. Sometimes, the lymph conduits become inflamed, and the inflammation is visible as fine red lines on the inside of an arm, for instance.

Examining the lymph nodes in a breast cancer patient is an important procedure to determine whether the cancer has progressed. It saves lives by tracking the movement of cancer cells and helping to determine the most appropriate treatment. Cancer cells like to migrate through the lymph channels into lymph nodes in other areas of the body, says Dr Keith Berndtson, medical director at Integrative Care Centers in Chicago and Glenview, Illinois. For this reason, it is standard practice to remove the lymph nodes in the region nearest a source of cancer and analyse them for evidence of malignant cells. If malignant cells are present, the treatment strategy shifts from purely local to local and systemic anti-cancer approaches.

After cancerous lymph nodes are removed, lymphatic fluids may tend to back up in the tissues drained by those nodes, causing swelling in the area. But this does not appear to interfere with overall immune system performance, says Dr Berndtson.

Lymphatic Flow

Unlike the bloodstream, the lymphatic system does not have a heart to act as a pump. Lymph fluid flows very slowly, pushed along gently by the movement of muscles, pressures within our chests as we breathe and the pulses of nearby arteries. Muscles in the walls of the larger lymph ducts also help move the fluid along.

Movement in the muscle tissues closest to the ducts is important in lymph transport. When we are very active, lymph flows more rapidly and returns to the bloodstream more quickly, easily maintaining blood vessel volume. On the other hand, when part of the body is severely infected, it is helpful to immobilise that area to slow the spread of material from the site of the infection.

Other Organs of the Lymphatic System

In addition to nodes that filter lymph fluid, there are several other organs composed of lymph tissue that help protect us against disease.

Spleen. Because this organ is designed to cleanse blood supplies, blood is carried to it by a large artery that branches into smaller vessels within the spleen. Fist-size, spongy and deep red, the spleen is located on the left side of the abdominal cavity, just behind the lower ribs.

Along with filtering out used-up and defective red blood cells, the spleen is home to cleansing phagocytes that fight infection by foreign substances and other debris from the blood. Large numbers of lymphocytes and antibodies also reside here, ever watchful for invaders.

If the spleen has to be removed, its functions are taken over by other parts of the immune system; nevertheless, we become more vulnerable to infection.

Thymus. The thymus is located behind the breastbone in the upper part of the chest. Its main function is to transform white blood cells into the various types of T-cells able to mount an attack against disease organisms. The thymus is most active from childhood into adolescence, after which time it begins to grow smaller.

Tonsils. Lymph tissue forms a ring of small, oval masses around the entrance to the throat. The ones we are likely to notice are our tonsils. These are the most visible, and they can be painful if they become red and sore and swollen with bacteria, a condition called tonsillitis.

Tonsils are built to trap and destroy bacteria, which protects us against a lot of the germs we inhale or swallow. If the tonsils have white patches or a pale yellow substance covering them, they may be infected with streptococcus or another type of bacteria. Since these can be serious infections, a visit to the doctor and a throat culture are good ideas. In young children, tonsillitis is usually caused by a virus; in older children and adults, the cause is more likely to be bacteria.

Before antibiotics were available, removing the tonsils (known as a tonsillectomy) was a common childhood surgery. It was performed if a youngster had frequent bouts of tonsillitis, and is still done today if the infections are severe as well as frequent, since each time the tonsils become inflamed, scar tissue forms on them. However, it is not performed as frequently because of the important function the tonsils play in trapping bacteria and keeping them from entering the rest of the body.

With its three defensive systems and their interconnections, the immune system is complex, mysterious and amazing. When it is working properly, it fights off potential diseases and infections to which we never even know we have been exposed. To a great extent, if our immune systems are healthy, so are we.

Chapter

3

THE IMMUNITY AND AGEING CONNECTION

Eighty years old. Eighty. 80. LXXX. The number is the same no matter how you write it, but the meaning has changed. To some researchers, you are in your prime.

Young may be a stretch of the imagination, but not for long. With promising results from scientific breakthroughs, age 80 soon could be the halfway point in your life span.

These are not romantic notions of the Fountain of Youth. One of the most significant breakthroughs has come out of MIT (Massachusetts Institute of Technology), where Leonard Guarente, MD, professor of biology, is in the early stages of developing a drug that slows down ageing.

After years of research, he has found longer-lived yeast strains that could have a connection with human longevity. While yeast is way down on the evolutionary scale, it possesses a protein found in humans, called SIR2, which counters the ageing process. This remarkable protein is involved in helping low-calorie diets stretch our life spans.

Research has shown that consuming fewer calories reduces the free radicals that attack our immune cells, enabling us to maintain stronger immune systems so that we can live longer. Free radicals are oxygen molecules that because of various sorts of wear and tear have lost an electron. In order to regain their missing electrons, they steal electrons from other molecules wherever they can. The molecular victims of these raids are damaged in the process and become free radicals themselves. The free radical attacks on our cells have a cumulative effect. As time goes on, our immune systems become less and less vigorous in their response to diseases and infection.

'If the mechanism is the same in humans as it is in yeast, we could think about designing drugs that mimic the benefits of caloric restriction,' says Dr Guarente. 'That's the most exciting possibility.'

The prospect of taking a single pill to guarantee a long, healthy life is indeed enticing. If only it were that simple. 'There will be no pill that says you don't have to take care of yourself,' warns Dr Guarente. 'You'll have to take care of yourself to appreciate any benefit of a drug like this.'

Luckily, it is never too late to start.

Controlling the Clock

If I'd known I was going to live so long, I'd have taken better care of myself.
JAMES HERBERT BLAKE

For the most part, we are born with a kind of internal time clock, scientists say. Think of it this way: no one lives forever.

Fortunately, however, in many ways we have control over how we age.

Scientists do not have to tell us that over time, our bodies wear out. Our energy levels drop with our muscle tone and strength. Fat accumulates in our abdomens. Our hair thins, our bones weaken and we are confronted with sagging, wrinkled skin and fading memories.

Most scientists attribute these changes to the oxidative damage caused by free radicals attacking the cells. Another prominent theory involves a process called glycosylation, which causes glucose to bind with amino acid groups of proteins, altering the structure and functioning of the proteins themselves. The result: stiffening of the blood vessel walls and connective tissue.

For the most part, we assume that the rate at which this occurs depends on our heredity, or genes. We reason that we are destined to this fate, just as our parents and grandparents were. If we had been more intelligent, perhaps we would have picked different parents – the ones with stronger genes that could withstand the damage.

However, while our genetic makeup plays a role in longevity, it takes a lot more than good genes to determine the quality and length of our lives, says Robert Butler, MD, president and CEO of the International Longevity Center in New York City. For example, you are predestined by your genetic makeup to live to 110, but you smoke, drink and eat too much. You stay out in the sun too long. You worry needlessly, causing stress on your system. Your chances of reaching that age are diminished.

In addition, 'There may be those people who have much more limited protection from the longevity genes,' says Dr Butler. 'By maintaining good health habits, they can help their genes.'

One of the most significant studies by an international team of researchers reports that it is our lifestyle choices, much more than heredity, that determine our health and longevity. John W Rowe, MD, and Robert L. Kahn, PhD, two of the researchers involved with this 10-year study by the MacArthur Foundation Research Network on Successful Aging in Chicago, wrote *Successful Aging* based on its results. 'Research shows that it is almost never too late to begin healthy habits such as smoking cessation, sensible diet, exercise and the like. And even more important, it is never too late to benefit from those changes. Making these changes can mark the transition from the risky state we call "usual ageing" to the goal we share: "successful ageing" – growing old with good health, strength and vitality,' they write in the book. 'We can, and should, take some responsibility for the way in which we grow older.'

GROUP OF PENSIONERS DISCOVERS NOVEL WAY TO BEAT AGEING

'Dreams I discarded 9 months ago are now the objectives I want to achieve,' says Herb Nicholas, age 78. 'I'm healthier physically and mentally. I have more energy. It has a multiplier effect.'

And to think that all Herb did was respond to a letter from Bruce S Rabin, MD, PhD, director of the Brain, Behavior, and Immunity Center at the University of Pittsburgh School of Medicine. In the letter, Dr Rabin asked the retired management consultant to join a group of older people once a week at the Carnegie Library of Pittsburgh.

Older people need more than good nutrition for a strong, vital immune system, says Dr Rabin. We can counter the functional decline of our cells – and their increasing inability to fend off disease – as we age by staying active in a variety of ways, believes Dr Rabin, who is the author of *Stress, Immune Function, and Health: The Connection*.

Spending time with good friends, having a sense of humour, and exercising are among the strategies we can use to keep our immune systems strong, Dr Rabin says. Do you consider the glass to be half-full or half-empty? If you're the optimist, you are giving your immune system a good jolt.

Another tip from Dr Rabin: stop to say a prayer now and then. With spirituality comes a calmness that has a positive effect on the immune system. 'These behaviours help improve the quality of your health,' he says.

Age is only a number, Dr Rabin points out, and that number tells us nothing about how physically or mentally fit we are. He explains this point every week to the dozen men and women between the ages of 70 and 83 who meet at the Carnegie Library to learn about computers and to work out a way to teach what they've learned to others.

At first, the group thought it would prepare a manual, but the participants realized that if it was hard for them to read directions, it would be hard for others, too. Instead, they decided they would become tutors. That way, they could get out of the house and socialise more.

This project has been fun for Dr Rabin, who wanted to check out his thesis without a formal study. Anecdotally, he sees a difference in how the participants act and feel. And the participants' comments about the project seem to confirm Dr Rabin's findings. 'Doing this, I'm healthier physically and mentally,' insists Herb.

Never Act Your Age

How old would you be if you didn't know how old you was?
LEROY (SATCHEL) PAIGE, who at age 42 in 1948 was the first
African-American pitcher in the American Baseball League

What many people forget is that your chronological age is merely a number. 'A person can be 70 years old and physically and mentally fit, or age 70 and debilitated,' points out Bruce S Rabin, MD, PhD, director of the Brain, Behavior, and Immunity Center at the University of Pittsburgh School of Medicine.

Anne Taylor of Pittsburgh understands. At 82, the grandmother of five and great-grandmother of three planned to work as a receptionist forever. She had taken the job in a doctors' office shortly after her husband died 30 years earlier, and had thrived. She exercised by walking to work. She relished the camaraderie of colleagues and patients.

Then one day the doctors said they had to cut back, and Taylor was made redundant. Within a few weeks, she could not shake the lethargy that overcame her. She became increasingly worried that she would become forgetful, and the arthritis in her knees flared up. She stayed at home. 'It was such a shock. What could I do at my age?' she says.

Until then, she had done a good job of keeping her immune system strong and healthy. 'The mind and body have an impact on a person's health, particularly as they age,' says Dr Rabin, author of *Stress, Immune Function, and Health: The Connection*.

Taylor's family felt helpless as they watched the once energetic woman become sedentary. Finally, her granddaughter took the initiative and encouraged her grandmother to sign up for a water aerobics class at the YMCA. She reluctantly agreed, but then found that she liked the classes so much that she now goes 3 days a week. A friend joined her. Afterwards, they may go out to lunch, then to a film or shopping.

TAKE THE **FIRST STEP**

To begin to slow the effects of ageing *today*, get out of your chair and do some light exercise. You can boost your immune system, and slow key aspects of ageing, simply by following a moderate exercise programme, such as walking 30 minutes a day. Even better, add some weight-lifting to your workout during the week.

She renewed her library card and started doing crossword puzzles again. She is energetic and active once again. Taylor is living proof that age does not preclude health and vitality.

Keeping Your Immune System Strong

*In sum, how successfully one ages is largely determined by
how hard one works at it throughout life.*
FROM *SUCCESSFUL AGING*

In 2000 14.8 per cent of the European population was over the age of 65, a figure that is expected to rise to 19.3 per cent by 2020. Worldwide, more than 700 million people will be over the age of 65 by 2020. What can these people do to keep their immune systems strong so that they remain healthy and vital?

'As far as studies show, it's never too late to start, and it's always too soon to stop,' says Dr Butler. 'That doesn't mean if you do all good things that you're going to live forever. But you're going to be healthier.' No matter how old or young you are, you have control over keeping your immune system strong.

Shake a Leg

A number of studies have demonstrated that regular exercise can slow key aspects of ageing, such as loss of muscle and bone. In many ways, you can say that exercise keeps you young. In one significant study, researchers at the University of Pisa in Italy found that the blood vessels of vigorous older people functioned as well as those of athletes half their age.

With exercise, the immune system experiences a decrease in the production of stress hormones, and lymphocytes work better – a sure way to boost resistance to viral infections. A moderate exercise routine – walking 30 minutes a day, for instance – enhances the immune system, helping it become a kind of buffer between disease and stress.

Even people in their nineties can reap the benefits of lifting weights. When they pump iron, their muscles get bigger and stronger. Drs Rowe and Kahn tell of frail older people in a nursing home who performed three sets of exercises for their arms and legs on weight machines over the course of 8 weeks. 'The results were astounding,' they write. 'Muscle strength increased 174 per cent on average, and the walking speed of individuals increased by 50 per cent.' And these were people up to age 98. Dr Rabin stresses that it is not safe to exercise so hard that you risk hurting yourself. For beginners, a gentle exercise routine will accomplish a lot to improve both your mental and physical health.

Share with a Friend

A simple gardening project at the University of Texas in Galveston produced uplifting findings among 24 volunteers ranging in age from 63 to 90. These volunteers experienced an improvement in their overall feeling of well-being, specifically their psychological well-being.

The participants did more than just create flower beds and vegetable gardens: they shared stories about the spirituality experienced when working with the earth and stories about their favourite trees – ones they climbed, or planted or sat under – as children. 'It was the sharing of those childhood memories that enhanced their well-being,' says Diane Heliker, RN, PhD, assistant professor at the university's school of nursing, and the study's lead researcher. There was no physical decline among the volunteers after 4 months, she reported.

'Social support can modulate immune function,' explains Dr Rabin.

In addition to the benefits of a social support system, William Thomas, MD, a geriatrician in Sherburne, New York, believes he has proof that people live healthier and longer with easy daily access to plants, animals and children. 'Human beings were meant to live in a garden,' he insists.

The founder of the Eden Alternative, Dr Thomas has taken his philosophy to 300 nursing homes across the country, where residents keep their own pets, cultivate their own gardens and participate in programmes with children. 'We've found that residents have fewer infections, fewer falls and fewer skin wounds,' he says, adding that in most cases he has observed, the amount of medications required also dropped.

What about Those Calories?

Though Dr Guarente's work with yeast cells has shown incredible promise, it is only the beginning of what Roy Walford, MD, professor of

LIVING TO 150

Dixie Griffin Good is in her early forties, the mother of a boy and a girl barely out of nappies. She wants to be there for them as they grow up, marry and have children of their own. 'Then I can have time with my grandbabies – all before I become a really old, decrepit lady,' she says. 'I want a full range of physical and mental options as I age.'

It is for those reasons that Good, an education policy writer who lives in Denver, has been subsisting on an extremely low calorie, yet highly nutritious, diet espoused by Roy Walford, MD, professor of pathology at the UCLA School of Medicine, who all but promises up to 120 years of the good, healthy life.

Dr Walford, a member of the National Academy of Sciences Committee on Aging, believes it is possible to extend the human life span. Much of his work so far has applied to mice, but he became convinced his plan would work for humans after his experience in Biosphere 2 – a microcosm of the world, separated from the outside – when he subsisted with seven others on no more than 1,800 calories a day. 'I did the experiment in Biosphere 2, and we showed the exact same bio-chemical changes (drops in blood pressure and cholesterol as well as drops in the levels of indicators for diabetes) found in rodents and monkeys,' he says.

Several thousand people around the world are counting on Dr Walford's premise that the biomarkers of ageing are changed by caloric restriction. This was observed during laboratory tests that evaluated intellectual functioning and physical agility tests in older mice fed a calorie-restricted diet and younger mice fed a normal diet. Dr Walford observed that the older mice did just as well as the younger mice on both tests.

Even for the highly motivated like Dixie Griffin Good, however, such extreme caloric restriction can be hard to follow. At first, eating 1,200 to 1,400 calories a day left Good much too hungry. 'It's especially challenging when it gets cold,' she says. In addition to filling her plate with lots of vegetables, she added some more protein to her diet, and she says she now feels better. 'This is systematic under-eating,' she notes. 'It's not starvation.'

Good has dropped from 9 st 8 lb to 8 st 11 lb, but she wants to weigh around 8 st 3 lb. She is 5 ft 6½ in tall. 'Exercising is more pleasurable when you're not carrying around a lot of extra weight,' she says. 'Sometimes, I run or swim. And I do a lot of yoga and a little bit of weight-training. I feel confident I'm going in a positive direction.'

Dr Walford agrees. 'It will take 50 years for this to prove itself, but the evidence is overwhelming,' he says.

pathology at the UCLA School of Medicine, views as the key to extending our lives. A leader in the life extension movement, Dr Walford contends that we will be able to live to 120 and beyond by following a nutritionally dense, low-calorie eating plan that results in sustained weight loss.

Dr Walford notes the success of calorie-restricted diets on rodents, worms, flies, spiders and monkeys – and how their lives have been extended and disease incidence greatly reduced. But the evidence that caloric restriction works for humans was demonstrated when Dr Walford was a doctor inside Biosphere 2, a group that volunteered to live for 2 years in a 3-acre glass enclosure. The volunteers subsisted on a low-calorie, nutrient-dense diet that consisted mostly of vegetables, whole grains, some fruit and very little meat.

During the experiment, Dr Walford measured the physiological changes among the participants. He says that he found drops in blood pressure and cholesterol as well as drops in the levels of indicators for diabetes. The participants also lost 10 to 18 per cent of their body weight.

In his latest book, *Beyond the 120 Year Diet: How to Double Your Vital Years*, Dr Walford describes, based on laboratory tests, how the 'calorie restriction with optimal nutrition', or CRON, diet can slow down the ageing process. 'The rate of ageing on calorie restriction, depending on how rigorous it is, is cut by about a third to 50 per cent,' he estimates. 'Instead of ageing 10 years in 10 years, you'll age 5 or 6 years.'

Dr Walford has a following, though it is far too early to know just how successful they will be. No matter. He is optimistic. 'If you want to take advantage of things in the future, this is what you do now,' he says.

In fact, Dr Walford has been following his own plan for almost 16 years. Except for some muscle aches, he says he feels good. 'You slow the ageing whenever you start,' he says. 'I started at 60. I can't reverse my age to be 40 or 50, but I can stay at 60 for longer.'

Chapter 4

IS YOUR IMMUNE SYSTEM IN BALANCE?

How do you know whether this invisible thing called your immune system is healthy? If your dog's nose is cold and moist and his tail is wagging, you know he is feeling fine, even though he cannot say the words. If your computer does what you expect it to, you know it is working well. If it tells you, 'An illegal operation has been performed', you can do some diagnostic tests to find out what went wrong and how you can fix it.

You can do diagnostic tests to assess your immune system's function, too. If you know what to look for, your body can tell you that it needs looking after. Take this series of short quizzes and give your immune system its own diagnostic exam.

But first, how are you feeling right now? Fine? If so, that's a miracle, because at this very moment you probably have a billion viruses, bacteria, toxic chemicals and who-knows-what-else invading your body like the Mongol hordes. They want to give you a cold, the flu, a heart attack, even cancer, and the only thing standing in their way is your immune system.

Made up of unassuming little organs such as your spleen and thymus, and microscopic cells that go by their initials (T-, B- and NK, for example), your immune system is the only thing in the world more complicated than tax laws.

Despite all that complication, you can help make your immune system stronger. There are plenty of simple things you can do to raise and arm your own personal, internal militia to fight off everything from colds to cancer, and you can save yourself a lot of time and effort by focusing on shoring up your own particular weaknesses.

That is where this series of short quizzes comes in. Here you will find questions on nutrition, sleep, exercise, even your relationships and attitude toward life, because they all affect how well your immune system works.

Answer the questions and score yourself. Then turn to the particular chapters mentioned for more information and specific advice for giving your immune system a boost where it needs it most.

In addition, be sure to read the MaxImmunity Plan, beginning on page 305, to find out about the Six-Facet Vitality Diamond. There, you will learn how to maintain your immune system in the luxurious style that it deserves.

The Seasonal Sniffles Test

How often do you succumb to an illness during the cold and flu season?
   A. Never
   B. Once or twice
   C. Three times or more
   D. I seem to pick up every bug that comes along.

How do you usually handle a winter cold or flu bug?
   A. I barely notice it.
   B. I'm off sick for a day or two.
   C. I'm off for a week or more.
   D. Slip my post under the bedroom door; I'll see you in the spring.

How frequently do you experience the following? (score yourself on each one):

Skin rash **A.** Rarely or never **B.** Occasionally **C.** Often

Vaginal thrush **A.** Rarely or never **B.** Occasionally **C.** Often

Swollen glands (under the armpits or in the neck) **A.** Rarely or never
   B. Occasionally **C.** Often

Runny nose/postnasal drip **A.** Rarely or never **B.** Occasionally
   C. Often

Dark circles under the eyes **A.** Rarely or never **B.** Occasionally
   C. Often

Scoring: Give yourself zero points for each A, 1 point for each B, 2
   points for each C, and 3 points for each D.

Zero: Apparently, you're from the planet Krypton.

1 to 5: Your immune system seems to be in good shape, but turn to
   Colds and Flu on page 168 for some tips to get you through the flu
   season.

6 to 10: You may have a problem. Take the rest of the tests to help
   pinpoint your weaknesses.

11 to 16: Get away, you're probably contagious! Perhaps you should
   memorise the 20 Immune Boosters starting on page 106.

What's Going On?

'Multiple upper respiratory infections are a classic sign of lowered immunity,' says Kenneth A Bock, MD, co-founder and co-director of the Rhinebeck Health Center in Rhinebeck, New York, and author of *The Road to Immunity*.

Low-grade, long-lasting infections that cause nasal or sinus problems as well as swollen lymph nodes may mean that your system is struggling to do its job. Skin rashes or recurrent vaginal thrush could also mean that your immunity is impaired.

If all is as it should be, you will not get as many infections, and the ones you do get will not last as long.

If you scored high and wish that you did not have to waste so many days being ill, your immune system may need some pampering. Look at Immune Boosters and Busters on pages 106 and 134, and get some specific strategies for dealing with your illnesses on pages 155 and 168.

The Sneeze Test

Are you bothered by any of the following? (score yourself on each one):

Seasonal allergies **A.** Not at all **B.** An occasional sniffle **C.** Please pass the tissues. **D.** Leave the box.

Allergies to dust or mould **A.** Not at all **B.** An occasional sniffle **C.** Please pass the tissues. **D.** Leave the box.

Pet allergies **A.** Not at all **B.** An occasional sniffle **C.** Please pass the tissues. **D.** Leave the box.

Scoring: Give yourself zero points for each A, 1 point for each B, 2 points for each C, and 3 points for each D.

Zero to 3: You can breathe easy.

4 or 5: You probably have your allergies under control, but to find out how to protect your immunity when they do flare up, read The Top 20 Immune Boosters on page 106, and Allergies and Asthma on page 179.

6 or 7: Bless you! Is that the cat or a cold? Allergy attacks *could* be weakening your immunity.

8 or 9: Your allergies need attention. Once you have got them under control, you may find that, as a bonus, you have improved your immunity.

What's Going On?

Allergies do not mean that your immunity is weak. Rather the reverse: they are, in fact, more like a sign that your immune system is a little *too* alert. An allergy attack occurs when your body overreacts to something in the environment, such as pollen, dust or animal dander.

Over time, repeated allergy attacks can contribute to what Dr Bock describes as immune load, or overload. An immune system that is constantly using almost all its resources during allergic reactions may well, as you can imagine, be less effective when it has to deal with a real threat, such as a cold virus.

Pay particular attention to Allergies and Asthma on page 179, and follow the MaxImmunity Plan starting on page 305.

The Motion and Rest Test

Which of the following best describes your exercise routine?

A. Non-existent, except for jumping to conclusions and running late.

B. Once a week, if I have the time, I'll do some light walking or the equivalent.

C. I work out two or three times a week, doing a light to moderate workout.

D. I exercise as often as I can and don't stop until I'm sweaty and totally exhausted.

How much sleep do you get?

E. Plenty. I never miss out on my Zzzs.

F. Not enough. I'm exhausted by the end of the day and feel like a zombie when I wake up.

G. It varies. I often stay up later than I should, but I usually catch up within a few days.

H. I couldn't identify my pillow in a police line-up.

Scoring: Give yourself zero points for C or E; 1 point for B or G; 2 points for A, D, or F; and 3 points for H.

Zero or 1: You know when to move and when to stop, and your immune system appreciates it.

2 or 3: You're in pretty good shape, but you may have some bad habits that need correcting.

4 or 5: It's time to take a hard look at what you've been doing – or not doing.

What's Going On?

Both exercise and sleep are good for your immune system – in the right amounts. 'Moderate exercise is an immune booster,' says Dr Bock, who notes that it takes half an hour of aerobic exercise to sweep back into circulation the white blood cells – key immune system components – that are stuck on the blood vessel walls. Studies also show that the amount of certain types of immune system cells increases, at least temporarily, following exercise.

Beyond any direct effects that exercise may have on the components of the immune system, it also helps you sleep and reduces stress, both big pluses. Poor sleep can actually reduce the activity of so-called natural killer cells that fight germs and cancer; stress hormones bind to your immune cells, hampering their ability to fight off illness.

Look at the exercises in the MaxImmunity Exercise Plan, starting on page 331. For tips on getting restorative sleep, turn to the MaxImmunity Stress Relief and Sleep Plan, on page 347. Even more sleep tips appear in The Top 20 Immune Boosters on page 106.

The Game of Life Test

How would you describe your interactions with other people?
> **A.** I have friends and/or family, but I rarely have time to keep in touch with them.
>
> **B.** I'm very close to a few friends and/or family members.
>
> **C.** I have close friends and/or family, and I also spend time with acquaintances at work or in voluntary/interest groups.
>
> **D.** Shut up and leave me alone.

People who know you would most likely describe you as a . . .
> **E.** Realist
>
> **F.** Pessimist
>
> **G.** Optimist
>
> **H.** Motorist

Scoring: Give yourself zero points for D, E, or H; –1 point for F; 1 point for A or G; 2 points for B; and 3 points for C.

–1 or zero: The good news is, you have plenty of friends. The bad news is, most of them are germs.

1 or 2: Be careful. You may be exposing yourself to unhealthy amounts of stress.

3 or 4: You're probably friendly and positive, which is healthy in more ways than one.

What's Going On?

It's no news flash that stress is not healthy. But what exactly does your social and family life have to do with how often you become ill? More than you might think. One review of 81 published studies found that social support – the network of friends and family that helps you cope with stress – had a measurable effect on several benchmarks of immune system function.

Experts think the reason is that positive relationships can prevent the immune-dampening impact of stress hormones such as cortisol. 'It's also possible that the relaxing psychological states people feel when they're not stressed – being in a positive mood, feeling satisfied with life – have an immunity-promoting effect,' says Bert Uchino, PhD, associate professor of psychology at the University of Utah in Salt Lake City, who directed the review. Dr Bock puts it more strongly: 'Love is an immune system nutrient, while isolation and loneliness are counter to a healthy immune system.'

Just as your attitude toward life can mean the difference between a clogged nose and clear sinuses, it can also mean the difference between life and death. Studies show that optimists live longer, and when pessimists put a more positive spin on the calamities in their lives, they have less stress and better health. In part, it is because optimists take better care of themselves, and, in part, it is because anything that mitigates stress can prevent damaging changes to your immune system – such as your faithful bodyguards, the natural killer cells, suddenly becoming pacifists. In one study, cancer patients who completed a special course designed to make them more optimistic had stronger immune systems than those who did not.

You need not be stuck with the attitudes you were born with. Give yourself a full-blown attitude adjustment with the inspiration and tips in Enhance Immunity with the Power of the Mind (page 96) and the Max-Immunity Emotional Quotient Plan (page 356).

The Healthy Eating Test

Which of the following combinations would you be most likely to bring back from the salad bar?

A. Pasta salad, lettuce, sweetcorn

B. Melon slices, tomatoes, walnuts

C. Cream crackers, celery, pineapple chunks

D. Pudding, potato salad, brownie

Do you take a multivitamin every day?

E. Yes

F. No

Scoring: Give yourself zero points for A, D, or F; 1 point for C or E; and 2 points for B.

Zero: Oh dear. Your immune system may be running on empty.

1: Your dietary instincts could use some fine-tuning.

2 or 3: Congratulations! Your internal army is probably well-fed.

What's Going On?

'We've known for some time that when a person is malnourished, her immune system is weakened,' says Jeffrey Blumberg, PhD, chief of the antioxidants research laboratory at the USDA Human Nutrition Research Center on Aging at Tufts University in Boston. 'When you restore the person to normal nutrition, the immune system improves, which is no surprise. But what we're just learning is that when you continue to improve nutrition beyond mere adequacy, the immune system continues to improve, even in healthy people.'

How much of an impact can nutrition have? In one study, Dr Blumberg and his colleagues discovered that boosting the vitamin E intake of a group of 70-year-olds seemed to make their immune systems function more like those of 40-year-olds.

Make permanent changes in your daily eating habits that will help you maintain a healthy weight and avoid disease. Each week, adopt a few of the suggestions that start on pages 51 and 308.

Strengthening

Your

Immune System

for Optimum

Health

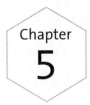

ACTIVATE YOUR BODY'S IMMUNE POWER WITH THE MAXIMMUNITY DIET

E<small>AT WORMS.</small>

Eat worms? Although worms may not be on the top of your shopping list, once upon a time they were essential to our digestive systems.

For thousands of years, our immune systems were used to having worms in our guts, says Joel Weinstock, MD, professor in the division of gastroenterology at the University of Iowa in Iowa City. Over time, as our lives have become more antiseptic – breathing clean air in airtight buildings, drinking pure water, eating refined and artificial foods – the worms have died off. Our immune systems may have suffered as a result.

It appears that our immune systems are now overproducing powerful inflammatory agents, such as gamma interferon, that are important for the control of harmful bacteria and other pathogens. For some people, as

SUCCESS STORIES

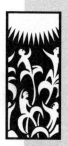

Her Packed Lunch Was the Key to Newfound Energy

Sometimes, a little menu adjustment is all you need to boost your energy levels all day long. Consider Mary Elizabeth Welling, a lawyer in Pittsburgh.

Mary was tired. Very tired.

'Of course, I wasn't surprised,' she says. Her life was busy: work, family, volunteer activities through her church, taking care of her ailing father. 'I was dragging all the time,' she recalls.

Mary tried to find time for breakfast before catching the bus in the morning, and she grabbed whatever fast food was available for lunch. By late afternoon, hunger pangs set in, but she tried to ignore them. She was famished by the time she got home for dinner.

Then she thought back to a time when her office was across town, not far from a deli that offered individual servings of vegetables, fruit and nuts for snacks. Every afternoon, she would take a break, walk to the deli for some fruit and nuts, and then take a longer walk before returning to work. 'I felt so much better then,' she remembers.

So, Mary began packing her own lunch: a peanut butter sandwich, some fruit and some cut-up vegetables. When she could, she found a park bench to sit on while eating her lunch, then took a walk along the Allegheny River. Within a few weeks, she was more energetic. If anything, she is busier than ever.

Since then, she has learned about the power of nuts, thanks to *Prevention* magazine's MaxImmunity Diet. She is sure to incorporate nuts and seeds into her family's diet, often sprinkling sunflower seeds on salads or mixing chopped walnuts into oatmeal.

In addition to walking at lunchtime every weekday, she now walks to church on Sundays, enjoys digging in her garden, and takes the family dog, Lily, for long walks in the park.

'I have to incorporate everything I do into my lifestyle. Otherwise it wouldn't get done,' Mary says. 'I'm not as tired anymore. I feel so much better.'

many as 1 million a year, this overproduction has resulted in severe chronic intestinal inflammation, which we call inflammatory bowel disease, for which there is no cure.

Noting these problems, Dr Weinstock thought that perhaps the people most severely afflicted would respond to worms. He found patients willing to swallow 2,500 worm eggs (they hatch and settle in the intestines). The initial small, controlled study was a success: the participants' immune systems got stronger. However, no one is suggesting you actually eat worms. For most of us, there are much tastier solutions.

Research scientists agree that much more palatable fruits, vegetables, grains, proteins and fats will keep your immune system healthy. They know that with just a sprig of broccoli, a sip of skimmed milk, a bite of an apple, a forkful of tuna, or a spoonful of whole-grain cereal, we are on the way to enhancing our immune systems.

'Good, healthy food in the gut produces hormones and proteins to keep us healthy,' says Paul Lebovitz, MD, medical director for the Allegheny Center for Digestive Health in Pittsburgh. 'There's no getting around that.'

Starting with the Cells

The human immune system depends on thousands of nutritional elements found in the foods we eat. Each nutritional element has a distinct role, but its influence comes with the synergy created.

We are made up of about 75 trillion cells, each one getting something from all the nutrients found in what we eat. By working together, these nutrients energize our cells. To keep this complex network of cells strong and intelligent the nutritional supply must be plentiful.

It's easy to understand strength, but intelligence, too? Absolutely. The immune system is clever enough to know instantly which cells belong to the body and which are harmful invaders. Further, it is programmed to react: It can help heal something as simple as a nasty shaving cut or help to destroy something as potentially dangerous as viruses, bacteria or parasites all before they can hurt us. 'The immune system has circuits upon circuits that sense its environment,' says Dr Weinstock.

Just as our brain cells give us the ability to identify and remember, our immune cells hunt down the invaders, or antigens, and keep them from coming back. To do the job well, our immune cells voraciously consume carbohydrates, fats, protein, water and, most important, vitamins and minerals.

If the immune cells do not get the proper amounts of these nutrients, however, they can be thrown off balance. Think of your immune system as a tightrope walker performing a high-wire balancing act. Without the right amount of vitamins, minerals, proteins, carbohydrates and fats, it can fail to work properly.

Malnourished immune cells become weak, inefficient and powerless. On the other hand, a well-nourished body can realise what may seem miraculous: good health, always. 'Food creates a composite of everything your body needs for a strong immune system,' says Leslie Bonci, RD, MPH, spokeswoman in Pittsburgh for the American Dietetic Association and the director of the sports medicine nutrition programme at the Center for Sports Medicine at the University of Pittsburgh Medical Center Health System. 'So, if anything, getting enough good, healthy food is more critical than anything else.'

TAKE THE **FIRST STEP**

To start eating more healthily today, think 'variety.' The best way to ensure that you get the largest possible number of different phytochemicals – compounds that fortify our cells – is to eat a wide range of different fruits and vegetables. One easy way to do this is to strive to eat foods that are different colours – orange sweet potatoes, red tomatoes, green spinach and pink grapefruit, for example.

Fortunately, even if you have eaten unsoundly in the past, your immune system can still regain its balance. 'Immune cells are constantly being formed,' says Namanjeet Ahluwalia, PhD, assistant professor of nutrition at Pennsylvania State University in State College. 'You have to think of the body as being in a constant state of flux in terms of the immune response.' This gives us an opportunity to repair and improve the immune response by maintaining our nutritional status.

Furthermore, age is no excuse, Dr Ahluwalia says, just as long as you do not let down your nutritional guard. In a study comparing older women with younger women, she found that the older women who ate healthy diets kept themselves as immune-system-sound as their younger counterparts.

Pile Your Plate with Phytochemicals

Phytochemicals are the very reason people should start eating a diet top-heavy in fruits and vegetables now, says Paul Lachance, PhD, executive director of the Nutraceuticals Institute at Rutgers University in New Brunswick, New Jersey. 'You name it. They prevent everything from gastrointestinal cancer to heart disease to infectious diseases,' he says.

For years, scientists have known which basic vitamins and minerals are in fruits and vegetables and other plant foods. They have learned, however, that the food system is not that simple; there are literally thousands upon thousands of compounds in the foods and beverages we consume, all interacting with our cells in ways still being discovered.

These compounds are phytochemicals, substances found in the plant system with the strength to ward off fungi, insects and viruses. When we consume fruits, vegetables and other plants, those same compounds fortify our cells. They become boosters of our immune systems, operating like antioxidants, the molecules that protect our cells from harmful oxygen substances known as free radicals.

In the herb basil, for instance, phytochemicals known as terpenoids detoxify cancer-causing substances. The selenium in Brazil nuts is also a cancer-fighting element, and the lycopene in a glass of tomato juice helps prevent heart disease as well as decrease cancer risks.

Researchers are hot on the phytochemical trail, continually uncovering them in foods and learning more and more about their roles in boosting our immune systems. Consider that almonds, a source of monounsaturated fat and sterols, help reduce cholesterol, or that watercress contains cancer-fighting compounds, including isothiocyanate. The list goes on.

'Nature has devised brilliant ways of presenting phytochemicals and nutrients in fruits and vegetables. For that reason, it's beneficial for us to consume a wide variety of them,' says Ranjit Kumar Chandra, MD, PhD, research professor at Memorial University of Newfoundland; director of the World Health Organization's Center for Nutritional Immunology in St. John's, Newfoundland; and author of *100 Percent Healthy in 100 Days*.

Furthermore, the immune system strengthens within only a few weeks of healthy eating.

So, how do you take advantage of the abilities of phytochemicals? The easiest way is to first understand the different, broad categories into which they fall. You do not have to remember the seemingly unpronounceable names of each group, but by remembering to eat brightly coloured foods in a wide variety, you will be able to choose a more varied and healthy diet. These foods also contain compounds that have a profound effect on health maintenance and disease prevention.

Terpenes. Found in everything from broccoli and oranges to soya and grains, these phytochemicals act as antioxidants. Terpenoids also have a subclass, known as carotenoids. These are the ingredients that give fruits and vegetables their colours, like the red in tomatoes, the green in spinach and the pink in pink grapefruit. But not all phytochemicals are colouring pigments; some carotenoids are found in the whites of citrus.

Phytosterols. These substances are related to cholesterol, yet they are the ones that are powerful enough to block bad LDL-cholesterol, helping to lower the risk of heart disease and inflammation. Pumpkins, rice, green peppers and summer squash are all rich in this element.

Phenols. These potent antioxidants protect our cells against infections and inflammatory conditions such as arthritis and allergies. The deep blue and violet colours of berries, grapes and aubergine are clues that they contain these powerful antioxidants. Scientists also are intrigued by the phenols' ability to block the conversion of precursor molecules into carcinogens; this might hold promise in learning how to prevent cancer.

AND THEY SAY SWEETS AREN'T GOOD FOR YOU

A study conducted by the Harvard School of Public Health has shown that sweets are not only mood boosters but may also help you live longer.

Researchers followed a group of Harvard graduates for 5 years and discovered that those who ate sweets were likely to live significantly longer than non-consumers. Mortality was lowest in those who consumed sweets one to three times a month, though it rose in more frequent consumers.

That's right. Researchers speculate that chocolate has a lot of phenols, antioxidant chemicals that boost the immune system.

More studies are being carried out. Until then, enjoy.

Flavonoids. There are close to 4,000 flavonoids, all with powerful abilities to enhance the effects of vitamin C. Found in foods such as camomile (apigenin), apples (quercetin) and grapefruit (hesperidin), they are a mighty bunch, protecting blood vessels and strengthening tiny capillaries so that oxygen and essential nutrients can get to all cells.

Isoflavones. These substances, which are concentrated in soya-based foods, have received a lot of publicity because they have been found to block enzymes that promote tumour growths. Studies show that Asian women who consume diets rich in tofu and soya milk have lower incidences of breast and uterine cancers.

The Ayurvedic Way

Balance, variety and moderation are integral to the philosophy of Ayurveda, which uses a holistic system of medicine, meaning that our minds, bodies and spirits are all taken into consideration in the diagnosis and treatment of any illness.

Many practising Ayurvedics are delighted that Western scientists are validating what they have been claiming for thousands of years. They believe in the immune-enhancing effects of phytochemicals in fruits, vegetables and grains. After all, food is the key to a healthy, vital life for those who practise Ayurveda. They believe that wholesome food is responsible for happiness, or health, while unwholesome food brings on misery, or disease.

'Ayurveda is the science of life,' says Sada Shiva Tirtha, DSc, director of the Ayurveda Holistic Center in Bayville, New York, and author of *The Ayurveda Encyclopedia*. 'We look at everything in moderation.'

In Ayurveda, each food plan is personalised to fit an individual's needs. 'Common sense and intuition will guide you,' says Dr Tirtha.

Clearly, much of what is being learned in laboratories confirms what has been practised for centuries in India, particularly in regard to the use of Indian herbs to boost our immune systems.

Stock Up on These Nutrient-Rich Foods

As scientists have learned more and more about the specific roles of nutrients, they have discovered which vitamins and minerals are vital in the making of a strong immune system. Dr Lachance suggests that you include some of the following vitamin- and mineral-rich foods in your diet.

- Leeks, chives, garlic, onions, shallots: they contain at least 200 phytochemical compounds that boost the immune system.

IMMUNE-FRIENDLY SNACKS (THAT EVEN CHILDREN WILL LOVE)

Boosting your immune system can be as tasty as an ice lolly or as satisfying as some chips. Try out the following sampler of snacks that are not only delicious but also give your immune system added nourishment.

Honey-flavoured sesame seeds (90 g/3 oz). These seeds are filled with magnesium, an immune-boosting mineral that helps in the regulation of calcium in the blood and is vital in controlling blood pressure.

Orange juice (240 m/8 fl oz). A refreshing drink, orange juice is packed with vitamin C, an antioxidant that helps tissue growth, promotes healthy gums and protects against the harmful effects of pollution. Many brands of orange juice include calcium, an important mineral that keeps bones strong and is a protective factor against high blood pressure and colon cancer.

Frozen fruit bars (230 g/8 oz). Look for those made with fruit juices. Whether they are raspberry, cherry, grape or papaya, these are delicious sources of phytochemicals, the immune-boosting plant compounds that protect our cells.

Chips (115 g/4 oz). Fry them in olive oil or safflower oil, and you have a favourite snack that's high in potassium, a high-powered nutrient.

Sweet potato (one medium). Sweet potatoes are naturally high in vitamin A, which has compounds known to be resistant to cancer.

Dry-roasted sunflower seeds (90 g/3 oz). These tasty seeds with the nutty flavour are high in vitamin E, an antioxidant good for circulation, and selenium, a cancer-fighting mineral.

Oysters (75 g/3 oz cooked). This tasty food is high in zinc, an important cancer-preventing mineral.

Dried apricots (45 g/1½ oz). High in beta-carotene, this sweet treat also contains potassium, a key mineral in keeping blood pressure down.

Papaya (one medium). This juicy fruit is high in vitamin E, folate, magnesium and potassium, all of which help keep your circulation strong and blood pressure down.

• Soya beans: their immune-enhancing effects are legendary – they protect the heart, lower bad LDL-cholesterol levels and suppress growth of cancer cells.

• Bok choy, broccoli, brussels sprouts, cabbage, cauliflower, kohlrabi, mustard greens, watercress: all cruciferous vegetables are rich in phytochemicals and contain anti-cancer antioxidant compounds. They also have folic acid, vitamin C, fibre and alpha- and beta-carotenes, which are converted into vitamin A by your body.

• Apricots, carrots, green peppers, leafy greens, sweet potatoes: these foods contain many carotenes, which are members of the carotenoid family. The carotenoids are responsible for giving many fruits and vegetables their vibrant colours.

Think 'Variety' for Optimum Nutrition

Your mother may have told you to eat your vegetables, but did she also encourage you to eat an apple or a pear for dessert? If so, she couldn't have been more right, says Dr Lachance.

To emphasize this point, Dr Lachance agrees with the plan advocated in the MaxImmunity Pie shown on page 60, which sounds and is delicious. In addition to including a few select supplements, the pie graph illustrates variety, moderation and servings for the MaxImmunity Diet. This exclusive vegetarian diet is composed of six mini-meals a day that are balanced and healthy. For those unwilling to take the plunge into a vegetarian diet, you may add up to 90 g (3 oz) – the size of a deck of cards – of cooked meat or poultry per day to your diet. If you desire, you can also eat up to seven eggs a week; if you have diabetes or high cholesterol or are overweight, however, you should limit yourself to no more than four eggs a week. But, of course, this is not part of the basic plan – you will get enough protein on the MaxImmunity Diet without adding meat.

Every day, we should eat a minimum of nine servings of vegetables and fruit, because these foods have the power to enhance the immune system. 'There's nothing mysterious about this,' Dr Lachance says. 'We can't pick a food and say, "This is the answer." It's the combination of things over time. With this plan, you double or even triple the effects on boosting

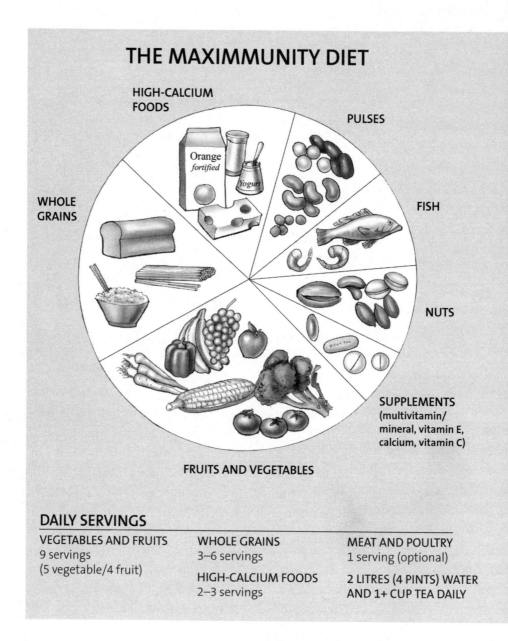

THE MAXIMMUNITY DIET

HIGH-CALCIUM FOODS

PULSES

WHOLE GRAINS

FISH

NUTS

SUPPLEMENTS
(multivitamin/
mineral, vitamin E,
calcium, vitamin C)

FRUITS AND VEGETABLES

DAILY SERVINGS

VEGETABLES AND FRUITS 9 servings (5 vegetable/4 fruit)	WHOLE GRAINS 3–6 servings	MEAT AND POULTRY 1 serving (optional)
	HIGH-CALCIUM FOODS 2–3 servings	2 LITRES (4 PINTS) WATER AND 1+ CUP TEA DAILY

your immune system. There's no such thing as too much fruit, or too many vegetables. That's the beautiful thing about this food system. You can't overdose when you eat the right foods.'

Some people may question the fact that seeds, nuts and pulses have a significant 'slice' on the pie graph. They should note, however, that the

WEEKLY SERVINGS

PULSES	NUTS	FISH
5+ servings	5 servings	2 servings

SERVING SIZES

VEGETABLES AND FRUITS
1 serving = 60 g (2 oz) chopped fruit
60 g (2 oz) cooked or raw vegetable
115 g (4 oz) raw green leaves
80 ml (3 fl oz) vegetable or fruit juice
1 medium piece of fruit

WHOLE GRAINS
1 serving = 1 slice wholemeal bread
115 g (4 oz) brown rice or bulgur
60 g (2 oz) whole wheat pasta

HIGH-CALCIUM FOODS
1 serving = 240 ml (8 fl oz) skimmed or
semi-skimmed milk
240 ml (8 fl oz) fat-free or low-fat yoghurt
240 ml (8 fl oz) calcium-fortified orange juice
1 ounce reduced-fat cheese

PULSES
1 serving = 115 g (4 oz)
cooked dried pulses/lentils

NUTS
1 serving = 30 g (1 oz) ,
chopped

FISH
1 serving = 90 g (3 oz), cooked

MEAT AND POULTRY
1 serving = 90 g (3 oz), cooked

SUPPLEMENTS

MULTIVITAMIN/MINERAL
100 per cent RDA for most nutrients a day

CALCIUM
Under 50 years old: 500 mg a day
Over 50 years old: 1,000 mg a day

VITAMIN E
70–250 mg a day

VITAMIN C
100–500 mg a day

omega-3 fatty acids in seeds and nuts, as well as in fish, provide energy and protect our cells by helping to lower blood fats. This means that 2 tablespoons of nuts five times a week is both a tasty treat and an immune system booster. Equally important are the soluble fibre and folate found in pulses, which lower blood cholesterol levels.

The Key Nutrients

To be sure that you are getting enough of the key vitamins and minerals, read this list of the essential nutrients.

Beta-carotene. Beta-carotene is found in dark green, leafy vegetables and fortified milk. Your body converts it into vitamin A on an as-needed basis. Vitamin A enhances white blood cell function, increases resistance to infection and carcinogens and helps maintain skin and mucous membrane defences to infection.

B vitamins. Boost your intake of B_6 and B_{12} with turkey, prune juice, chickpeas and bananas. Vitamin B_6 is needed for white blood cells to ensure that they are ready to defend our immune systems, while vitamin B_{12} governs cell division and growth. Other sources include eggs, cheese, milk, poultry, tuna, beef liver and cod. The Recommended Daily Allowance (RDA) for vitamin B_6 is 2 mg. The RDA for vitamin B_{12} is 1 mcg.

Vitamin C. Our white blood cells depend on this vitamin to combat infections. It also keeps intact the defences of our mucous membrane, which is one of the immune system's physical barriers. Vitamin C is found in citrus fruits, strawberries and raw red peppers. The suggested daily intake for vitamin C is 100–500 mg.

Copper. The richest food sources are pulses, whole grains, nuts, shellfish, organ meats and seeds. This trace mineral turns white blood cells into aggressive attack forces against invading germs. The suggested daily intake for copper is 1.2 mg.

Vitamin D. It was not known until recently just how critical vitamin D is in helping the thymus gland generate a sufficient number of immune system cells. Though it is found in eggs, butter and fortified milk, you also get vitamin D each time you walk in sunlight. The RDA for vitamin D is 5 mcg. If you are over 50, however, some experts recommend you take at least double this amount.

Vitamin E. Scientists have long promoted the E vitamin as a powerful antioxidant, shielding immune cells from abuse by free radicals. Wheatgerm provides a powerful dose, as do molasses, whole grains, nuts and seeds. The RDA for vitamin E is 10 mg.

Folate (Folic acid). This vitamin functions well with vitamin B_{12} and is critical in the development of the nervous system of the foetus. Its name comes from the Latin word *folium*, which means 'leaf'. Kale, asparagus, cabbage, whole grains, beetroot and root vegetables are good sources. The RDA for folate (folic acid) is 200 mcg.

Iron. Found in red meat, green leafy vegetables and raisins, iron is used to produce haemoglobin in the blood. The RDA for iron is 14 mg.

Selenium. Good sources of this trace element are whole grains, nuts, seeds, broccoli and fish. It acts as an antioxidant and is associated with lower rates of cancer. The suggested daily intake for selenium is 75 mcg.

Zinc. The best sources are turkey (dark meat), ham, sirloin steaks and seafood: you get five times the amount you need by eating only six steamed oysters. Without zinc, your immune cells would not have the strength to

SIMPLE SECRETS FOR HEALTHY EATING

A quick rule of thumb for healthy eating is to eat fruits and vegetables of different colours. Since the different colours often indicate different compounds, just having a colourful diet can ensure that you are eating the healthiest combination of foods. For example, orange and yellow foods such as carrots, melons and sweet potatoes contain beta- and other carotenes. Blueberries and aubergines contain phenols, and ruby red tomatoes and grapefruit contain terpenes.

In addition to turning your dinner plate into a rainbow of colours, think about the timing of your meals. What you eat, how much you eat, and when you eat can help – or hurt – your immune system.

To keep your immune system strong, eat small meals every few hours, recommends Leslie Bonci, RD, MPH, spokeswoman in Pittsburgh for the American Dietetic Association and director of the sports medicine nutrition programme at the Center for Sports Medicine at the University of Pittsburgh Medical Center Health System. 'You need to keep your body on an even keel, and you do that by eating smaller, more frequent meals,' she explains. 'You want to minimise excess. An immune-enhancing plan is one that takes into account your energy level, and you get energy by eating every few hours.'

You may think that you're eating too much when you consume frequent meals, acknowledges Paul Lachance, PhD, executive director of the Nutraceuticals Institute at Rutgers University in New Brunswick, New Jersey. 'But it's possible to consume all the necessary nutrients in as few as 1,800 calories a day – as long as you start with breakfast,' he says.

ward off antigens. This is one of the reasons why some researchers believe that zinc may shorten the duration and severity of colds, says Bonci. The RDA for zinc is 15 mg.

So, now that you have been introduced to the basic essential vitamins and minerals, you might be wondering what is the most efficient way to get the powerhouse of elements you need to boost your immune system. Fortunately, the answer is simple: consume a wide variety of foods because synergy among the various components of food is essential. After all, if you ate the same foods day in and day out, you would quickly be bored. Well, our cells react the same way. To get the benefits of all the compounds, they need variety. Instead of having an orange at breakfast every day, try having a bowl of mixed berries on Sunday morning, half a melon on Monday, and a sliced kiwi fruit on Tuesday, all with yogurt or skimmed milk, suggests Dr Lachance, who never has the same breakfast 2 days in a row.

Why Not Just Swallow Vitamin and Mineral Supplements?

Considering our frenetic lifestyles and mile-long 'to do' lists, shopping for fresh, colourful produce and then making sure that we eat numerous servings of it each day might seem like a daunting prospect. Surely it would be easier to forget that and just pop a multi-supplement?

Unfortunately, multivitamins are no substitute for a healthy, varied diet. First of all, our natural food system, as it exists in nature, is so complex that even the best manufacturers cannot create pills or powders with all the immune-enhancing benefits our immune cells demand, says Dr Lachance. Second, extremely large doses of vitamins and minerals can do more harm than good. Too much vitamin C, for example, can mask subtle bleeding of precancerous polyps, and an excess of vitamin E can cause undue blood thinning.

Nevertheless, studies show that people who take a multivitamin have better health. 'I'm totally convinced that senior citizens – and I'm talking about people 60 and up – need vitamin and mineral supplements,' says Dr Chandra. He believes that at least one-third of that population has deficiencies because of poor eating habits, and that they need to boost their immune systems with vitamin and mineral supplements.

Chapter 6

BODY BASICS: KEYS TO A BALANCED IMMUNE SYSTEM

THE SISTERS OF THE DIVINE PROVIDENCE MAY WELL HOLD THE key to a strong, healthy immune system.

In a study at the University of Pittsburgh, researchers found that the group of Roman Catholic nuns fell asleep more quickly, were less likely to awaken in the early morning, and spent more time in the deep sleep stage than a control group of women the same age. In addition, they possess a 'younger-looking sleep', one that keeps them vital and energetic for their daily chores and prayers.

As any sleep-deprived person can confirm, a good night's rest is an elixir – and so is exercise, a jolly belly laugh and good friends. Research has found that going on a long walk, watching a funny film, or visiting family and friends strengthens the immune system for overall good health. The feel-good feeling we get from these activities enhances the immune system's ability to stave off disease and illness, says Bruce S Rabin, MD, PhD, director of the Brain, Behavior, and

Immunity Center at the University of Pittsburgh School of Medicine.

When we are at ease and relaxed, we help calm down the parts of our brains that produce stress hormones. At that time – whether we are feeling optimistic, enjoying a good joke or just generally feeling good about ourselves – we are in essence 'buffering' our immune systems, protecting them from suppression and from being unable to function normally, says Dr Rabin, author of *Stress, Immune Function, and Health: The Connection*.

To understand the importance of buffering the immune system, we first need to take a look at the damage that occurs in our bodies when we are feeling stressed. After that, we shall explore some ways to strengthen our natural defences against stress and its ill effects. After all, the Sisters of the Divine Providence are not the only ones with the power to improve their immune systems.

The Havoc Stress Wreaks

Every time we become tense and anxious from lack of sleep, job and family pressures and yes, even loneliness, stress hormones attach themselves to our immune cells, inhibiting their ability to fight off illness. Scientists say, too, that stress hormones kill brain cells, which is why we may become forgetful and distracted when we cannot handle the pressures we face in our daily lives.

It is during these times that areas of the brain become activated to produce higher concentrations of stress hormones, or cortisol, putting us at risk of disease, says Dr Rabin. In turn, the higher secretion of stress hormones impedes the body's ability to fight infections, leading to problems such as high blood pressure, heart disease and diabetes.

Take Advantage of the Healing Power of Sleep

Like the nuns in the study, we can give our immune systems the strength they need by first getting a good night's sleep, says Charles F Reynolds III, MD, professor of psychiatry and neuroscience at the University of Pittsburgh and director of the university's Sleep and Chronobiology Center.

HERBS THAT HELP US SLEEP

Quality of sleep plays a big part in keeping your immune system strong, says Charles F Reynolds III, MD, professor of psychiatry and neuroscience at the University of Pittsburgh and director of the university's Sleep and Chronobiology Center. 'Good sleep helps us cognitively and emotionally, so we can better solve the day-to-day problems that face us,' he says.

Here are some herbs that promote stress relief by helping us to relax and get some sleep, suggested by David Winston, founding member of the American Herbalist Guild and president of Herbalist & Alchemist, Inc., in Washington, New Jersey. Because herbal preparations can vary slightly from manufacturer to manufacturer, Winston advises us to follow the dosage instructions on the label.

Valerian root. This herb is a reliable treatment for nervousness and insomnia. It acts as a sedative but doesn't cause dependence or addiction. Because it is so potent, however, it should not be used with sleep-enhancing or mood-regulating medications. Valerian is available as a tablet, capsule, tea or tincture. Be aware that it has a mildly unpleasant odour and bitter taste, so some people may want to avoid it as a tea. High doses can cause nervousness in a small percentage of people.

Hops. Generally known as a flavouring in beer, hops helps relax the nervous system. Those who are seriously depressed, however, should avoid them, as should pregnant women. Dried strobiles, or flowering parts, can be used to make a bitter-tasting tea, though it isn't as effective as a capsule or tincture.

Camomile. This is a gentle herb that soothes the nerves and promotes relaxation. Most commonly available as a tea, it also comes in pill form or capsules. To make a tea, steep 1 teaspoon of camomile flowers in 240 ml (8 fl oz) of hot water, covered, for 20 to 25 minutes; drink 2 to 3 cups a day. People with severe hay fever allergies (ragweed, asters and chrysanthemums) should avoid this herb because it could cause similar allergic reactions.

California poppy. Not only is this California's state flower, it's also an excellent sedative and painkiller, and you can use the whole plant, especially the root. It's used primarily as a tincture.

'Poor sleep interferes with protein synthesis in the brain, and that in turn can have an impact on our ability to remember and learn,' says Dr Reynolds, who was a researcher on the nuns' sleep study. He suggests that we prepare for the optimal 7 to 8 hours of sleep a night by 'winding down' 15 to 30 minutes before bedtime with, perhaps, a warm, relaxing bath or calm, soothing music.

School administrators in Edina, Minnesota, witnessed the power of sleep first hand in 1996 when they decided to delay their high school's first class by an hour to give their teenagers and teachers an extra hour of sleep. Since the school bell started ringing at 8:30 a.m., students have missed fewer days of classes because of illness, and they are getting better grades, says Kenneth A Dragseth, PhD, superintendent of the Edina Public Schools.

There are tangential benefits, too. 'Before, everyone had to rush out of the house. Now, parents can have conversations with their kids in the morning. All around, it's a nicer environment,' Dr Dragseth notes. As the Edina model demonstrates, we often fail to step back and examine our options for creating a strong, healthy immune system.

TAKE THE **FIRST STEP**

To help balance your immune system and keep it strong, make a point of getting 7 to 8 hours of sleep tonight. If you usually have trouble falling asleep because you can't stop worrying, try taking a warm bath or listening to soothing music half an hour before going to bed. Or try praying or meditating to release the worries of the day from your mind.

Calm Down

'Just as stress affects our hormones, so does relaxing,' says Dr Rabin. 'The relaxing things you do calm down the areas of the brain that produce the stress hormones.'

This means that we have control over creating the foundations for a strong immune system with even the simplest of actions, such as painting, gardening, reading or taking a holiday.

In fact, holidays can mean the difference between life and death, according to researchers who looked at the holiday patterns and causes of death among more than 12,000 middle-aged men at risk of heart disease. The more times the study's participants – aged 35 to 57 – skipped their annual holidays over 5 years, the more likely they were to die in the next 9 years.

Those who took regular, annual holidays had a 21 per cent lower risk of death and a 32 per cent lower risk of heart disease.

'People who don't take vacations may be chronically on guard. This sort of vigilance has been shown to be associated with elevated blood pressure,' says Brooks B Gump, PhD, assistant professor of psychology at the State University of New York at Oswego and a researcher on the study. 'These spikes in blood pressure may be the mechanism whereby arterial walls are damaged and atherosclerosis develops.'

Think about your last holiday and how much you enjoyed being with family and friends. Perhaps you played tennis, swam and went for bike rides. While you were having fun, you gave your immune system a much-needed break by limiting the amount of stress hormones your body produced. Now, instead of feeling guilty about taking time away from work and other responsibilities, do your immune system a favour and line up a holiday for this year.

Light Up Your Social Life

Your immune system could use a friend, or two or three. For good reason: the more gregarious you are, the less chance you have of getting a cold.

Over a number of years, David Skoner, MD, chief of allergy and immunology at Children's Hospital of Pittsburgh, and his colleagues have injected more than 1,000 men and women with cold viruses to see who is most susceptible to the sniffles.

Before sequestering the participants in hotel rooms for a week of reading, TV watching and rest, the scientists administer psychological tests to determine personality types. Over the course of the week, some of the participants come down with the sniffles; others do not. Time after time, it has been the ones classified as loners who get sick, says Dr Skoner. The conclusion is obvious: the stress of isolation in loners' lives has a negative impact on the immune system, while positive relationships prevent the immune-dampening effect of stress hormones such as cortisol.

The researchers have found that those who socialise with up to only three people – including spouses, parents, children, friends or colleagues – at least once every 2 weeks are four times more likely to develop colds than those who spend time with at least six people. 'This demonstrates how important it is to strive for a stress-free life,' says Dr Skoner. 'It's so important to make lots of friends – through work, church, school.'

There are other things you can do, however, if making friends is not one of your favourite pastimes. 'Even if you don't make friends easily, you can help your immune system by becoming more active,' notes Dr Rabin.

Get Moving

People who exercise regularly are less likely to become ill when confronted with stressful situations. This is because the areas of the brain that are provoked by stress are the same ones activated by exercise. 'When you continually turn those parts of the brain on by exercise, it becomes harder and harder to turn them on by stress,' Dr Rabin says.

Think of exercise as preventive medicine for the immune system, says Dr Rabin. To get the full benefits of exercise, strive to do something to boost your heart rate for 30 to 45 minutes 5 days a week. Simply going for a walk or taking a bike ride will do the trick.

Look on the Brighter Side

Jeweller and storyteller Cathy Raphael, author of *It's Our Turn to Play!!!*, finds that when she speaks gibberish to make others laugh and replaces her dreary brown and navy blue clothes with hot pink, purple and other cheerful colours, she feels better. She believes the people around her do, too.

In a study by Lee S. Berk, MPH, DrPH, a neuroimmunologist and laughter expert at Loma Linda University School of Medicine in California, 10 healthy men who watched a self-selected funny video for an hour showed significant increases in cytokine gamma interferon, a booster to the immune system.

The late author Norman Cousins may have predicted the study's result more than 20 years ago. In his book *Anatomy of an Illness As Perceived by the Patient*, he wrote that '10 minutes of genuine belly laughter' gave him 'at least 2 hours of pain-free sleep'.

Stricken by a disease of the connective tissues, Cousins described how much his positive outlook helped him overcome pain during his recuperation. He watched the spoofs on old television episodes of *Candid Camera*, and the outright slapstick of Marx brothers' films. A nurse read amusing books to him. 'I was greatly elated by the discovery that there is a physiologic basis for the ancient theory that laughter is good medicine,' he wrote.

If anything, the Cousins model demonstrates that 'there truly is magic in play and laughter,' says Raphael.

Go Hands-On

Chinese medical texts discussed it 4,000 years ago. Western health care has advocated it as a form of therapy for centuries, too. Recent studies confirm its stress-busting benefits to the immune system. There is no doubt about it: massage has helped people for centuries.

In one trial, 20 men with immune systems weakened by HIV demonstrated less anxiety and improved immune functions after undergoing 45-minute massages 5 days a week for a month. Their number of cytotoxic T-cells, which help in the regulation of the immune system, increased – as did their number of cells that annihilate viruses and tumours, according to researcher Gail Ironson, MD, PhD, professor of psychology and psychiatry at the University of Miami in Coral Gables.

Dr Ironson and two colleagues with the Touch Research Institute in Miami have just completed a study that looked at the effect of massage on women with breast cancer. Thirty-four women with stage I and stage II breast cancer, post-surgery, received two massages per week for 5 weeks. At the end of the study, the women reported a decrease in depressed mood, anxiety and anger and an increase in natural killer cells as well as dopamine and serotonin, brain chemicals involved in regulating mood.

Write Creatively

Putting your thoughts on paper can help you look at your problems in a less stressful way.

At the University of Texas at Austin, James W. Pennebaker, PhD, a psychology professor, found that people who wrote about traumatic events for 20 minutes a day, three to five times a week, had half as many visits to their doctors as people who did not write. Once on paper, those stressful issues seem to dissipate, reducing your stress hormones.

Another encouraging finding of the study was that the antibody response to bacteria and viruses was more vigorous in the participants who wrote than in those who did not write. Therefore, pick up a pen and start putting your thoughts on paper instead of keeping them bottled up.

Drink Up

You know how uncomfortable a dry mouth can be. Well, that is how your immune system's cells feel when they are dehydrated. Without enough water, your system becomes parched and sluggish and your cells draw water from your bloodstream, leaving you feeling tired and sluggish. Your body is forced to work harder to pump the blood, which is now thick and sludgy. So drink 2 litres (4 pints) of water a day to keep your cells plump and healthy.

Daydream, Meditate or Pray (or Try All Three)

Imagery is a relaxation technique similar to daydreaming. As you allow images to drift through your mind, you heighten your immune response to disease. Again, you are calming down that part of your brain that otherwise would produce stress hormones.

Studies have demonstrated that both prayer and non-religious meditation elicit relaxing effects. Harold G Koenig, MD, director of Duke University's Center for the Study of Religion/Spirituality and Health in Durham, North Carolina, urges his patients to keep an open mind about the existence of God, but agrees that non-religious meditation can be effective. In his book, *The Healing Power of Faith*, he urges readers to pray or meditate – whatever works for them. He stresses, however, that you should have some kind of belief system for the meditation or prayer to boost your immune system most effectively.

In fact, studies at Duke University have found that religious people live longer. Those who attended religious services regularly had lower blood levels of interleukin-6 – a hormone that rises with stress, leading to greater infections and disease. 'The element of getting your eyes off of yourself and being with others, praying with others, serving others, relating to others – that may be the key in helping your immune system,' Dr Koenig says.

The Sisters of the Divine Providence would have been the first to agree with Dr Koenig's findings. While the University of Pittsburgh researchers attributed the nuns' solid sleeping habits to their highly regulated, busy schedules that leave no time for daily worries, the sisters disagreed.

They told the scientists that their untroubled sleep comes with the territory. They are the ones who go to bed each night with clear consciences enhanced by their religious calling, the nuns explained.

'I liked both explanations – the scientific and the theological,' says Dr Reynolds, who conducted the research. 'Either way, they proved to be active, engaged and vital.'

Chapter

7

PROTECT YOURSELF FROM ENVIRONMENTAL HAZARDS

WHERE ARE POLLUTANTS LURKING IN OUR ENVIRONMENT? A better question might be where *aren't* they. Consider:

• Factories, cars, power plants and other sources release millions of tons of toxic pollution into the air each year, according to the US Environmental Protection Agency (EPA). These pollutants can float in the air that we then breathe, or they can drift down to contaminate our food, drinking water and soil.

• In 1995, world pesticide consumption reached 2.6 million metric tons of active ingredients. You can be exposed to these chemicals by using them around your home – as 85 per cent of families in developed countries do – or by consuming pesticide residues in your food and water.

• Data from the mid-1990s found that more than a quarter of the British population were drinking tap water polluted with various toxic

74

chemicals, lead, bacteria and other potentially harmful ingredients.

Pollutants that enter our bodies can cause many types of health problems, including diarrhoea, fertility problems, nerve damage and cancer. But just what marks are they leaving on our immune systems?

According to the watchdog organisation Environmental Working Group, federal government studies indicate that all people in the United States are carrying around at least 100 chemical pollutants, pesticides and toxic metals in their bodies. It is not known just how all these get into our bodies, and it is virtually impossible to study all of their health effects. When a toxin is studied, it is often just in terms of its relationship with cancer.

'The fact is that we understand relatively little even today about the immune responses to various environmental toxins. There aren't that many researchers in the world conducting that kind of research,' says Lee Newman, MD, an immunotoxicologist and head of the division of environmental and occupational health sciences at the National Jewish Medical and Research Center in Denver. 'And there are many chemicals in use today for which there are no data in terms of their human toxicity, let alone their human *immune* toxicity. There's a lot that is just not known.'

Dr Newman and fellow immune system researchers know that certain substances can trigger autoimmune diseases. For example, excessive exposure to hydrazine (a jet fuel ingredient) has been associated with lupus. But these kinds of situations generally are the result of an intense exposure to the toxin in the workplace, which would be more likely to happen to specific workers than to average people in their everyday lives, Dr Newman notes.

While it is hard to generalise – and he acknowledges that there will be exceptions – 'It's pretty hard in scientific studies to demonstrate much of a long-term effect from passive environmental exposures,' says Dr Newman. 'As a general rule, John Q Public shouldn't be worried about his general environmental exposures, until he gets into places of high concentrations.'

Dr Newman does, however, stress the importance of 'sensible living'. For some doctors, this means being vigilant in avoiding *any* unnecessary exposures to potentially unhealthy chemicals, for the simple reason that we know so little about so many of them.

'Since World War II, how many tens of thousands of industrial chemicals have been produced that didn't have wartime uses anymore?' asks Keith Berndtson, MD, medical director at Integrative Care Centers in Chicago and Glenview, Illinois. 'Since manufacturers were making these things, they had to come up with peacetime uses for them, and so we were delighted to learn that we could use them to destroy roaches in our

THE MOST UNWANTED LIST

The US Agency for Toxic Substances and Disease Registry maintains a priority list of its top hazardous substances of concern. The list is decided in part by considering how toxic the substance is and how often it's found on hazardous waste sites around the country. Here are the top five substances on a recent list published by the agency, along with some of their health effects.

1. Arsenic. Found naturally in water, air and soil, arsenic is also present in wood preservatives, insecticides and weed killers. Ingesting some forms of it increases the risk of skin cancer and bladder, kidney, lung and liver tumours.
2. Lead. Mostly as a result of activities such as mining and manufacturing, lead is found throughout our environment. It can damage the kidneys, nervous system and immune system when it is breathed in or swallowed.
3. Mercury. This metal may be found in contaminated seafood and in fumes from industrial combustion. It can damage the nervous system, including the brain.
4. Vinyl chloride. Long-term exposure to this gas used in making plastic products has mainly been studied in workers who make or use the substance. It can cause liver cancer, immune reactions and nerve damage.
5. Benzene. Widely used in manufacturing, benzene is also found in glues, paints, lubricants and dyes, among other products. Levels of it are usually higher in indoor air than in outdoor air. Long-term exposure can damage bone marrow and can harm the immune system, increasing the chance of infections. It's also a known human carcinogen.

houses, kill weeds and any number of other uses.'

While our bodies have slowly adapted to cope with toxins found naturally in the environment, these new chemicals might 'throw a different type of curve,' Dr Berndtson says. 'This is speculative; let's be honest about it. But it sometimes is worth speculating in the name of preventive medicine.'

One general guideline to remember when considering chemicals you want to avoid is this: if a chemical has been shown to cause cancer in the laboratory, there's a good chance that it's harmful to your immune system, too, says Samuel Epstein, MD, professor emeritus of environmental medicine at the University of Illinois at Chicago School of Public Health, author of *The Politics of Cancer Revisited*, and co-author of *The Safe Shopper's Bible*.

How Pollution Leaves Its Mark

Toxins can alter the immune system in two divergent ways: by suppressing it or by causing it to overreact, Dr Newman says.

A toxin that suppresses the immune system can do it by killing cells in the system – such as the lymphocytes and macrophages we discussed on page 24 – or by interfering with the way those cells do their jobs. For example, the heavy metal cadmium stops macrophages from being able to gobble up bacteria, weakening your ability to fight off infection, Dr Newman explains.

On the other hand, isocyanates – chemicals used in painting, plastic making and many other manufacturing roles – are probably the leading cause of asthma in the industrialised world, reports Dr Newman. They cause the immune system to go into hyperactive mode. Asthma is a sign of an overactive immune system, and when it begins in adulthood, 25 per cent of the time it is because of exposure to an occupational toxin, such as isocyanates.

Pollution may damage your immune system in other ways, too. Toxins that enter your body can send more free radicals – oxygen molecules that have lost an electron – racing through your system, where they steal electrons from other molecules and leave a trail of damage that your defence

RID YOURSELF
OF ENVIRONMENTAL TOXINS

If you'd like to clear toxins out of your system, a good sweat might be a good place to start.

Your liver is responsible for most of your body's detoxification chores, but different people are genetically equipped with a varying ability to flush out toxins. In addition, sometimes the liver's detoxification processes fail to work properly, causing toxins to build up and creating the potential for cell and tissue damage. To combat these problems, Charles Hinshaw, MD, a retired environmental physician in Wichita, Kansas, and former president of the American Academy of Environmental Medicine, has used intensive sauna treatments for patients who have significant toxins in their bodies. These treatments, which are supervised by a nurse, are designed to rid a patient's system of pollutants.

The results can be dramatic. For example, one of Dr Hinshaw's patients who followed this sauna regimen was a printer. 'He was actually sweating printer's ink out on his skin surface,' Dr Hinshaw remembers.

If you have a known heart condition, talk to your doctor before using sauna treatment. If you experience dizziness or any other symptoms while using the sauna, leave the sauna immediately. Dr Hinshaw doesn't advise women who are pregnant to use sauna treatment, but with a doctor's approval, they can use the hot bath or shower treatment described below.

mechanisms (the immune system) have to clean up. This can take an added toll on your immune system.

Doctors with an holistic viewpoint, such as Dr Berndtson, use the analogy of a waste disposal system to describe how many toxic demands the immune system can handle. In this analogy, the lungs, lymph and blood may be delivering five lorries of rubbish (toxins) to the liver, but the liver can process only four during that time. When this 'toxic noise' backs up in the system (in this case, your body), it can jam metabolic pathways and circuits throughout your body, including your immune system.

To begin to approach the problem, we need to understand that it is important both to decrease the entry of toxins *into* the system and to boost our ability to clear toxins *from* the system.

For the average person with limited chemical exposure who just wants to act preventively to keep any toxins flushed out, 20 minutes in a sauna once a week for as long as you're exposed to toxins will do the trick. (If you don't have access to a sauna, soak in a hot bath or hot shower for 10 to 30 minutes.) The first step is to engage in some type of aerobic exercise for about 20 minutes. 'For some reason, when people are exercising outside when the sun is shining, such as gardening or yard work, they tend to sweat more,' says Dr Hinshaw. Most toxins are stored in your body's fat, and aerobic exercise helps break them loose. Then, as you relax in the sauna for about 20 minutes, your sweat glands pick up these oils and usher them out to your skin's surface. Those of you who are already experiencing toxic complications (including respiratory problems such as wheezing or asthma, or reduced fertility) can follow this routine daily for 3 to 6 months, Dr Hinshaw says. For more serious detox needs, you may want to consult with a doctor familiar in these matters, suggests Dr Hinshaw. Symptoms such as inexplicable fatigue, mental confusion and difficulty thinking, and joint aches and muscle pain may be signs that you should see a doctor.

Be aware that you may need to follow a somewhat complicated nutritional regimen under a doctor's care to ensure that you detoxify safely, since the process can cause you to feel even worse before it's over, cautions Dr Hinshaw.

Here are guidelines on how to avoid toxins when they enter your body from the air you breathe, the water you drink, the food you eat and the products you use.

Gasping for Breath

The 20,000 breaths you take on average each day – give or take a few – suck about 13,500 litres (3,000 gallons) of air into your body.

'Anything you're inhaling is going to reach your lungs. They're directly involved with the external environment. And because the lungs are exposed to a high degree to the external environment, in some ways they're most vulnerable,' says Judith Zelikoff, PhD, an immunotoxicologist and associate professor at the Nelson Institute of Environmental Medicine at the New York University School of Medicine in Tuxedo.

Some of the leading metal pollutants in the air that can affect your immunity are cadmium, nickel and manganese, Dr Zelikoff says. Manganese, for example, is sometimes added to petrol. Lead, however, has declined as an airborne problem in developed countries with the demise of leaded petrol.

Another big threat is particulates – tiny bits of carbon particles that may carry other chemicals on their surfaces. These may come from sources of combustion, such as exhaust from diesel engines and smoke from chimneys, states Dr Zelikoff.

Also associated with immune dysfunction, she says, are sulphur dioxide, which can result from coal and oil combustion and industrial processes, and nitrogen dioxide, which comes from sources such as vehicles and electric power plants.

Another serious airborne health problem is ozone, a form of oxygen that brings about a chemical change in the lung tissue that causes negative health effects. The main ingredient of smog, ozone forms when sunlight encounters certain pollutants emitted from vehicles, power plants and other sources. It can irritate your lungs, making you wheeze and cough, and it has been shown to increase bacterial pneumonia in animals. Stay indoors if you can when smogs are really bad.

Even when you are indoors, toxins still pose a threat to health. In fact, many types of pollutants are thicker inside than outside. Because today's houses are much more efficiently insulated and therefore more airtight than in generations past, indoor pollutants become trapped.

The airborne stew of pollutants in your home can include particulates from gas stoves and fireplaces, tobacco smoke, radon and volatile organic compounds, or VOCs – gases that waft from certain items in the household such as MDF furniture and cleaning products. This is *in addition* to the other toxins that can get into your home from the outdoors.

While these are chemicals everyone should try to avoid when possible, people at extra risk – young children and the elderly, and those with asthma or other chronic diseases – should be especially vigilant in avoiding them, Dr Zelikoff says.

SUCCESS STORIES

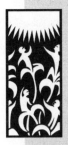

Changing Her Environment Improved Her Health

One woman's story shows that your environment can play a huge role in how well you feel.

Charles Hinshaw, MD, a retired environmental physician in Wichita, Kansas, has had 'hundreds' of patients who began feeling better after bringing down the amount of pollutants and toxins in their lives, he says. One particular patient complained of fatigue and problems with her memory, until she came to understand how important a clean environment was for her, says Dr Hinshaw, who is also former president of the American Academy of Environmental Medicine.

This patient made some dramatic changes in her life. For example, she now lives in a home built with materials that are low in toxins. The house is also heated and cooled only with electric appliances, which eliminates potential pollutants from gas, wood and coal heat. In addition, 'She eats the right foods and she avoids chemical exposures not only in her home but in the surrounding environment,' Dr Hinshaw says.

As a result, she reports that she's now feeling much healthier.

Turn Down the Toxin Level in Your Home

To limit your exposure to potentially harmful toxins in your residence, keep the following pointers in mind.

• Ban smoking in your home, since merely trying to ventilate it fails to get rid of all the smoke. Tobacco smoke contains more than 4,000 chemicals, many of which can cause cancer. About 3,000 nonsmoking Americans die each year of lung cancer caused by secondhand smoke.

• Consider testing the air in your home for radon. Radon is a naturally occurring radioactive gas given off by decaying radium in the soil, rock and building materials around your home, or in well water. You cannot see it or smell it, but radon is the second leading cause of lung cancer, after smoking. If you live in an area where much of the underlying rock is granite, such as the Scottish highlands or southwest England, seek advice from your local council or a specialist in radon protection. It is not possible to radon-proof your home but you can reduce the risk of exposure by keeping your home well ventilated and by sealing cracks in walls and floors. For further advice, contact the Department for the Environment, Food and Rural Affairs, at *www.defra.gov.uk*.

• If you are especially sensitive to particles in the air – for example, if you have asthma or are elderly and/or have chronic obstructive pulmonary disease – avoid using a fireplace in your home, Dr Zelikoff suggests. In fact, you might want to consider not living in an area where lots of neighbours heat their homes with wood-burning devices that give off smoke. A gas fireplace is safer than a wood-burning one in that it reduces the amount of particles to practically nothing. Wood pellet stoves are also safer in terms of particulate emissions.

• Have any gas-burning boilers, water heaters, fires and other equipment inspected periodically. Also, have your fireplace chimney and flues to your wood stove or coal stove cleaned and inspected before each heating season.

• Use your kitchen exhaust fan while cooking, and make sure that it is vented outside.

• One of the best-known VOCs is formaldehyde. This is found in permanent-press fabrics and some MDF furniture. Wash permanent-press clothes before you wear them and avoid ironing them, to minimise the gas they produce. If you must buy MDF furniture, ask about the formaldehyde content first, and try to choose types sealed with polyurethane or other waterproof sealant to cut down on the gas they emit.

For more information on VOCs, which are released by many cleaners, air fresheners and other household products, see 'Run a Safe Household' on page 91.

• Carpets can also emit VOCs, especially when they are new. The next time you buy a new carpet – if you must have one – tell your carpet retailer that you want a carpet and adhesive that produce low levels of VOCs. Also, ask the carpet fitters to unroll the carpet and air it out for a few days before they bring it into your home. Afterwards, for a few days, get as much ventilation through your home as you can.

• If you live in an area where the air is not heavily polluted, and you do not react to airborne allergens, allow your home to breathe. Open the windows when possible, and keep the doors between the rooms open so that the air circulates. If you have airborne allergies, or if you live near a busy road, you should consider placing a high-efficiency particle arrestor, or HEPA, filter in your home. This will trap most of the particulate irritants circulating in the room in which it is placed.

Special Advice for People with Allergies

To best control your allergy symptoms, you need to limit or eliminate the allergy triggers that your immune system faces each day. So, while you are trying to cut down on the levels of toxins in your home, also work to reduce the number of allergens found there.

• Keep the humidity in your home between 30 and 50 per cent to keep down the level of mould and dust mites, which can aggravate asthma and other allergic attacks. You may need to dry out your home with exhaust fans in the kitchen, bathroom and utility room and a de-humidifier in the basement.

• To cut down on allergy and asthma attacks, allergy-proof your bed, where you spend one-third of each day. Encase your mattress and pillows in allergen-proof covers, and clean them weekly according to the manufacturer's directions. Wash your sheets weekly in hot water.

• Keep your house free from clutter to reduce dust. Clean weekly with a HEPA-filter-equipped vacuum cleaner.

• Lay heavy-duty doormats outside your entryways and use them before entering. When you go indoors, remove your shoes. That will reduce the levels of pesticides and other toxins that you bring in from outside.

Exercise Caution When You Head Outdoors

By taking a few simple steps, you can limit your exposure to outdoor toxins such as car exhaust and ozone.

• Avoid exercising on congested streets and at times of the day when traffic is heavy, so that you do not breathe in as much vehicle exhaust.

• If you live in an area with lots of air pollution, avoid exercising in the afternoon, since that is when levels are usually highest. Also, check your local paper for reports on pollution levels.

• Stay aware of the ozone levels in your area. They are usually worst from May to September.

• Limit your exposure to the sun. While some sun is life-giving and critical in manufacturing vitamin D, too much sun can increase the risk of numerous problems, including macular degeneration and skin cancer. To protect your eyes, wear sunglasses designed to block ultraviolet A and B (UVA and UVB) rays. To protect your skin, always wear a sunscreen with an SPF of at least 15 (or 30, if you will be out in the sun all day) and apply it 30 minutes before going out in the sun – even on cloudy days.

TAKE THE **FIRST STEP**

Since some household products release chemicals into the air even when you're not using them, now is the time to clean out that shelf in the back of your cupboard where you store all the cleaners and aerosol sprays you use infrequently. Take a hard look at the air fresheners, paints, aerosol sprays and cleaning products that you've accumulated, and throw away any that aren't absolutely necessary. Be sure to read the label to find out how to dispose of them in an environmentally friendly way. The next time you go shopping, replace the products you've got rid of with non-toxic, biodegradable cleaning supplies.

Be a Wise Worker

An educated worker is a healthy worker. Know the facts about any chemicals with which you come into contact on the job, and measure the risks carefully.

• If you can, avoid working around harmful chemicals.

• If you must work around dangerous chemicals, be sure to educate yourself about them, and take all the necessary precautions to protect yourself, Dr Newman urges.

Businesses are required to keep Control of Substances Hazardous to Health (COSHH) sheets for the potentially harmful chemicals used in their workplaces. These contain information about the chemicals, including their health effects and protective recommendations. Read these carefully.

Water, Water Everywhere, but Not Always Safe to Drink

If you saw your drinking water before it was cleaned and treated, the sight might just make staying thirsty sound like an attractive alternative. The average water treatment plant will clean out 250 cubic feet of sludge from each million gallons of water it processes, which is enough to fill three large lorryloads.

Chemicals can soak into your water supply from waste disposal sites. Pesticides can wash off fields and lawns, where they flow into lakes and streams. Animal and human wastes can bring dangerous bacteria into the water supply.

Arsenic, a cancer threat, is swimming in the drinking water of millions of people. Lead may be leaching from the pipes that bring water into your home. The chlorine used to disinfect the water can combine with organic compounds in the water to produce potentially cancer-causing chemicals called trihalomethanes (THMs). These have been linked with bladder and colorectal cancer in humans.

Roughly a quarter of all British tap water contains pesticides at levels above Maximum Admissible Concentrations set by the EC for public safety. Contaminants range from antimony (which comes from oil refinery discharge and can make your cholesterol go up) to xylenes (which also comes from oil refinery discharge and can cause nervous system damage), along with the previously mentioned substances.

• If you get your water from a public water utility, you can obtain a Consumer Confidence Report (CCR) from your water supplier. Protecting yourself from waterborne hazards starts with obtaining this information. It will tell you where your water comes from and what contaminants (if any) were found in it.

• If you aren't satisfied with the information you get from your water supplier, you might want to have it tested on your own. Of course, if you get water from a well or other private water supply, your only option is to have it tested on your own.

According to a US Physicians for Social Responsibility report on drinking water, if your well is in an agricultural area, it's more likely to contain pesticides and nitrates. Groundwater may also be contaminated with radon. If your water source is in an industrial area, you should have it checked for petroleum products and VOCs.

Depending on how many substances you're looking for, the cost of testing your water can vary. Contact DEFRA for information on water testing laboratories in your area (*www.defra.gov.uk*).

• When shopping for a water filter, use the knowledge of what contaminants, if any, are in your water, since not all filters strain out different impurities equally well. Even if your water seems safe, remember that if you have a poor immune system – for example, if you're undergoing chemotherapy for cancer or have AIDS or a transplanted organ – you're more vulnerable to the risks of contaminated water than the general population. Speak to your doctor about whether you need to take special precautions with your water, particularly regarding cryptosporidium, a microbe that can travel in drinking water with deadly results for people with such health problems. It can also cause diarrhoea in babies and in healthy people.

• Bottled water isn't necessarily cleaner or safer than tap water. It may not even be any different: some companies put municipal water into a jug with a pleasing, natural-looking label and resell it. A study by the US Natural Resources Defense Council tested 103 brands of bottled water and found that while most of the samples were clean, one-third contained chemical or bacterial contaminants at levels that exceeded government or industry standards. If you want specially handled water, you'll probably find that using a filter on your own water is a much more affordable way to get a drink.

• Drinking water is not the only way to ingest potentially cancer-causing THMs: you can inhale them or soak them up through your skin, too. A recent study compared groups of people who drank a litre

CHOOSE THE RIGHT FILTER FOR THE JOB

Not every water filter sifts the same contaminants out of your drinking water, so the first step in choosing the correct filter is to have your water tested privately or to study the results given in the water test report provided by your water supplier. When you have this information, you'll be able to determine which contaminants you should be concerned about filtering.

Keep these pointers in mind.

• A point-of-use filter will handle water at a particular location, such as on your kitchen tap. A point-of-entry filter treats all the water that enters your home and goes to your sinks, showers, dishwashers and other water-handling devices.

• Filters using activated carbon are effective for removing chlorine, radon, some volatile organic compounds (VOCs), pesticides and trihalomethanes (THMs). Some also reduce lead and mercury. The carbon filters must be replaced regularly according to the manufacturer's instructions. These filters can be used in a variety of locations, such as at the point of entry, connected to your tap, or in a special container that you fill with water that then filters through.

• Reverse osmosis filters, in which water passes through a cellophane-like membrane, are useful for filtering out bacteria and bringing down levels of chemicals such as cadmium and chromium and some pesticides. But these filters waste a lot of water for each litre they treat. In addition, you may want to use a carbon filter in conjunction with a reverse osmosis filter to remove more pesticides, THMs and VOCs.

• Distillers boil water into steam, which then condenses back into water, leaving behind some contaminants in the process. These are good for removing arsenic and some pesticides. They may not be so good for removing THMs and VOCs, since these turn to vapour near the same temperature as water and can travel along with the steam into the treated water.

• Ion exchangers replace contaminants in water with safer chemicals such as sodium or chloride. These may help reduce the levels of radium, arsenic and some heavy metals in your water, but some of these devices, like the so-called water softeners, may produce too much sodium in the water for people on sodium-restricted diets.

• Look for filters that display an EC kitemark, and carefully read the package to learn what the filter is built to handle.

of tap water, sat in a bath for 10 minutes, or took a 10-minute shower. Those who took the shower had the highest levels of THMs in their blood. Those who drank the water had the lowest. You can cut down on your exposure by making sure that your bathroom gets plenty of ventilation while you shower, and by buying a showerhead with an activated-charcoal filter to trap these chemicals.

• Most of the lead in your water will probably be from your home's plumbing system rather than from your water supplier. Lead solder may be used to connect the pipes, whether you have lead pipes or not. If a tap has not been used in at least 6 hours, turn on the cold-water tap and, before drinking any water, let it run until it turns as cold as it will get. As the water waits in your pipes, lead may leach out into it. Running the tap will flush out this leaded water.

• Use only cold water from your tap for drinking and cooking. Hot water from the tap is more likely to contain higher levels of lead and some other toxic metals.

Choose Environmentally Friendly Food

These days, when you glance at the list of ingredients on a package of processed food, it often looks less like a recipe than like a chemistry student's thesis paper. Food manufacturers may add a variety of chemicals to their products to ensure that they have a pleasing colour, texture and freshness when we toss them into our shopping trolleys. But those chemicals may have a less pleasant effect on us when we eat them.

Processed foods are not the only grocery items with man-made ingredients, though. The fruits and vegetables in the fresh produce aisle may be laced with pesticides, and the meat counter may offer products containing antibiotics, pesticides and other unwholesome chemicals.

Here are some ways to trim unwanted chemicals from your diet.

• Cut down on meat. The farther up the food chain an animal is, the higher the concentrations of toxins it contains – even if the animal is a plant eater. Eating less meat will expose you to smaller amounts of environmental pollution, according to Andrew Weil, MD, director of

READ THE LABELS

If you see any of these ingredients on a food label, put the product back on the shelf.

• Acesulfame K. This sweetener, which is found in chewing gum, puddings, gelatine and non-dairy synthetic cream, causes cancer in animals and may increase the risk in humans.

• Artificial colours. Most of these are synthetic dyes, and some that are suspected to be toxic have been banned. Since they're chiefly in foods with low nutritional value, it's best to avoid foods containing artificial colours.

• BHA and BHT. These are added to foods containing oils as preservatives. They are possible carcinogens.

• Potassium bromate. This ingredient is added to bread to improve its volume and texture. Bromate causes cancer in animals, and the small amount in bread holds a small risk for consumers.

the programme in integrative medicine and clinical professor of medicine at the University of Arizona College of Medicine in Tucson and author of *Eating Well for Optimum Health*.

When you are feeling carnivorous, consider buying organic meat and chicken. Always trim the fat away from meat, and the skin from poultry and fish, since some pesticides accumulate in fat.

• Limit barbecued food. Charring meat over flames creates carcinogenic chemicals called polycyclic aromatic hydrocarbons. If you must barbecue, cut away the blackened layers before you eat the meat, and avoid breathing the smoke while barbecuing.

• Curb your cravings for swordfish. It's wise to limit your intake of swordfish, tuna, shark and marlin to one serving a week, since some studies have found that they can contain high levels of mercury. Women who are pregnant should avoid swordfish.

• Fill your diet with whole, natural foods that are minimally processed and have a minimum of added colours and preservatives, urges

Dr Berndtson. Cured meats such as bacon and salami, for example, may contain preservatives called nitrites, which can form carcinogens in your stomach after you eat them.

• When you buy fruits and vegetables, choose those that have been grown organically, as much as your budget and their availability allow. Buy locally grown produce that is in season. Out-of-season fruit is usually imported and is more likely to carry chemical contaminants than domestic varieties.

• When you get home with your produce, take the extra time to get rid of pesticide residues. Food growers may spray chemicals on their crops to combat insects, rodents, weeds and fungus. Wash all your fresh fruits and vegetables thoroughly under running water, which helps loosen the pesticides from the foods, and use a scrubbing brush when feasible. Also, discard the outer leaves of vegetables such as lettuce and cabbage, and peel vegetables such as cucumbers, apples and carrots.

• Milk can contain any number of industrial pollutants, carcinogens, pesticides and other toxins, says Dr Epstein. Try to buy organic milk if you can.

• Components from plastic can migrate into the foods they contain, particularly if the food is hot and has a high fat content. Therefore do not use empty margarine tubs or similar containers to microwave food; use microwaveable dishes instead.

• Never forget that microbes in the kitchen present an environmental threat to your immune system, too. To help protect yourself from nasty bacteria, use a different cutting board for raw meat than you use for other foods. In addition, always wash your hands, cutting boards, utensils and other surfaces with hot, soapy water. Then, disinfect the cutting boards and utensils in the dishwasher or by rinsing them in a dilute chlorine bleach solution (15 ml/1 tablespoon bleach to 4.5 litres/1 gallon water) after they touch raw meat.

Remember that roasts and steaks should be cooked to at least 62°C/145°F, minced beef to 70°C/160°F, and whole poultry to 80°C/180°F. Use a clean food thermometer to check. Fish should be cooked until you can flake it apart easily with a fork, and eggs should be cooked until the yolks and whites are firm.

Finally, if you intend to keep leftovers, freeze or refrigerate them within 2 hours. Keep them in small, shallow containers that will cool quickly.

Run a Safe Household

Household products such as paints, aerosol sprays, cleaners and air fresheners release chemicals into the air when you are using them – and even when they are in storage. Studies from the US EPA have found about a dozen common organic pollutants at levels up to five times higher inside homes than outdoors.

The agency acknowledges that we do not know much about what health effects such levels can cause, but many of these chemicals are known to cause cancer in animals, and some are known to cause it in humans. Read on to learn how to protect yourself.

Around the House

A home scrubbed with harsh chemical cleaners and scented with artificial air fresheners may seem clean, but it may also be contaminated with toxins. To help protect yourself and your family, follow these tips.

• Avoid artificial air fresheners. Products with artificial scents merely cover up odours, and many of them do it with chemicals that can cause cancer when you inhale them.

• Try to avoid highly toxic products that say 'Danger' or 'Poison' on the label. Those labelled 'Warning' are moderately toxic; those marked 'Caution' are less toxic. This labelling goes for all products, not just air fresheners.

• Whenever you can, use non-toxic, biodegradable cleaning supplies around the house. These are available at health food shops and supermarkets. You can also make some cleaners from safe ingredients: for instance, instead of harsh oven cleaners, make your oven shine by

THE PROBLEM WITH CLEANLINESS

We may be too clean for our own health.

Our zeal for cleanliness may, in fact, be the reason for the emergence of anti-biotic-resistant strains of bacteria. When we use antibacterial products that kill most of the harmful bacteria, we're also eliminating more than one-third of the good, resident bacteria vital to the health of our skin.

'The hard part to get across is that a little dirt is a good thing,' says Stuart B Levy, MD, director of the Center for Adaptation Genetics and Drug Resistance at Tufts University School of Medicine in Boston. 'You should wash after normal activities, where you come in contact with microbes and dirt, especially before you eat. But you don't have to clean every 5 to 10 minutes.'

We've become so obsessed with cleanliness that we seem to sterilise everything in our paths with products that contain antibacterial agents such as the chemical triclosan. The problem is that triclosan may be a culprit in the creation of superbugs – bacteria that have changed so much that they can no longer be killed off by anything. In a study at Tufts University, Dr Levy found five strains of *Escherichia coli*, or *E. coli*, that are immune to triclosan. Triclosan kills off most of the normal bacteria (95 per cent), but a few bacteria have mutations that enable them to resist triclosan. These bacteria don't get killed; they reproduce. Although the number of mutations per generation is very small, bacteria reproduce quickly, so many mutations can occur in a short time. The 5 per cent of each population that survives triclosan will result in mutations that are better and better at resisting the effects of the chemical. If these mutants are also resistant to antibiotics, you've got superbugs.

scrubbing it with steel wool and a paste of baking soda and water. Clean your toilets with a toilet brush and 115 g (4 oz) of baking soda. Use undiluted white vinegar as a household disinfectant. To avoid using caustic chemicals, flush drains weekly with hot water, 115 g (4 oz) of baking soda, and 120 ml (4 fl oz) of white vinegar.

• If you must use potentially hazardous products in your home, follow the label closely. If a product's label recommends using it in a well-ventilated area, bring in as much outdoor air as you can by opening windows and turning on exhaust fans.

When he served as president of the American Society for Microbiology, Dr Levy organised a symposium that was designed to educate people about the good of bacteria. 'Little did I know that this cleanliness craze was going to get out of hand. We need bacteria. If we destroy them, we're going to destroy ourselves,' he cautions.

Take a look at the soaps and cleaners in your kitchen and bathroom. Many of the labels may be screaming 'antibacterial!' at you. Check the cleaning sprays for worktops, hand soap, laundry and dishwasher detergents, toothbrushes, toothpaste and cosmetics. Even your children's plastic toys and the plastic utensils we put in our picnic baskets are impregnated with triclosan. There are more than 700 products made with antibacterial agents. This widespread use ultimately could mean that antibacterials will become ineffective when we really need them, warns Dr Levy.

We need antibacterial products in hospitals and in the homes of people who have low immunity, acknowledges Dr Levy. 'When I send a patient home, I will often tell her to use an antibacterial cleaner until her condition is healed. I will say that she should cleanse with it for minutes, not seconds. But when I find out she has been using that same antibacterial product casually in the home, I worry whether it will do any good,' he says. 'Bacteria have likely already been selected that resist it.'

To stay clean and to do your part in keeping superbugs from taking over, Dr Levy recommends using fast-acting non-residues for cleaning: bleaches, peroxides, alcohols and the traditional soap and water. Also when you do wash your hands, wash them thoroughly for 15 to 30 seconds with plain soap and water.

• Buy only the amounts of potentially hazardous products that you are going to use soon. If you have unnecessary chemicals gathering dust around the house, dispose of them in an environmentally friendly manner. Call your local council's recycling or waste disposal department to find out your options.

• Keep your exposure to products with methylene chloride and benzene to a minimum. Methylene chloride, found in paint strippers, adhesive removers and aerosol spray paints, causes cancer in animals. If you must use it, go outside if you can, or bring in plenty of outdoor air if you must use it indoors. Benzene, which is found in sources such as tobacco smoke, stored fuels and paint, is known to cause cancer in humans. Get plenty of ventilation if you use paints with benzene.

For Your Appearance

Looking good should not mean having to expose yourself to potentially hazardous chemicals. To limit your exposure, take heed of the following tips.

• Since we tend to use many cosmetics, toiletries and other personal care products each day – and they tend to be riddled with all sorts of potentially unhealthy chemicals – Dr Epstein suggests that you stick with brands that are completely natural and organic.

• Be aware that an environmental pressure group found a chemical called dibutyl phthalate in 37 popular nail products. They also found many patents from manufacturers proposing to use the chemical in a range of shampoos, cosmetics and other personal care products. The chemical is linked with birth defects in animals.

• Think twice before using perfumes. In his book *The Politics of Cancer Revisited*, Dr Epstein writes that synthetic fragrances are composed of hundreds of chemicals, and there is no way for the shopper to know which perfumes contain carcinogens.

In the Lawn and Garden

If you use pesticides to keep your lawn and garden free of weeds and insects, you may be risking your health. Follow these tips the next time you are working outside your home.

• Keep your use of hazardous pesticides to a minimum. The only safe insecticide is pyrethrins.

• If you must use a pest-killing chemical, read the label on the package carefully before each use, and follow the directions for protective clothing and other precautions. Use the minimum amount necessary for the task, and afterwards, wash your hands and any other skin and clothing that came in contact with the chemical.

• Always use natural techniques to combat pests in your lawn and garden. Diatomaceous earth contains tiny algae skeletons that kill insects, most likely by cutting into their waterproof coating. You can also buy lacewings and ladybirds to use as predators against harmful aphids.

You can also naturally reduce the number of insects in your home by making it less inviting to them. Seal any cracks and holes in the perimeter of your home that would let them in, and keep the interior clean of food and sources of water. That means repairing leaky pipes, keeping your food in sealed containers and taking out the rubbish regularly.

Chapter

8

ENHANCE IMMUNITY WITH THE POWER OF THE MIND

Two men are sitting at a bar, bragging about their dogs, each trying to outdo the other.

First man: 'I taught my dog to read.'

Second man: 'I know. My dog told me yesterday.'

Granted, the joke isn't *that* funny – but it's certainly silly enough to elicit a chuckle or maybe even a fleeting smile.

Here's another one:

What do you get when you divide the circumference of a pumpkin by its diameter?

Pumpkin pi.

Joking aside, the point is that when you laugh, something physical happens to make you feel good, says humour expert Diana L Mahony, PhD, associate professor of psychology at Brigham Young University–Hawaii in Laie. Most important, comic relief is a key element in protecting and enhancing our immune systems, she says.

How Humour Can Improve Your Health

Scientists know that a specific part of the brain stimulates laughter, and a good hearty laugh, in turn, helps keep immune cell receptors from binding to stress hormones and lowering our defences. In addition, when we laugh, our heart rates and blood pressure levels drop and our muscles relax. These immune-enhancing changes are proof that the power of the mind can keep our bodies – specifically, our immune systems – strong, so that we can lead healthy, productive lives.

Consider the 10 healthy men who watched a humorous video for an hour in a study conducted by neuroimmunologist Lee S Berk, MPH, DrPH, and researchers at Loma Linda University School of Medicine in California. Dr Berk found that the men showed significant increases in gamma interferon, a hormone of the immune system that activates other components of the immune system such as natural killer cells, which help fight infected cells and some tumour growth.

Even serious types can benefit from looking at life in a slightly absurd way. Forty participants who normally did not cope well with humour narrated a serious film in a humorous way in a study at Pennsylvania State University in State College. That group received the same positive immune-boosting benefits as a second group of 40 who regularly use humour as a coping mechanism, reports lead researcher Michelle Newman, PhD, assistant professor of psychology.

In fact, laughter is just one of many immune-boosting activities being studied by scientists interested in the connection between the body and the mind. Other activities that also have powerful immune-boosting elements – described as the 'beneficial hormonal milieu' by Bruce S Rabin, MD, PhD, director of the Brain, Behavior, and Immunity Center at the University of Pittsburgh School of Medicine – include socialising with friends, optimism, physical fitness and religion or spirituality.

Regular Sex Boosts Immune Function

In one study, people who had sex once or twice a week showed an increase in immune function, according to Carl J Charnetski, PhD, the leader of the study at Wilkes University in Wilkes-Barre, Pennsylvania. He and his colleagues found higher levels of the antibody immunoglobulin A (IgA) in participants who engaged in sex once or twice a week than in those who had no sex, or sex less than once a week. This antibody is the first line of defence against most viruses and bacteria.

'We also found that the frequent-sex group had higher immunoglobulin A levels than the very frequent – more than twice a week – sex group,' reports Dr Charnetski, who is also co-author of *Immunity Pleasure Connection*.

In his book *Stress, Immune Function, and Health: The Connection*, Dr Rabin emphasises how much the mind 'can influence the hormonal composition of blood' and in turn influence the function of the immune system and our health. 'A common emotional after-effect of sexual fulfilment is a feeling of relaxation and peace,' he says.

Our Minds Matter

The study of the relationship between the mind and the body is known as psychoneuroimmunology. The term was first coined in 1980 by Robert Ader, PhD.

Dr Ader, director of the division of behavioural and psychosocial medicine at the University of Rochester, New York, and co-author of *Psychoneuroimmunology*, conducted experiments in which he was able to condition the immune systems of animals. He concluded that if animals can learn to alter their immune responses, so can people. 'It never occurred to me that there might not be a connection between the brain and the immune system,' he says. 'You can't separate one system from another system. There is only one integrated system.'

He insists that additional research is critical to determine the science behind the connection between the mind and the body. He is concerned that psychoneuroimmunology is being embraced by people who refuse to understand the science on which it is based – science that requires an integration of the physical and psychological aspects of the person. Certain mind–body responses, such as 'spontaneous healing', may indeed occur, he agrees, but without clinical research, spontaneous healing is nothing more than 'a description of somebody getting better for reasons you can't explain.'

Dr Ader also believes in the power of the mind-body connection to help strengthen our immune systems, though he remains cautious about some of the practices that people adopt for this purpose. 'If somebody came into my office rubbing stones, I may think that's nonsense,' he explains. 'But I won't make him stop if I have nothing better to offer. If this is what makes him comfortable, then why not? I'm not saying you should not do this. I'm saying there's no evidence it works.'

Scientists may not have all the answers, but they are not sitting still. They realise that if we can better understand the relationship between the mind and the body, the potential for improving the health of our immune systems – indeed, the health of our entire bodies – is limitless.

For example, researchers in Bristol studied the psychological burden of people who were caring for spouses with dementia. The scientists found that the chronic stress took a toll on the caretakers' immune systems. 'This is representative of what could happen to people who are under a great deal of stress,' says Dr Rabin.

Try to have a positive outlook. Believe that the glass is half-full rather than half-empty. Find comfort engaging in religious activities, and incorporate time for fitness into your schedule. Laugh. Make friends – and reach out to them when they need help, says Dr Rabin.

TAKE THE **FIRST STEP**

This weekend, search your local bookshop for a collection of amusing stories or jokes. Then try reading a story or joke a day, and don't feel ashamed about letting out a roar of laughter after you've read it. Alternatively, stock up on some comedy videos and pull them out when you're feeling particularly stressed.

Enlisting the Power of Prayer

'Prayer gives people a sense of purpose, vision and meaning for their lives, and rituals to deal with stress,' says Harold G Koenig, MD, director of Duke University's Center for the Study of Religion/Spirituality and Health in Durham, North Carolina, and author of *The Healing Power of Faith*.

SUCCESS STORIES

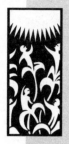

Drumming Helped Her Focus on Healing

Marla Downing attributes her new sense of calmness – and her health – to the beat of drums. 'The drumming is so soothing. I feel better doing it,' she says. 'It takes me into a relaxed state where I can focus on healing.'

Marla, who lives in Oil City, Pennsylvania, with her husband and two daughters, took part in drumming sessions conducted by Barry Bittman, MD, chief executive officer and medical director of the Mind-Body Wellness Center in Meadville, Pennsylvania. The treatment is part of the centre's Insights for Living Beyond Cancer programme. The drumming sessions are the result of research Dr Bittman has done. He says that the study's findings are an important first step in understanding the relationship between the mind and body in fighting disease. 'I am not suggesting that drumming is a cure for cancer, but rather that it may reverse the components of the classic stress response that can have a nega-tive impact on our immune system,' says Dr Bittman.

Marla did not have a good health history. A smoker since she was 15, she became very ill at 30 with kidney disease, followed by complete failure of her right kidney. She survived, but began taking antidepressants and anti-anxiety drugs.

Within 2 years, surgeons discovered that the incessant headaches she was experiencing were caused by a brain tumour. The tumour turned out to be benign, but doctors prescribed medication to prevent possible seizures.

'They watched the tumour in my head for a year, and then they removed it,' says Marla, a secretary. 'I was a

In a groundbreaking Duke University study that measured the immune systems of 1,719 religiously active people, Dr Koenig and his colleagues found that those people who regularly attended religious services had lower levels of a protein called interleukin-6 than those who did not. A high level of the protein, which is produced by your body in response to walking zombie. I was on so much medication for seizures, for anxiety, for I don't know what.'

Still, she continued to smoke. 'I went to counselling. I saw lots of doctors. No one told me to stop,' she remembers.

Then she met Dr Bittman. He immediately gave her three prescriptions. One: keep a journal. Two: start walking daily. Three: start cutting back on the number of cigarettes smoked each day.

She did all three, and was feeling better. Dr Bittman also took her off all seizure medication at that point. Doctors, however, soon found a mass in her lungs. 'I would have given up had I not already been taking some steps to get better,' she says. 'I wrote down my thoughts, how afraid I was, how much I wanted to be here to watch my daughters grow up. I got my thoughts out. I felt better from walking, and I was already cutting down on cigarettes. I said right then that if my surgery was successful, I'd never pick up a cigarette again.'

It was, and she has not smoked since.

Just as important, Marla, who is in her forties, believes that she was taking control of her life, even while having to deal with lung cancer.

She began meditating and listening to music. 'Anything instrumental. Listening to music is so important to me,' she notes. She listened to classical and Celtic music through 28 treatments of radiation and 12 weeks of chemotherapy. 'Meditation and music gave me a positive focus, a chance to relax and focus on healing,' she says. In addition, she started adding more fruits and vegetables to her diet.

And then she joined Dr Bittman's drumming sessions.

She's convinced that the drumming gave her additional cancer-fighting strength. She now listens to guided imagery tapes, which help her keep calm. 'As with the drumming, I feel my body calming down from head to toe,' she says. 'When I was first diagnosed with cancer, I thought, this was it. I'm not afraid anymore. Now, I have control.'

inflammation, may be a sign of a weakened immune system and is linked to some autoimmune diseases, cancer and heart disease.

A believer in the power of faith in enhancing our immune systems, Dr Koenig feels that in order to qualify for the benefits, 'you have to buy the whole (religion) package.' He notes that 'there's something about traditional religion that combines lots of things.' For example, people who regularly attend worship services almost always have more social contacts and seem to be better able to cope with stress than those who don't. 'Those kinds of things are all very, very positive in terms of social contact, sense of purpose and meaning,' he says. 'All of those things may impact immune functions.'

Even the simple act of saying a prayer, wherever you happen to be, may serve as a form of meditation, which could help to relieve stress. 'The

THE AMAZING POWER OF DREAMS

'Dreams try out things the waking mind hasn't thought to try,' says Deirdre Barrett, PhD.

Dreams can be sources of inspiration and can help us to solve problems. They can also warn of impending illness, and let you know that all will be right with the world in a matter of time, says Dr Barrett, a Harvard Medical School psychologist, former president of the Association for the Study of Dreams, and author of *The Committee of Sleep: How Artists, Scientists, and Athletes Use Dreams for Creative Problem-Solving — and How You Can, Too*.

'In our sleep, some sensation from the body reaches consciousness that has not been in our awareness while we were awake,' Dr Barrett notes. She tells of a woman who dreams about a bank cheque. 'At first, in the dream she's talking about the need to get a cheque. And then, she says in her dream that she needs to get a check for cancer. She went for a check-up and found she had a tumour. It could be that cancer can be slow in developing, and our body senses it before we know about it in a clinical way.'

Dreams may also have another important benefit. According to Dr Barrett, dreams are similar to visualisation, which athletes have long used to focus on their goals. In a study with competitive swimmers, Dr Barrett taught 'dream incubation' techniques that produced many dreams about swimming in the 2 weeks between their last practice and their competition. She found that the swimmers had better times in that competition than in previous races.

Dr Barrett says that if you 'incubate' your dreams, you are more likely to remember them and to learn to understand them. Here are some tips for doing just that.

reaction is exactly opposite to the fight-or-flight response we have to stress,' says Dr Koenig.

'I think we're going to find that there are very clearly defined biological changes with prayer – more so than with any social or psychological phenomenon that we've examined to date,' he adds. He emphasises, however, that prayer is no substitute for traditional medical care, such as immunisations, antibiotics, surgery or drugs to control major disorders.

• First, be sure to get enough rest. 'Sleep is as important to your dream recall as it is to your immune system,' says Dr Barrett. 'People who are sleep-deprived lose stages of sleep and more of their dreaming time. They're not having as many long dreams, and they're dramatically less likely to remember them.'

• Write down your problem as a brief phrase of a sentence and place this by your bed. Keep a pen and notepad, and perhaps also a torch or a pen with a lit tip, on your bedside table. Look for these pens at office supply stores and some department stores.

• Review the problem for a few minutes before going to bed.

• Once in bed, visualise the problem as a concrete image if it lends itself to this. If not, visualise yourself dreaming about the problem, awakening and writing on the bedside notepad. Perhaps arrange items connected to the problem on the night table. (An artist might place some sketches, a poet some poems.)

• Tell yourself that you want to dream about the problem just as you are drifting off to sleep.

• When you wake up, lie quietly before getting out of bed. Note whether there is any trace of a recalled dream, and invite more of the dream to return if possible. Write it down.

Don't be discouraged if you don't remember your dreams after the first night of trying these tips. Dr Barrett notes that it could take a week or so before you're able to remember your dreams. When you do, though, you're bound to be amazed at the work your mind is doing while you are asleep.

The Health Benefits of Making Music

Much of what has been learned about the function of the immune system focuses on areas of the brain that play a key role in releasing hormones when we are stressed. 'When this cascade of hormones occurs, there are a series of happenings that can diminish the immune function,' says neurologist Barry Bittman, MD, chief executive officer and medical director of the Mind–Body Wellness Center in Meadville, Pennsylvania, and co-author of *Maze of Life*.

He says that the harmful surges of stress hormones can sometimes be ameliorated with music. While many individuals are familiar with a theory called the Mozart effect, which maintains that certain music can improve health, memory and awareness, Dr Bittman turns to an even older form of music to improve immune system function: the ancient rite of drumming.

Dr Bittman found that the 61 men and women who participated in his experimental group drumming circles showed significant increases in cytokines, the protein substances secreted by cells that help direct and regulate immune responses, and natural killer, or NK, cells, which seek out and destroy cancer cells and virally infected cells. 'The results are incredible,' he says. 'Here we have an activity that is joyful. Group drumming is a delight. People just love to do it.'

The group used a special kind of drumming, called composite drumming, to create the effect. This included several steps using 'shakers' made from plastic Easter-type eggs filled with seed or gravel. First, the shakers were passed around in the group as an icebreaker activity. Second, the participants used the shakers, one at a time, to rhythmically drum the syllables of their names. This was done to create unique and individual rhythms. Next, the members drummed their names in unison. The tempos and rhythms varied. Finally, a facilitator led the group in a guided imagery activity, telling a story while the participants drummed along, adding sound effects that matched the spoken descriptions.

Blood samples taken from the participants showed that they had significant chemical changes that are known to strengthen the body's natural immune response. The drummers had also improved their ratios of dehydroepiandrosterone (DHEA) to cortisol, a condition considered beneficial to immune function.

'My feeling is that in an age like this – where we're focused on using computer technology, and e-mail and voice mail, and distancing ourselves from each other – creating fun-filled activities that bring people together and exercise our minds, bodies and spirits in a creative fashion is the essence of what wellness is all about,' says Dr Bittman. 'This is the first step in proving what our ancestors knew all along, that making music is good for you.'

The study of the way in which the body and the mind interact is still a relatively new one, and there will probably never be a set equation for improving your immune function. But that is a good thing, since it opens the door to allowing us to freely enjoy – even pamper – ourselves without feeling guilty. The key is to incorporate positive activities into your life each day: laughing at the ludicrous tabloid headlines instead of grumbling when waiting in a long queue at the supermarket; meditating or saying a silent prayer at breakfast before a particularly stressful day; making it a priority to reconnect sexually with your partner. No matter what methods you choose – humour, a healthy sex life, prayer, even music – remember that the mind influences the body in mysterious and amazing ways.

Chapter 9

THE TOP 20 IMMUNE BOOSTERS

THE IMMUNE SYSTEM IS EXTREMELY COMPLEX, WHICH IS WHY this book, basically an immune system manual, is such a big one. You will not find out everything you need to know by reading just one chapter. But you will find here some essential nuggets of information that represent many key ideas explained more fully elsewhere in the book. Consider this chapter and the next as a salad bar of crucial information: full of nutrients and wonderful for a quick snack, but just one element of many in your search for the Immune Advantage.

'If you do just take these 20 steps, you'll go a long way toward boosting your immune system,' says Keith Berndtson, MD, medical director at Integrative Care Centers in Chicago and Glenview, Illinois.

1. Put Some Colour on Your Plate

Eat 9 to 10 servings of fruits and vegetables each day.

This may seem impossible to do. The average person subsists on a paltry four servings of fruits and vegetables a day. But the average person is also 3 kilos (7 pounds) overweight and so tired that she can barely keep her eyes open to watch her favourite weeknight drama. The good news is that meeting the '9 to 10' goal is really very much easier than you think.

Make them more palatable. You don't need to eat them plain, the way you did as a child. Add butter and cheese if it will help you eat them. Many experts say that the healthiest way to eat vegetables is by preparing them in any fashion that tastes good enough to make you eat them. (Except for deep-fat frying.) One study conducted at the University of Washington in Seattle found that women who dislike green vegetables such as broccoli are particularly sensitive to the taste of a chemical in these foods called propylthiouracil, or PROP. They concluded that these women should seek to reduce the bitter taste by adding fat, sugar or salt. As the French do, use butter, oil or nuts to make vegetables taste seductively rich. A major bonus: adding some fat to your vegetables means that you'll absorb more of the carotenoids, which are fat soluble.

Mix them up. Think about a fast food meal. It's a beige meal: beige chips, beige bun-covered burger, beige apple pie. Now, think of a healthy meal, a rainbow of fruits and vegetables: red peppers, orange cantaloupe melon, yellow squash, green broccoli, blue berries, purple onions. Adding the vibrant colours and flavours of fruits and vegetables makes any dish more appealing.

Try different vegetables. Tired of spinach? Try some pak choi, a favourite of the Chinese. These delicious greens are perfect with a little soy sauce and mushrooms. Broccoli make you yawn? Try some turnip tops. The Italians use them to make a pasta sauce.

Whip up a smoothie. Try this classic recipe recommended by *Prevention* magazine, which offers two servings of fruit in one glass. Mix the following ingredients in a liquidizer until smooth: 240 ml (8 fl oz) skimmed milk; half a frozen banana or 115 g (4 oz) frozen mango slices; 1 teaspoon sugar and 230 g (8 oz) frozen fruit such as strawberries, pineapple chunks or blueberries. Feel free to experiment by adding a touch of vanilla, cinnamon or other favourite flavours to taste. Each milkshake has about 220 calories, 1 g of fat, 4 mg of cholesterol, 5 g of fibre and 130 mg of salt.

2. Take the Supplements

Take a multivitamin plus vitamin E, vitamin C and calcium.

The vast majority of the population does not take supplements, assuming instead that nutritional needs will be met from a balanced diet. However, even if you are generally healthy and eat well, taking a supplement may act as an insurance policy against any nutritional shortfalls. Your nutritional needs vary throughout life and are also affected by lifestyle factors such as stress, smoking and drinking alcohol. Taking supplements might be the most practical and efficient way of meeting your nutritional requirements.

Here are our solutions to your most common excuses for not taking your vitamins.

'It's too confusing. I don't know what to take.' In fact, increasing your odds for better health is easy, in just seconds a day, with these four supplements.

- Multiple vitamin and mineral formula
- 70–270 mg of vitamin E
- 100–500 mg of vitamin C
- 1,000 mg (if you're 50 or under) or 1,200 mg (if you're over 50) of calcium

'I get all the nutrients I need from food.' Do you routinely drink 840 ml (28 fl oz) of olive oil? That's how much you would have to drink each day to get 70 mg of vitamin E.

'I can't remember to take my vitamins.' Make it easier by putting them in a place where you'll see them each day, such as next to the kettle. Also, take them at the most convenient time for you. Experts say that for most people, the best time to take your vitamins is simply the time of day when it's easiest to remember them faithfully.

'They're too expensive.' Just a few pence a day can buy you the assurance that you're getting the immune-enhancing minerals and other vitamins that you need most. When you're choosing between the many brands, remember that the most expensive brands aren't necessarily the best ones. Labelling laws vary from country to country, but a reputable product should always give you information on dosage, how and when to take it, chemical names and amounts of different vitamins and a list of other substances (such as fillers, binders and lubricants) that have been used to make it.

3. Discover the Wonders of Working Out
Get moving for 30 minutes a day.

Just do it. It sounds so simple, yet only a fraction of the population actually exercises five times a week for 30 minutes. Here are some ways to motivate yourself to get moving.

Exercise makes you feel great. Sometimes it's hard to start, but think about how wonderful it is to see subtle changes as you walk through your neighbourhood, smell spring in the air, feel your muscles working in concert and hear sounds of nature or the bustling city all around you.

Exercise is an excellent way to make friends. If you have a dog, walk him. People always seem to smile and say hello to someone with a dog. If you do exercise in a group, whether it's taking a guided nature walk or canoeing, you'll reap the bonus of a friend-making opportunity.

It's also a good way to spend time with the friends you already have. Rather than meeting a friend for a calorie-laden lunch, why not meet her for a calorie-burning walk?

Exercise is play for adults. The best exercise is one that you will continue to do. So think of enjoyable, active things to do, such as hitting a tennis ball against the house, kicking a ball around the park with your children, or dancing to a golden oldie on the radio. If you find something that you like, incorporate it into your daily workout.

Exercise can be an excuse to go shopping. If you buy yourself a new piece of exercise equipment, the expense may help motivate you to use it and exercise. It doesn't have to be expensive, though. A skipping rope, for instance, costs little.

Exercise can also be an excuse to reward yourself. Changing habits is hard work, so reward yourself along the way for sticking with your exercise programme. Didn't miss a single walk last week? Treat yourself to a manicure. Made it all the way through an hour-long step class? Buy yourself a bunch of flowers. Choose anything that feels like a reward – except food.

Exercise is time spent on yourself. A few years ago, the slogan for one popular American soap opera was 'My Time for Me'. Even better than spending an hour watching your favourite soap opera, spend that amount of time on yourself. Give yourself the gift of more energy and better health.

4. Enjoy the Power of Sleep
Get your 8 hours.

At the end of the day when the chores are done, the children are in bed, and the house is still, it's finally time for you to do what *you* want. The TV beckons; so does the unread novel and your partner from the other room. Sleep can wait, you think.

The average person faces this choice nightly, and sleep often gets the short end of the stick. Most of us get only 6 hours and 41 minutes of sleep during the working week. That's more than an hour less than the 8 hours that sleep experts recommend to function at our best.

Often, in our busy lives, sleep is the first thing sacrificed. It's almost a badge of honour these days to proclaim, 'I'm so tired – I only got 4 hours' sleep last night!' It's time to take back the night and get the sleep you deserve.

'Get plenty of sleep. Not just sleep, but restorative sleep,' says Dr Berndtson. 'If this is hard to come by, seek medical help.'

Here's how to get the sleep you need.

First, make your room conducive to sleep. Move the papers and clutter to another room, or at least hide them from sight. It will be easier to relax if you cannot see the pile of laundry or work. Then invest in soft sheets and fluffy pillows. Think of your bed as your nest, and make it so.

Second, make your night clothes conducive to sleep. Besides comfortable pyjamas, consider slipping into some woolly socks. One Swiss study found that warm feet and hands may help you nod off. Your partner may think you've gone mad, but you could even try wearing gloves or mittens to bed.

Next, make your body conducive to sleep. Avoid caffeinated beverages and exercise late in the day. Also, if certain TV programmes overstimulate and energise you, consider turning off the set 20 to 30 minutes before bed.

Instead, prepare for sleep and soothe yourself with a warm bath or a mug of herbal tea. Camomile is especially calming. Crush 1 to 2 teaspoonfuls of dried camomile flower heads between your fingers to release their oils. Then place them in a tea strainer. Add a cup of boiling water and steep in a covered vessel for 15 minutes. Or, take a shortcut and buy camomile teabags; they are available in most supermarkets.

5. Raise Your Emotional Quotient
Pay attention to your psychological health.

Few people would deny the link between mind and body: just think of how our faces pale when shocked and redden when enraged. Elsewhere in this book, we talk about the strong link between emotional well-being and immunity. Emotional honesty and self-awareness are highly important. If these are hard to come by, seeing a therapist or counsellor is a wise health investment.

Whether you're working through an issue, fighting your way through a crisis, or even just dealing with the struggles of daily life, having an empathetic friend or relative can be a great source of comfort, but therapists and counsellors are *trained* to be good listeners.

Studies show that opening up to people boosts immunity. One study conducted at the University of Colorado at Colorado Springs found that the people who repressed their emotions after a disaster had altered immune systems, compared with the people who openly shared their feelings.

Other strategies that people have found useful include joining an informal women's or men's group (or other form of support group), participating in chat rooms online (of the supportive and informative variety), taking the dog to the park, pursuing favourite hobbies, doing some voluntary work, going to church, communing with nature, and keeping a diary.

6. Listen to Your Body and Learn Your Family History

Study your family tree to target your disease prevention.

Sometimes our bodies whisper – a tiny rumble indicates hunger – and sometimes they scream – a blinding pain signals a broken bone. Often, we are too busy to heed our bodies' calls. But since our body signals offer important information about illnesses, perhaps we should start paying attention.

To our credit, sometimes our bodies speak to us less directly than other times. Anxiety, for example, can cause symptoms as diverse as lower back pain, chest pain, shortness of breath and loss of sexual function. So, until someone invents a universal translator for our bodies, we need to work out for ourselves what our symptoms are trying to tell us. Pay close attention to your body and try to determine what it's saying. For example, a headache could be triggered by many things, including stress, depression, environmental changes and certain foods. It can be helpful to track your symptoms in a diary, as many experts recommend for headaches. The diary can be as informal as noting your symptoms on a calendar until patterns emerge. If you are unable to unravel a mystery, consult your doctor.

Another, much subtler way that your body communicates with you is through your genes. Scientists are busy mapping the human genome, but you don't need that much detail, and you don't need to wait for the results. Just learning your family history will tell you the diseases for which you could be at risk. Scientists have so far found 4,000 diseases with a genetic component. Of those, the two most likely to affect us are heart disease and cancer. Of course, most cardiovascular diseases and cancer are triggered by accumulated damage to body cells from bad habits such as eating too much fast food or smoking, but other risk factors are due to a set of genes in which one part of the genetic instructions to your cells is missing, altered, or out of alignment. For a simple and potentially life-saving way to get in touch with your genetic heritage, look at 'Record Your Own Family History' on page 114.

7. Wet Your Whistle

Drink eight to ten 240 ml (8 fl oz) glasses of water and one cup of tea a day.

It's not included in the Recommended Dietary Allowances, but water is one of nature's most important nutrients – and one of which most people don't get nearly enough. Nothing is better than water when it comes to beverages. It has no calories, no sugar and no caffeine. On average, women drink 4.7 cups of water-based liquids – juice, soda, coffee and so on – a day. People should be drinking twice that amount: eight to ten 240 ml (8 fl oz) glasses a day.

Count a cup of coffee, tea or cola as half a glass, since the caffeine in these drinks acts as a diuretic. Also, drink an additional glass of water for every alcoholic beverage that you drink, since alcohol has a significant diuretic effect. Steer clear of exceeding four or more alcoholic drinks at a time.

Water does so much more than quench your thirst. It keeps you alert, cools you down, makes your skin glow and helps prevent diseases ranging from cancer to kidney stones. It can even help you lose weight.

When you don't drink enough, your cells start drying out. They suck fluid from your bloodstream, which leaves your blood thicker and more sludgy. That makes your heart pump harder to push your blood, which in turn wears you out.

Drinking more water has a direct immune advantage. When you're drinking enough water and properly hydrated, the mucus that coats your throat contains antibodies and can trap cold viruses. But if you are even slightly dehydrated, the viruses have a better chance of survival because your dried-out tissues aren't producing enough mucus.

Once you start drinking more water, it becomes a habit, and once you feel the health benefits, you'll start to crave it. It helps to put a slice of lemon or lime in a glass of water to give it some flavour. One great advantage: drinking water can make you look thinner. The body retains fluid when it begins to get dehydrated.

In addition to your water, drink one relaxing cup of tea each day. Every cup of tea provides a strong jolt of antioxidants that help keep blood from clotting too easily and may help lower your risk of cancer and

(continued on page 116)

RECORD YOUR OWN FAMILY HISTORY

A study presented at the American Society of Human Genetics found that few of us really know our family disease risk. Maren Scheuner, MD, director of the GenRisk Programme at Cedars-Sinai Medical Center in Los Angeles, developed this survey to help you calculate yours. On the chart, indicate whether you

CONDITION	YOU	YOUR FATHER	YOUR MOTHER
1. Early-onset heart disease (heart attack, angina, bypass surgery, or angioplasty) up to the age of 60	Y N ?	Y N ?	Y N ?
2. Heart disease after the age of 60, or if age of onset unknown	Y N ?	Y N ?	Y N ?
3. Any type of stroke	Y N ?	Y N ?	Y N ?
4. Vascular disease (blockage of a major artery)	Y N ?	Y N ?	Y N ?
5. Abnormal blood cholesterol or triglycerides	Y N ?	Y N ?	Y N ?
6. High blood pressure	Y N ?	Y N ?	Y N ?
7. Diabetes (a major risk factor for heart disease) onset in childhood	Y N ?	Y N ?	Y N ?
8. Diabetes onset in adulthood, or if age of onset unknown	Y N ?	Y N ?	Y N ?
9. Early-onset breast cancer up to the age of 50	Y N ?	Y N ?	Y N ?

or your biological parents have had any of the conditions listed. Circle '?' if you don't know. Relatives include sisters, brothers and parents. Your half-brothers and -sisters should be included in the brothers or sisters column. Then, take the results to your doctor, who can monitor your health to catch any genetic glitches that may be working against you.

HOW MANY OF YOUR CHILDREN?	HOW MANY OF YOUR BROTHERS OR SISTERS?	HOW MANY OF YOUR FATHER'S RELATIVES?	HOW MANY OF YOUR MOTHER'S RELATIVES?
0 1 ≥2	0 1 ≥2	0 1 ≥2	0 1 ≥2
0 1 ≥2	0 1 ≥2	0 1 ≥2	0 1 ≥2
0 1 ≥2	0 1 ≥2	0 1 ≥2	0 1 ≥2
0 1 ≥2	0 1 ≥2	0 1 ≥2	0 1 ≥2
0 1 ≥2	0 1 ≥2	0 1 ≥2	0 1 ≥2
0 1 ≥2	0 1 ≥2	0 1 ≥2	0 1 ≥2
0 1 ≥2	0 1 ≥2	0 1 ≥2	0 1 ≥2
0 1 ≥2	0 1 ≥2	0 1 ≥2	0 1 ≥2
0 1 ≥2	0 1 ≥2	0 1 ≥2	0 1 ≥2

(continued)

RECORD YOUR OWN FAMILY HISTORY (CONT.)

CONDITION	YOU	YOUR FATHER	YOUR MOTHER
10. Breast cancer after the age of 50, or if age of onset unknown	Y N ?	Y N ?	Y N ?
11. Ovarian cancer	Y N ?	– – –	Y N ?
12. Early-onset colon cancer up to the age of 50	Y N ?	Y N ?	Y N ?
13. Colon cancer after the age of 50, or if age of onset unknown	Y N ?	Y N ?	Y N ?
14. Endometrial (uterine) cancer	Y N ?	– – –	Y N ?
15. Early-onset prostate cancer up to the age of 50	Y N ?	Y N ?	– – –
16. Prostate cancer after the age of 50, or if age of onset unknown	Y N ?	Y N ?	– – –

rheumatoid arthritis. Both green and black tea contain powerful antioxidants, so drink whichever you prefer.

8. Remember, Variety Is the Spice of Life
Eat a wide variety of foods.

The vast majority of the population fails to follow that advice. In one American study, researchers examined data from the second National Health and Nutrition Examination Survey (NHANES II). They found

HOW MANY OF YOUR CHILDREN?	HOW MANY OF YOUR BROTHERS OR SISTERS?	HOW MANY OF YOUR FATHER'S RELATIVES?	HOW MANY OF YOUR MOTHER'S RELATIVES?
0	0	0	0
1	1	1	1
≥2	≥2	≥2	≥2
0	0	0	0
1	1	1	1
≥2	≥2	≥2	≥2
0	0	0	0
1	1	1	1
≥2	≥2	≥2	≥2
0	0	0	0
1	1	1	1
≥2	≥2	≥2	≥2
0	0	0	0
1	1	1	1
≥2	≥2	≥2	≥2
0	0	0	0
1	1	1	1
≥2	≥2	≥2	≥2
0	0	0	0
1	1	1	1
≥2	≥2	≥2	≥2

that only one-third of adults ate at least one food each day from five food groups: dairy, meat, grains, fruits and vegetables. Delving further, they found that *less than 3 per cent* ate at least two servings each day from the dairy, meat, fruit and vegetable groups and four servings from the grains group.

Of course, it's easier to fall into patterns of eating the same thing for breakfast every day or the same vegetables to accompany your evening meal. But a little more planning is beneficial. Simply put, the more varied the foods you eat, the more varied the nutrients you get.

Researchers from Queens College of the City University of New York and the National Cancer Institute found that, compared with the women who ate the least diverse diet, the women who ate the most varied diet had at least a 30 per cent lower risk of dying of cancer, heart disease and stroke.

Here's another major bonus: eating a wide variety of foods will also help you lose or maintain your weight. If you get bored with your food, you won't stick with a healthy diet, and you'll start to crave junk food. Buy at least one new healthy food every time you go shopping. Try an exotic grain such as quinoa or interesting produce such as Jerusalem artichoke. If you like it, incorporate it into your usual meal plans. If not, try something else next time.

Broadening your culinary horizons can be difficult as an adult. It may feel like a struggle for you, but you can help your future children like a wider range of foods. A study at the Monell Chemical Senses Center in Philadelphia found that babies whose mothers drank carrot juice while pregnant and breastfeeding preferred cereal prepared with carrot juice to cereal made with plain water. The researchers say that this demonstrates that early exposure to a taste can affect a person's preference for it later.

9. Be a Fat Detective

Eat the good fats, not the bad.

Eating the right kind of fat is absolutely essential for health. You need to investigate which are the ones to eat and which ones to avoid.

Calculate your fat budget. Fat should not exceed 25 per cent of your total calories. See 'The Tax-Free Fat Budget' for help with how to calculate this.

Avoid trans fats. Avoid products with the words 'partially hydrogenated oil' on the label. This means that trans fats are present. Margarine, for example, contains hydrogenated or partially hydrogenated fats. It's made from solidified vegetable oil, and in addition to damaging your immune system, it's bad for your heart. These fats are bad because they promote the formation of trans fatty acids in the body, which raise blood

THE TAX-FREE FAT BUDGET

First, determine your activity level from the following choices:

Sedentary = You have a life that involves a lot of sitting and you exercise rarely, if ever.

Active = Your daily routine requires more activity than light walking, or you exercise aerobically for 45 to 60 minutes three times every week.

Very active = In addition to an active daily routine, you exercise aerobically for 45 to 60 minutes at least five times every week.

Next, determine the activity factor below that corresponds to your activity level and gender:

Sedentary woman = 12
Sedentary man = 14
Active woman = 15
Active man = 17
Very active woman = 18
Very active man = 20

Now, calculate your caloric needs by multiplying your activity factor by your healthy target weight in pounds. For example, a 140-pound active woman who wants to lose 10 pounds would multiply 15 (her activity factor) by 130 (her target weight). She would need to eat 1,950 calories each day.

Next, you need to work out how many of those calories can be from fat. So, multiply your calorie needs by 0.25. The 140-pound woman could eat 487.5 calories each day from fat.

Last, translate calories from fat into grams of fat. Since each gram of fat contains 9 calories, divide the number of calories above by 9. The 140-pound woman can eat 54 grams of fat each day and stay under 25 per cent of calories from fat.

cholesterol levels and increase the risk of breast cancer. If you use a spread, be sure to buy brands that specifically say that they are free of trans fats. Or better yet, try one of the newer spreads that contain cholesterol-lowering plant sterols or stanols. These are expensive, but they can lower your cholesterol anywhere from 7 to 14 per cent.

Cut down on polyunsaturated fats, like the ones in meats and full-fat dairy products. These fats, especially polyunsaturated fats, tend to suppress the immune system.

Use olive oil instead. Substitute olive oil for butter or margarine at the table, drizzle it on salads and use it to replace vegetable oils in baking wherever possible. Buy only cold-pressed, extra-virgin oil. It retains more of the olive's heart-healthy antioxidants than other forms.

Opt for omega-3s. There is scientific evidence that omega-3 fats help prevent or treat a host of illnesses, including asthma, attention deficit hyperactivity disorder, cancer, cystic fibrosis, Crohn's disease, heart attacks, manic depression, rheumatoid arthritis, schizophrenia and severe menstrual cramps. It's simple to get more omega-3 fats into your diet: eat more fresh oily fish, like salmon or tuna.

Of course, you have to take care to avoid methyl mercury exposure from eating too much of certain types of fish. For up-to-date advice on contamination levels for different varieties of fish, contact the Food Standards Agency (*www.foodstandards.gov.uk*).

In a study of more than 20,000 male doctors, researchers found that eating 115–170 g (4–6 oz) of fish just once a week reduces your risk by 52 per cent of dying of a heart attack within an hour of the onset of symptoms. Scientists speculate that the omega-3 fatty acids in fish are responsible for this statistic. The richest source of omega-3 fatty acids is salmon. A 170-g (6-oz) cooked serving provides about 3.7 grams, which is what the experts recommend you consume in a week.

10. Exercise Kitchen Care
Use safe cooking methods.

Taking some simple precautions in the kitchen can have a dramatic impact on your health. Food poisoning hits the headlines when people come down with salmonella poisoning from eating at the local fast-food outlet. But still, about 20 per cent of the yearly millions of cases of food-borne illness start in the home, where you have complete control over the cooking and cleaning. Low levels of exposure to many germs help your immune system train itself to keep you well-defended against infection. But exposure to high concentrations of germs (especially the more aggressive ones) can overwhelm your immune system and make you ill. If you take steps to limit your exposure to the germs in the first place, you can help protect your immune system. Here's how to keep bacteria at bay.

Wash produce, even the pre-washed kind. Hold firm products such as carrots and peaches under running water, and rub them all over with your hands or a brush. Discard the outer leaves of lettuce and cabbage, then swish the remaining leaves around in a colander under running water. Place berries in a large bowl and soak them in several changes of cold water.

Make sure your food stays at the proper temperature. Use an instant-read thermometer, sold at kitchen supply shops or in the kitchenware departments of larger stores, to make sure that your cooked food reaches the following safe temperatures.

- Whole cuts of beef, veal and lamb: 63°C (145°F)
- Minced beef, pork and casseroles with eggs: 70°C (160°F)
- Leftovers or takeaway food, or minced poultry: 73°C (165°F)
- Chicken breasts: 75°C (170°F)
- Whole poultry and thighs: 80°C (180°F)

Don't let food sit at room temperature for more than 2 hours, or 1 hour on a hot day or in a very warm room.

Defrost foods in the refrigerator or in the microwave oven, but never at room temperature.

Use a clean sponge or cloth to mop up. Everything from worktops to refrigerator handles can be blanketed in a coating of bacteria after a wipe with a germ-laden sponge. Moist sponges provide the perfect petri dish for microbes – a surface to cling to, moisture and a steady supply of nutrients. Experts say that the kitchens that look the cleanest can actually be the opposite because their owners are always wiping everything down, spreading germs around. Disinfect your sponge each day by putting it in the dishwasher with your dishes.

11. Hold Hands with a Friend

Be sociable, stay connected, have fun.

The benefits of being connected and happy keep adding up.

One review of 81 published studies found that social support had a measurable effect on several benchmarks of immune system function. Experts think that positive relationships can prevent the immune-dampening impact of stress hormones such as cortisol.

A 1997 study of 276 people conducted at Carnegie Mellon University in Pittsburgh found that those who had a variety of social relationships were better able to fend off colds and had 20 per cent greater immune function than more introverted people. Researchers speculate that social ties may help us cope with the stresses that lower immunity. Surprisingly, many people do not understand this. According to a survey by Oxford Health Plans, one in six Americans say that they're too overworked to take a holiday with their families. *Nearly one-third* say that they eat lunch at their desks, instead of out with friends.

Surely, there are millions of ways to remedy this, to make more connections and have more fun. Here are just a few ideas.

Spend more time with your family and friends. Plan at least one recreational activity every weekend that is shared with others. Studies consistently show that the people who are the best able to manage stress are those who have the strongest network of family and friends. Research also indicates that married people are more likely to have shorter hospital stays than unmarried people. A happy, stable marriage can make you years younger.

Volunteer. People who do voluntary work on a regular basis report feeling a 'helper's high'. Studies show that volunteers reap health benefits from giving to others.

Take up a hobby. Activities such as reading or running can become opportunities to make new friends by joining a book discussion group or a running club.

Attend religious services. In a series of famous studies, people who participated in religious groups were shown to live longer and healthier lives.

Get a pet. About half of all households have some kind of pet, and surveys show that many people view their pets as family members. A 1995 study of heart attack survivors showed that owning a dog significantly improved 1-year survival rates.

Exercise with a friend. Improve your health and be sociable at the same time.

12. Celebrate Your Sensual Side
Enjoy your sex life.

The average woman has sex less than once a week. Experts say that's not enough.

Researchers at Wilkes University in Wilkes-Barre, Pennsylvania, have shown that people who have sex once or twice a week produce more immunoglobulin A (IgA) than people who have sex less than once a week.

Researchers say the boost could be because sexually active people are exposed to more infectious agents than nonactive people. The immune system would respond to these antigens by producing and releasing more IgA.

But be warned: experts say that *the single most important* step you can take to protect your immune system overall, however, is to protect yourself from contracting HIV – the cause of AIDS. AIDS destroys the immune system and leaves the body open to fatal disease. One of the main ways it is transmitted is by having unprotected sex with someone who is infected. So, if you're not in a mutually monogamous relationship, insist on a condom.

That said, here are some ideas to spark up your sex life.

Give (and receive) a massage. In a *Men's Health* and *New Woman* magazine survey that asked readers about their sexual likes and dislikes, 50 per cent of the women said that a massage was a definite turn-on. Visit a department store cosmetics counter to check out the many massage oil scents available, such as cedarwood, sandalwood and ylang-ylang, and choose one that appeals to you. Don't use these oils on the sensitive genital area, however, because they might irritate the skin.

Go shopping. While most men find a nude woman arousing, one wearing lingerie is even more of a turn-on, they say. Old-fashioned lingerie, such as a basque, stockings and suspenders, or even pure white underwear, is more likely to cause a thrill than greying bras and big knickers.

Read a good book. While romantic novels aren't a substitute for a real relationship, the best ones can teach a woman about herself and her relationships. The passion between the hero and heroine can stoke some great fantasies. In one study, women who read romantic novels made love with their partners twice as often as women who didn't.

13. Discover the Dynamic D
Take 10 mcg of vitamin D a day.

Vitamin D is such a powerhouse, the *D* should stand for dynamite. It's the key to building strong bones, and it may also play a role in preventing breast cancer, keeping arthritis in check and fighting depression.

The mechanism behind all of these feats is the fact that vitamin D promotes cell differentiation. Like a teacher, it directs developing cells in the right direction, toward their proper mature form. In the skin, for example, it normalises the growth rate of cells called keratinocytes, which are produced at a rate of around ten times faster than normal in people with psoriasis, which causes the skin to flake.

Also, vitamin D almost certainly plays a role in the development of type 1 diabetes, and it may even help prevent the disease. Vitamin D is needed for islet cells in the pancreas to produce insulin, the hormone that allows cells to take up blood sugar. In animals with an inherited tendency to develop type 1 diabetes, supplemental vitamin D helps prevent the disease.

Experts recommend 10 mcg of vitamin D a day, the amount found in many multivitamins.

Since our bodies process vitamin D from sunlight, some people argue that we should get more sun exposure and not wear sunscreen. However, experts say this is not so.

Several studies prove that ultraviolet (UV) exposure is not required for maintaining vitamin D sufficiency, nor is UV a scientifically proven cancer fighter. Prospective sunscreen trials examining whether sunscreen contributes to vitamin D deficiency found that people who used sunscreen regularly were not deficient in vitamin D.

What's more, intense exposure to the sun can dampen immune function. Ultraviolet radiation from the sun causes the formation of free radicals, depleting the body of important antioxidants. UV radiation may also raise levels of stress hormones, which also dampen immune function.

For the first time, in the US Department of Health and Human Services' *Report on Carcinogens*, solar UV radiation, as well as exposure to sun lamps and sun beds, was listed as a known human carcinogen – right alongside tobacco.

People seem to be getting the message. Sales of sunscreens are rising significantly each year.

If you need a better reason for staying out of the sun, remember that sun exposure accounts for 90 per cent of visible ageing.

14. Seek Serenity

Practise stress reduction techniques.

Stress can affect your body, mind and spirit. Stress hormones compromise your health when they bind to immune cells and short-circuit their ability to fight off illness. A healthy body is the best defence. But even if you do the basics – exercise, drink plenty of water and get your rest – it is important to find ways to neutralise the stress that we all face in our fast-paced, often chaotic lives.

Create balance in your life by scheduling stress-relieving activities into your calendar. You deserve it, and your health demands it. Try meditation, or a yoga class. These can help you become more aware of stresses in your life and teach you how to intervene with deep breathing exercises.

Start a stress diary. A study by James W Pennebaker, PhD, professor of psychology at the University of Texas at Austin, found that writing down your worries may cut your visits to the doctor in half and increase your antibody response to bacteria and viruses. When you give perspective to worries, you won't automatically produce cortisol, the stress hormone. Another enjoyable way to ease your troubles is with music: it can heighten relaxation while increasing levels of antibodies in saliva that resist infection and cancer. Listen for 20 minutes a day to unwind, or get up and move to your favourite dance music to release bad energy and stir your soul.

If you can't take a break from the office, you can still free your mind with the restorative powers of the sights and sounds of nature. Get a fish tank, scenic artwork, plants, or a desk fountain. Do a little daydreaming. If you don't have a window, use imagery to relax and allow pleasant images to drift through your mind. Not only have daydreaming and imagery been found to reduce stress and heighten immune response to disease, but they can also help you to increase self-understanding, increase problem-solving abilities and explore real-life situations.

Most of all, keep your spirit healthy. Learn to adjust to life's events and regroup every day to be more resilient to stress. Find what you most enjoy, and do it with friends or family: confide in them, make plans together and have fun. Meet new people, try new things and cultivate a belief system. A positive outlook can mean the difference between life and death. Research shows that optimists live longer and pessimists who can find the bright side of problems have less stress and better health. Look for humour in everything. When it comes to reducing stress, make healing laughter, one of the most powerful Immune Boosters, a part of your life.

15. Experience the Magic of Touch
Get a massage.

Sometimes it's equally as good to give as to receive. Massage is a great example. Getting a massage can boost your immunity. Giving a massage can make you feel wonderful too, and may help you get one in return.

Research conducted at the renowned Touch Research Institutes at the University of Miami suggests that massage can boost the immune system and generally benefits the entire body. Several studies on adults with HIV and breast cancer who received regular massage showed an increase in natural killer cells.

In one study conducted at the University of Miami in Coral Gables, 20 men with immune systems weakened by HIV (the virus that causes AIDS) received 45-minute massages 5 days a week for a month. At the end of that time, they had less anxiety, and several of their immune functions improved considerably. For example, natural killer cells, important

HOW TO GIVE A MASSAGE

Have the person being massaged lie comfortably on his stomach. Wash your hands. Gently stroke downwards, using the flats of your fingers, along both sides of the back six times. Perform continuous hand-over-hand movements down the back, to the waist, beginning with one side of the back and moving to the other.

Next, use your palms to spread out the back from spine to sides. Work your way up and down the back twice. Perform circular motions with the flats of your fingers from the neck to the tailbone along one side of the spine. Cross over the spine and then go up the other side of the back toward the neck. Make two complete circles around the back. Rub and knead the muscles in the shoulders for about 10 seconds. Gently rub the neck for about 10 seconds using the flats of your fingers. Repeat the circular motions up and down the spine as described previously.

Never massage the spine directly. Do not exert pressure on the joint areas, such as the shoulders, or on the rib cage area. Enjoy.

in eliminating viruses and tumours, became more efficient and multiplied. Cytotoxic T-cells, a type of suppressor T-cell that helps regulate immune response, also increased. Researchers think that the relaxation effect of massage decreases stress hormones – in particular, cortisol.

So, here's the prescription: have a 15- to 20-minute back rub daily. It's best to wait at least 30 minutes after a meal.

16. Tap the Poet Within

Keep a diary.

'I think with my right hand,' said the writer Edmund Wilson.

Wilson was on to something. Pouring those thoughts from your brain, through your hand and on to a page can be therapeutic for many reasons. Studies show that people who write about their troubles have stronger immune systems and fewer illnesses than people who don't write. We may suppress certain thoughts to ignore negative feelings or to be tactful to others, but this takes a toll on our immune function. Keeping thoughts bottled up lowers levels of infection-busting lymphocytes and makes us more at risk for illness.

In one study, researchers found that people who wrote about traumatic events for 20 minutes a day three to five times a week had about half as many visits to the doctor as people who didn't write. Their antibody responses to bacteria and viruses were more vigorous than the control group's, too. Putting it all down on paper may help you to see your problems as less stressful, so that your body doesn't automatically produce stress hormones such as cortisol. Preliminary evidence also shows that writing improves function in the parts of the brain that control cortisol secretion.

Diary therapists believe that by recording and describing your issues, you can better understand them and eventually diagnose problems that stem from them. The Center for Journal Therapy, in Lakewood, Colorado, contends that diary therapy has been used effectively for dealing with grief and loss; coping with life-threatening or chronic illness; recovering from addictions, eating disorders and trauma; repairing troubled marriages and family relationships; increasing communication skills; developing healthier self-esteem; getting a better perspective on life and clarifying life goals.

Use your imagination to make writing easiest and most convenient for you. A diary can be as simple as an engagement diary where you write down a few words at the end of each day, or it can be as elaborate as a book that you hand-make. Another option is to search bookshops, both local and online, for a wide selection of blank books. You can even keep your diary on the computer. The tapping of the keyboard may be music to your ears and soothing to your senses. There are also versions of computer software that prompt you with quotes and ideas to inspire you.

17. Keep Clean

Practise good hygiene.

Below is a three-pronged assault on germs.

Wash your hands. Infectious diseases are the third leading cause of death in the United States. The US Centers for Disease Control and Prevention (CDC) call hand washing 'the most important means of preventing the spread of infection'.

Viruses are often passed from an infected person to a doorknob or other surface that other people then touch with their hands. In the case of the flu, viruses fly through the air and stick to things. To keep a virus from latching on to you, wash your hands often. Packaged hand wipes let you clean up without leaving your office. There is no need to become obsessed about it; just use common sense.

Make sure you wash your hands before you prepare food or eat, and after you use the lavatory or visit a public place such as the gym. Scrub under your nails, too: that's a favourite place for pathogens to hide. Avoid wearing false nails. Researchers discovered that artificial nails are more hospitable to microbes than natural ones.

There's no magic to washing your hands. Simply remove rings and bracelets and, using any kind of soap and warm, running water, thoroughly wash all surfaces of your hands for at least 20 seconds. Then dry them completely with a clean or disposable towel.

Brush teeth several times a day, and floss at least once. That's the best way to keep germs from settling in your mouth. Most adults have some degree of gum disease. Flossing for just 2 minutes a day may be even more important than brushing for preventing gum disease. This is important to your immunity because gum disease has been linked to an increased risk of heart disease. When you have gum disease, oral bacteria may enter your bloodstream through small ulcers that develop in the gum tissue. This may increase your risk for a heart attack by contributing to narrowing blood vessels and to blood clots.

Take your shoes off at the door. Not only will this simple step keep your home cleaner to the naked eye, it will also help keep microscopic germs and chemicals out. Put a mat at each entrance to your home. About 80 per cent of dirt on floors comes in through the doors.

18. Prevention is Better Than Cure

Get appropriate vaccinations and make doctor and dentist appointments.

At the beginning of the 20th century, infectious diseases were the leading cause of death in children and young adults, exacting an enormous toll on the population. With the introduction of immunisation programmes the incidence of a number of infectious diseases declined dramatically world-wide. Smallpox has been eradicated, polio has been virtually eliminated and measles has been reduced to a low number of cases.

Vaccinations are effective. However, if you have a history of severe reactions to prior vaccinations, or allergies to eggs, make sure you mention this to your doctor first. For adults, your best defence against influenza (which can be lethal) is to get a flu vaccination to prevent the disorder and its serious complications.

An annual flu vaccination is essential for the elderly and for those who have a condition that would make flu or its complications more likely, such as congestive heart failure, emphysema or asthma. But the flu shot is just one of several vaccines that experts recommend for adults. People over the age of 65 should also be vaccinated against *Streptococcus pneumoniae,* bacteria that can cause pneumococcal pneumonia or meningitis.

Even if you were vaccinated against diphtheria and tetanus as a child, you should have booster shots every 10 years. People who contract tetanus suffer from stiffness and spasms of the muscles, which can cause bones to break. It can cause their throats to close, making it difficult to eat and breathe. Some people go into a coma; thirty per cent die.

When you visit your doctor for routine immunisations, ask for a complete medical check-up as well. Ideally, you should have a complete check-up once a year.

Make regular appointments to see a dentist. As mentioned above in Booster 17, dental health is an important key to immunity. Getting regular dental check-ups is particularly important if a family member has had gum trouble.

19. Stop Sneezing
Protect yourself against allergies.

Allergies are what happens when your immune system runs amok. The reaction of your body to allergies is like its reaction to an unclean wound. If you fail to remove the dirt from the wound, it will not heal. Similarly, if you fail to remove the allergens, your allergy symptoms, which could be anything from a stopped-up or runny nose to itchy eyes and breathing problems, will not go away.

Here are a few ways to make your home an allergen-free oasis and keep your immune system in balance.

Make your bed a safe haven. You spend about one-third of your day burrowed into sheets, blankets and pillows on top of a comfortable mattress. But there are also about a million dust mites sleeping with you. To reduce your exposure to them and their wastes, slip allergen-proof covers over your mattress and pillows. These keep new dust mites from entering your bed and form a barrier between you and any allergens that may have already accumulated there. Covers are available at department stores and online. Wash all bedding at 60°C (140°F) if possible as this will kill off any dust mites making a home in it.

Keep your home dry. Most homes have three of the four requirements that mites need to thrive: nesting sites such as carpets and mattresses, human skin cells to eat and a comfortable temperature. The fourth variable – the humidity that gives them moisture – is often what determines whether they will multiply up to a problematic level in your home or not.

Another problem that dampness causes is mould. A study by the University of Maryland in College Park found that exposure to mould spores can trigger flu-like symptoms and may even weaken your immunity to other illnesses. Mould normally just causes allergies, but in extreme cases, inhaling it can lead to serious illness, such as bleeding in the lungs. Kill mould by wiping infested areas with a 1-to-5 solution of bleach and water. Dehumidifiers and frequent dusting prevent its return. If you keep the humidity in your home between 30 and 50 per cent, probably best accomplished with an air conditioner and possibly a dehumidifier, you can help keep dust mites and mould at bay.

Filter out allergens. Proper filtration in your home can snatch up even the smallest allergens. This could include a vacuum equipped with filters to keep it from spewing out allergens as fast as it sucks them up, clean and well-working filters on your boiler (if you have one) and a free-standing air filter in your bedroom to trap airborne allergens.

20. Treat Yourself to the Miracle Herbs
Try herbs to heal and protect your body.

Like it or not, many of us are exposed to a number of factors that can wear us down: poor diet, bad sleep habits, stress and daily exposure to micro-organisms, to name a few. For a two-pronged attack to boost low-performance immune systems, first, use herbal medicine to help speed your body's healing process, then, continue herbal therapy to arm yourself long-term.

Marticia Hall, PhD, conducted research at the University of Pittsburgh on stress-related sleep disturbances. She found that poor sleep could lower immune system function and decrease killer cells that combat viruses. There are several herbal teas, in addition to the soothing camomile tea, that can help promote sleep the natural way. To help you sleep through the night, place 2 tablespoons of dried valerian in an infusion ball with cloves and cinnamon bark, and then steep for 15 minutes in a covered container with 500 ml (16 fl oz) of boiling water. Remove the infusion ball and sip the tea as needed. Herbalists recommend passionflower, 1 teaspoon of dried herb per cup of boiling water, and find it especially helpful for insomnia caused by anxiety. Night sweats, another of the sleep bandits, can be eliminated with sage. Make sage tea by placing 4 heaped tablespoons of dried sage in a cup of boiling water. Strain the sage after steeping for 4 or more hours, then drink the tea at bedtime.

If you don't get sufficient rest, you may find yourself a candidate for taking drug-free remedies for the most common ailments: colds, flu and bacterial infections, says Dr Berndtson. In 32 studies, echinacea was shown to prevent colds, possibly by activating the white blood cells that then fight the cold virus. Take it in tablet, capsule or tincture form, as directed, at the first sign of a cold. For improved immunity, take it for 3 months. Arabinogalactan, or AG, a soluble fibre, helps stimulate the immune defence system and destroy invading micro-organisms. It can be taken as 1 teaspoon three times a day, dissolved in juice or water, or it can be combined with echinacea to enhance its effect. Many herbalists suggest that astragalus be taken regularly during the cold and flu season. It is available in capsule form and should be taken as directed. There are a number of additional herbs used by herbal practitioners to boost the immune system. Siberian or a combination of Korean/Siberian ginseng, for example, has been used for centuries to improve endurance. Echinacea may bring relief at the first sign of a cold or sore throat. Follow the directions on the label for dosage information.

Hawthorn may help lower blood pressure and help circulation. This herb contains rutin, which reduces plaque formation in the arteries, helping to stave off heart attacks or strokes. To try it, boil 1 tablespoon of dried hawthorn berries in 240 ml (8 fl oz) of water for 10 minutes. Strain and drink this once a day.

According to herbalists, herbs can also help people who have skin conditions, including some forms of psoriasis, eczema and acne, which are often signs of a weak immune system. Oregon grape, which contains two alkaloids, berbamine and berberine, helps clear up these chronic conditions. Add 15 ml (1 tablespoon) of dried root to 240 ml (8 fl oz) of boiling water. Boil for 10 minutes, strain and drink. To improve the flavour, you can add a handful of camomile, which is also a potent skin tonic.

Mushrooms may be fungi that live on dead wood in shady forests, but in doing so they compete with bacteria, viruses and other fungi to survive, giving them natural immune system enhancers. The maitake mushroom, when taken daily over a long period of time, may stimulate the immune system to fight any recurring bacterial or viral infection. As an Immune Booster, take 2 grams of maitake per day in capsule form, and 4 to 6 grams a day in capsule form when you are ill. You may consider adding shiitake mushrooms to your next Chinese stir-fry dish. Studies have shown that this mushroom may help fight bacterial infections and flu, fight cancer and lower cholesterol.

Chapter 10

THE TOP 10 IMMUNE BUSTERS

WE HOPE YOU ENJOYED OUR GARDEN SALAD OF SUPER IMMUNE Boosters. Just as there are simple steps you can take to boost your immunity, here are some simple ways to pull out the weeds that can bust your immunity, says Keith Berndtson, MD, medical director at Integrative Care Centers in Chicago and Glenview, Illinois, and primary consultant for this book.

1. Kick the Habit

Stop smoking.

'The effect of chronic exposure to cigarette smoke is tantamount to asking the immune system (and one of its chief allies, the liver) to clean up one toxic spill after another,' says Dr Berndtson.

Smoking, and breathing in secondhand smoke, are terrible for your entire body. Cigarette smoke contains more than 4,000 chemical compounds. Of these, at least 43 are known carcinogens. Here are just some of the ways it wreaks havoc: smoking causes heart disease, lung and oesophageal cancer and chronic lung disease. It contributes to cancer of the bladder, pancreas and kidneys. Women who smoke during pregnancy are more likely to have problems, including babies with low birth weights, which is a leading cause of infant death.

In fact, smoking kills more than two times as many people as AIDS, alcohol abuse, car accidents, murders, drugs and suicide *combined*. One out of every five deaths in America is smoking-related. On average, smokers die nearly 7 years earlier than nonsmokers.

The risk of developing lung cancer is up to one-third greater for non-smokers who are regularly exposed to tobacco smoke. Children whose parents smoke are twice as likely to develop asthma than those with non-smoking parents.

Nicotine is a very addictive drug, which is why it is so hard to stop smoking. For some people, nicotine can be as addictive as heroin or cocaine.

No matter how long you have been smoking, you can prevent further damage to your health by giving it up. As soon as you stop smoking, the risk of developing lung cancer and other respiratory disorders, stroke and cardiovascular disease lessens.

According to the US Centers for Disease Control and Prevention, studies have shown that these five steps will help you quit for good.

1. Get ready. First, set a quit date. Then, dispose of all cigarettes and ashtrays in your home, car and place of work. Once you quit, don't smoke – not even a puff.
2. Get support. You will have a better chance of being successful with support. Here are some ways to get it. Talk to your doctor. Tell your family and friends that you are going to quit and need their support. Get individual, group or phone counselling. Call your local health department for information about programmes in your area.
3. Take a whiff. One study found that sniffing strong smells can stop cravings. In a University of Pittsburgh study, 58 smokers rated their nicotine cravings on a scale of zero to 100 before and after they smelled scents such as coconut, peppermint and Vicks

mentholated rub. Researchers found that the strongest smells reduced cravings by 20 per cent, because the part of the brain that controls cravings also happens to be where you process smells.

4. Get medication and use it correctly. Your doctor may recommend prescription medications to help you stop smoking: bupropion (Zyban), nicotine inhalers and nicotine nasal sprays. Until more studies are done, Dr Berndtson recommends only Zyban. Nicotine gum and a nicotine patch may also be useful. Use the gum as directed until the craving ceases. A nicotine patch worn daily may be necessary for about 6 weeks, says Dr Berndtson, and you should take it off at bedtime. Do not use the patch if you are still smoking, and check with your doctor before using it if you have any medical problems. Taking any one of these medications will double your chances of quitting.

5. Be prepared for relapse or difficult situations. Most relapses occur within the first 3 months of quitting. Here are some difficult situations to watch out for: drinking alcohol, being around other smokers, gaining weight and experiencing depression.

The benefits of quitting are numerous and powerful. If you quit before the age of 40, you will add 5 years to your life. After 10 smoke-free years, you will have cut your risk of dying of lung cancer in half. After 15 years, your risk of heart disease will be almost the same as someone who has never smoked.

2. Steer Clear of PCBs

Avoid toxic chemical exposures.

In 1988, researchers identified the virus that was responsible for taking the lives of approximately 20,000 harbour seals in the Baltic and North Seas. Biologists reported that they had never witnessed such an enormous decline, and they thought that the devastation was over, but they were wrong. In less than a year, the same virus infected seals in Canada, but this time there were no casualties. Concerned for the seals' safety, scientists quickly began extensive research and discovered that seals found dead in northern Europe were from areas that were contaminated with toxic pollutants, particularly polychlorinated biphenyls (PCBs). Scientists were familiar with the suppressive effects that PCB had on the immune systems of fish and laboratory animals.

The National Wildlife Federation reported that the immune defences of wildlife species are being adversely affected by contaminants that are dispersed into our environment. The continuous accumulation of these contaminants may be responsible for the vulnerability of these species until either an environmental change or a pathogen creates another decline.

It takes just one exposure of less than one-millionth of a gram for immunotoxic contaminants such as PCBs, mercury, certain pesticides and dioxin-like substances to disrupt the immune function of innocent wildlife. Since these chemicals can stay in the environment for decades, vulnerable wildlife species have no escape from their devastation. Moreover, not only do these toxins become more concentrated as they move their way up the food chain, they can also cause life-threatening autoimmune reactions – the immune system's inability to tell the difference between the body's own tissues and foreign invaders.

Evidence suggests that some of these same chemicals may be putting us at risk. For example, in Aberdeen, North Carolina, scientists found that young adults were two times more likely than non-residents to have shingles, a painful condition caused by a herpes virus. In another study, researchers found that chlordane, a termite-killing substance, caused weaker immune responses in people who had been exposed.

Fortunately, the enforcement of national and international bans has resulted in the declining use of PCBs and dioxins. But the process is slow. Low-level chemical leakage from hazardous waste sites can linger for decades, and new industrial chemicals are not normally tested for their effects on the immune system. As a result, we are unaware of the potential threat that these chemicals pose to wildlife until massive problems begin to show up.

Therefore, you need to reduce your exposure as much as possible to unnecessary toxins. Stay away from cigarette smoke, excess alcohol and illicit drugs. Buy organic produce when possible. Rinse your fruits and vegetables thoroughly to remove pesticides. Switch to natural gardening methods and stay indoors or go away when your neighbours are using pesticides. Choose cleaners, paper goods and other products that are made with less toxic materials. Read food labels vigilantly and avoid products that contain unnecessary chemicals.

3. Avoid Sleep Deprivation
Give your body time to refuel and rest.

To your conscious mind, sleep is a restful time, as in 'to sleep, perchance to dream'. To your body, it is work time. During sleep the brain, liver and immune system conduct their strategic planning sessions for handling the onslaught of the upcoming day, says Dr Berndtson.

Sleep is as critical to our bodies as exercise and diet. While you sleep, your body is performing two essential tasks. First, it's resting and refuelling. During sleep, your heart rate and blood pressure drop and your metabolism slows. This allows your cells to concentrate on the second vital task: repairing and creating new cells in every system of the body, including your immune system.

Sleep deprivation has a powerfully detrimental effect on your immune system. The perfect example is college students who become ill after working all night cramming for exams.

Most people need between 6 and 8 hours a night, but consider the quality of your sleep time too. If you're tired when you wake up in the morning, you're not getting enough sleep, or maybe not enough quality sleep. Either way, your immunity is probably compromised. Poor sleep is associated with lower immune system function and reduced numbers of killer cells that fight germs. Killer cells are also the part of the immune system that combats cells that divide too rapidly, as they do in cancer. Lower their numbers and you may be at greater risk for illness.

Studies have shown that chronic sleep deprivation also contributes to heart disease, gastrointestinal problems and other medical illnesses. One study on the effects of sleep deprivation showed that a group of men restricted to 4 to 6 hours of sleep per night experienced changes in hormone function and carbohydrate metabolism that mimic ageing changes. The lack of sleep was making them age more quickly.

You are much more likely to have an accident if you drive when sleep-deprived. In one study, researchers gave driving performance tests to 39 people after they had stayed awake for 17 to 20 hours and again after they had drunk enough alcohol to raise their blood alcohol levels to 0.1 per cent. Half of the participants performed as poorly when sleep-deprived as they had when drunk.

If you could fall asleep sitting in a meeting or quietly reading in your office, you're overtired.

For tips on how to get better sleep, see Booster 4, Enjoy the Power of Sleep, on page 110.

4. Release Yourself from the Stress Trap

Reduce your stress levels to halt a harmful
chain reaction in your body.

There is no doubt about it, stress is an Immune Buster. We owe much of what we now know about the stress/immunity connection studying rats.

Back in the 1930s, Hans Selye, MD, PhD, DSc, an endocrinologist, was trying to learn about a hormonal substance that had been isolated from the ovaries of animals. Dr Selye injected one group of rats with the hormonal substance and another group with a placebo. Several months later, he noticed that the rats developed severely impaired immune systems. What was disturbing was that *all* of the rats were harmed, not just the ones injected with the hormonal substance. The rats given the placebo had impaired immunity, too. Dr Selye was puzzled: if it wasn't the ovarian extract that caused the physical changes, what could it have been? The only other factor affecting both sets of rats was the daily injections, which they all disliked. The rats hated the injections so much that often, he had to hold them down to inject them while they writhed and squirmed to get away.

Dr Selye conducted other experiments in which he created equally unpleasant conditions for rats, such as plunging them in cold water. In each case, he duplicated the results of his earlier experiment.

While we may not be plunged into cold water, everybody experiences stressful situations every day. We must put up with flight delays, bad weather, impatient bosses and deadlines. These normal stresses, however, are usually transient and do not exact a steep toll on us physically or emotionally. Other stresses can be more profound and long-lasting and hit us harder than the usual stresses of daily living. The loss of a job, the death of a spouse, the breakup of a marriage: these are all examples of situations that can trigger a vigorous stress response in the body.

When we encounter a stressful situation, our brains give our adrenal glands a signal to pump out stress hormones. These hormones trigger a chain of reactions that prepare our bodies for an emergency. Our blood pressure rises, our hearts pump faster, our pupils dilate and we are ready for fight or flight. A short time after the crisis passes, our bodies return to normal and we are none the worse for the experience. However, under constant stress, the sort a secretary who cannot escape the capricious whims of her demanding boss experiences, our bodies are always bombarded with stress hormones. These hormones can have a harmful effect on many different body systems, especially the immune system.

There is compelling scientific evidence that chronic stress causes a measurable decline in the immune system's ability to fight disease. Severe and chronic stress have a direct impact on the immune system that can cause disease or change the course of a pre-existing disease. For example, four studies have indicated that higher levels of stress hormones lead to more rapid cancer progression.

Several studies have linked stress to increased disease and ageing. In one study, stressful life events such as the death of a child or a major financial difficulty increased the risk of premature death.

Other research has shown that people who are stressed are more prone to developing cardiovascular disease. Studies show that women with cardiovascular disease who are better able to manage their stress live longer and remain healthier than women with cardiovascular disease who undergo a lot of stress and do not know how to manage it.

Periods of extreme stress can result in lower natural killer cell count, sluggish 'killer T-cells', and diminished macrophage activity that can amplify the immune response. In fact, widows and widowers are much more likely to become ill during the first year following the death of their spouse than their peers who have not experienced a major loss.

Knowing that stress is bad for your immune system and doing something about it are two different things. For tips on how to reduce stress, see Booster 14, Seek Serenity, on page 125.

5. Conquer Depression

Adopt an optimistic outlook for better health.

This Buster is especially important for women, since women are more likely than men to become depressed during their lifetimes.

Like many other illnesses, depression is a continuum. Everyone gets the blues now and then. Being down in the dumps over a period of time is not normal, however. When a person is clinically depressed, her ability to function is affected. Here are just some of the signs of clinical depression: an empty feeling, tiredness, lack of energy, sleep problems and loss of interest or pleasure in ordinary activities. If these symptoms last for more than 2 weeks, see a doctor.

Clearly, clinical depression is detrimental to immunity. But even subtler shades of sadness can weaken your immune system.

Studies show that pessimists who look at a half-glass of water and think that it's half-empty don't live as long as optimists, who see the same glass as half-full. When pessimists put a more positive spin on the calamities in their lives, they have less stress and better health. One reason for this could be that optimists take better care of themselves. It could also be due to less stress-related damage to your immune system, such as killer cells that suddenly become pacifists. In one study, cancer patients who completed a special course designed to make them more optimistic had stronger immune systems than those who maintained their bleak outlooks.

Other research supports the idea that having a negative outlook when under stress can make you and your immune system miss out. A 1998 study at UCLA found that the law students who began their first term optimistic about the experience had more helper T-cells mid-term, which can amplify the immune response, and more powerful natural killer cells. The reason is that they perceived events such as their gruelling first year as less stressful than did their more pessimistic classmates. Researchers say that this establishes the possibility that a person's outlook and mood when stressed might affect responses to common immune challenges such as exposure to cold viruses.

Here are some ideas to help you look on the bright side of life.

• Make three appointments. First, make a lunch or dinner date with your partner, best friend or a family member. Second, go to a meeting of a voluntary or interest group that you'd like to join. While loving and intimate relationships are important, so is variety. Third, make a date with yourself and treat yourself to something that will relax you, whether it's meditating in a quiet room or browsing in a bookshop.

• Change your attitude by changing how you respond to adverse events. When you lose an important client or break your diet for a day or two, avoid exaggerated, negative generalisations, such as 'I'll never get another client!' or 'Diets never work!' Those statements simply aren't true and just feed your feelings of hopelessness. It's more honest, and more productive, to remind yourself that you've lost clients before and always found another. And it's hard to stay on a diet during the holiday season. Also, when one thing goes wrong, don't assume that everything is wrong. Learn how to section off areas of your life. Your job may be terrible, but you still have your friends and family who make you happy.

• Change your vocabulary. Rid yourself of negative words such as *try* and *but* because they don't give you a sense of commitment to your goal. Focus instead on words like *will* and *can*.

• Try to talk more to cheerful people and shun unhappy ones. Notice how some people make you feel great while others sap your energy. It's your life: spend it with people who make you happy.

• Smile. Sometimes consciously doing happy things can make people respond positively to you, which can make you feel better.

6. Throw Out Your Couch

Avoid sedentary lifestyles.

'Death is very still, so keep moving,' says Dr Berndtson.

Exercise is an essential part of a healthy lifestyle, but the majority of people still do too little exercise. Women are even more likely to be inactive than men. Sedentary ways have a tremendous impact on health. The benefits of exercise are so great that choosing not to exercise is like throwing away a winning lottery ticket. Millions of people suffer from illnesses that can be prevented or treated through exercise, including high blood pressure, coronary heart disease and type 2 diabetes.

Studies show the dangers of a sedentary life. One study compared inactive people with those who walked briskly almost every day. Researchers found that those who didn't walk took twice as many days off sick in 4 months as those who walked.

Another study conducted by researchers at the University of Illinois at Urbana-Champaign found that when previously sedentary elderly people spent 6 months exercise-training, their immune function improved.

In yet another study, researchers at Temple University in Philadelphia found that light to moderate aerobic and resistance exercise helps to offset the apparent decrement in natural killer cell activity associated with weight loss.

When you begin an exercise programme, you should build up your activity level gradually. For example, begin slowly with a 10- to 15-minute walk, three times a week; if you're unfit, start at a slower pace. If you choose a more vigorous exercise than walking, such as squash, begin each session slowly. Stretch first for 5 minutes to give your body a chance to warm up. At the end of your workout, cool down for another 5 minutes with more stretching.

If you have or are at risk of chronic health problems such as heart disease, diabetes, or obesity, check with your doctor before beginning an exercise programme. It's also a good idea for all men and women over 45 to check with a doctor before beginning an exercise programme.

Over time, you should work up to the standard recommendation of five times a week for at least 30 minutes. Experts say that it takes half an hour of aerobic exercise to sweep white blood cells, key immune system components that are stuck on the blood vessel walls, back into circulation.

Moderate exercise is the key. If your exercise is too intense, it can actually suppress your immune system, which is why marathon runners often get colds after a race. What defines overexertion depends on your fitness level. Consult with your doctor to determine yours before starting an exercise programme.

The benefits of exercise stretch even beyond its direct immune effects. When you exercise, you're more likely to sleep better and reduce stress, effectively wiping out two other big Immune Busters.

Also, leading a sedentary life is likely to make you fat. Obesity is associated with alterations in immune function. Researchers at Appalachian State University in Boone, North Carolina, studied 157 women, some of whom were at their ideal weight and some of whom were obese. They found that the obese women had higher blood cell counts, a risk factor for heart disease. Weight loss is associated with a decrease in these blood cell counts, which boosts immunity.

One way to boost your exercise quota is to get a dog. Having a dog can give a double boost to your immune system. Besides encouraging you to exercise, dogs can boost your immunity in their own right. One study found that new dog owners had significantly fewer minor health problems than non-owners in the 10 months after getting their dogs.

For other tips on how to exercise more, see Booster 3, Discover the Wonders of Working Out, on page 109.

7. Escape from Your Home
Avoid social isolation.

We can chat, research and even shop without moving from our desk chairs. But people reduced to type on a screen cannot be touched. While they may be able to reciprocate our feelings, this is no substitute for friendly human contact.

'Feeling disconnected from others, or allowing things like excessive television watching and Internet surfing to interfere with cultivating one's important relationships, will work behind the scenes to weaken immune system function,' says Dr Berndtson.

The cost of social isolation may be higher than we think. Studies show that the fewer human connections we have at home, at work and in the community, the more likely we are to become ill, flood our brains with anxiety-causing chemicals and die prematurely.

One study in Sweden showed that those who frequented cultural events such as concerts, exhibitions and even ball games tended to live longer than their stay-at-home peers. The key factors could be increased social contact and reduced stress. Other studies have found that people who are isolated may live only half as long as those who have a lot of human contact. Love seems to be an immune system nutrient.

The good news is that these same studies also show that the more human connections we have, the more likely we are to live longer and healthier. Connectedness is the unacknowledged key to emotional and physical health. The more ties you have, the more likely you are to stay well in the first place. Researchers who monitored 276 people between the ages of 18 and 55 found that those who had six or more connections were four times better at fighting off the viruses that cause colds.

Here are a few ways to connect.

• Think of your favourite social events and make them a habit.

• Avoid those who oppose you. The only way to make room for meaningful relationships is to get rid of the connections that aren't re-warding for you.

• Renew your faith. Worship is an excellent way to get in touch with something greater than yourself and structure spiritual connections into your life. Even if you don't have a lot of faith, just sitting in church and thinking big thoughts for an hour a week is good for you.

QUIZ: HOW CONNECTED ARE YOU?

To find out how connected you are, take the following quiz, developed by Edward M Hallowell, MD, instructor in psychiatry at Harvard Medical School and author of *Connect: 12 Vital Ties That Open Your Heart, Lengthen Your Life, and Deepen Your Soul*. Answer yes or no to each of the 10 questions, then see below to determine your connectivity quotient.

1. Do you make time to be with members of your family of origin, even if it means giving up some activity that you might enjoy?
2. Do you eat family dinner together with the family you've created or joined, or do you spend time together with them in some other way?
3. Do you know the people who live next door well enough to ask them to do you a favour?
4. Do you sometimes get so interested in your work that you forget what time it is or where you are?
5. Do you know details about your parents' and grandparents' lives?
6. Are there special natural habitats that speak to you in ways that no other place can?
7. Can you understand intuitively why it is that older people do better if they have pets around?
8. Have you put up sufficient barriers so that unimportant messages, random data and useless information are not overwhelming you?
9. Do you feel a connection to whatever is beyond knowledge, whether you call it God, the cosmos, or some other name?
10. Do you feel happy about your body?

Now, add up your answers. The more 'yes' answers you have, the more connected you're likely to be. If your score is lower than you'd like, take a moment to review where you answered no. Then, think about putting a little extra energy into building new connections.

8. Avoid Junk Food

Fuel your body with the vitamins and minerals it needs.

The exponential growth in the availability and popularity of junk food has led to a corresponding rise in poor eating habits, obesity and the numerous health problems associated with being overweight. Junk food often contains large amounts of fat, salt and sugar that can be very damaging to health.

While junk food probably will never be a controlled substance, it is coming under increasingly critical scrutiny and some public health officials would like to subject junk food to special taxes in order to subsidise the cost of healthy foods such as fruits and vegetables. The money generated by the tax could also be used to fund health promotion programmes.

Experts believe that nutritional deficiencies are probably the greatest cause of immune system weakness. What you eat is vital because your immune system is a voracious user of vitamins and minerals. Every few days, your body feverishly replaces one-quarter of all your immune cells. For example, special cells called neutrophils, which swallow bacteria whole, live for only about 36 hours and then have to be replaced by fresh troops of new cells.

Experts have known for some time that when a person is malnourished, her immune system is weakened. When you restore the person to normal nutrition, her immune system improves, which is no surprise. But what they're just learning is that when you continue to improve nutrition beyond mere adequacy, the immune system continues to improve, even in healthy people.

One thing that a lot of junk food has in common is excess fat. Fats, especially polyunsaturated fats, tend to suppress the immune system. Make sure you cut your total fat intake to no more than 25 per cent of daily calories.

Another bad component of junk food is excess sugar. Sugar inhibits phagocytosis, the process by which viruses and bacteria are engulfed and then literally chewed up by white blood cells. Alcohol is in a class of its own. It's true that in moderation, alcohol can actually boost immunity. But as with junk food, the temptation to overimbibe is so great that we feel it belongs here in the Busters.

Alcohol is a double-edged sword. Red wine is a good source of anthocyanidins, which are important Immune Boosters. In fact, moderate drinkers (one or two drinks a day) tend to have lower levels of heart disease. A daily glass of wine may be great for lowering cholesterol. In general, some studies suggest that people who drink occasionally have lower death rates than teetotallers.

However, the case *against* drinking is still stronger than the one *for* it. Too much alcohol definitely does increase mortality. For more than 200 years, doctors have observed that excessive alcohol consumption can lead to increased illness and death from infectious diseases. Alcohol abusers suffer from increased susceptibility to bacterial pneumonia, pulmonary tuberculosis and hepatitis C.

What's more, compared with moderate drinkers, people who drink a great deal may be at increased risk for infection with HIV if they engage in unsafe sex practices while they are intoxicated. Researchers are also investigating whether alcohol consumption itself may increase susceptibility to HIV infection or hasten the progression from HIV infection to full-blown AIDS.

There is now quite a lot of evidence that in women, even moderate alcohol consumption can increase the risk of breast cancer. In excess, alcohol dampens immune function. Plus, alcohol can suppress the B-cells that make antibodies, which can leave you more prone to bacterial infection.

Furthermore, if you drink even a little within 3 hours of bedtime, it can disturb your most restful period of sleep, rapid eye movement, or REM, when most dreaming occurs.

Yet another reason to avoid alcohol is that it causes you to gain weight. In one study, Dutch researchers offered cocktails to 52 normal-weight to obese people. Compared with those who chose juice or water, the beer and wine drinkers ate about 200 more calories (plus the 240 calories they drank), they ate faster, they spent nearly 20 per cent more time eating, they took longer to feel full and they continued eating past the point of feeling full. To avoid all these unwanted effects, always order mineral water instead of alcohol. It's calorie-free, it fills you up and it helps curb your appetite.

For tips on how to improve your diet, see Booster 1, Put Some Colour on Your Plate, on page 106, and Booster 8, Remember, Variety Is the Spice of Life, on page 116.

9. Arm Yourself against Too Many Antibiotics

Do your part to keep bacteria from getting the upper hand.

A hundred years ago, infectious diseases were the leading cause of death in the world. In 1900, pneumonia and tuberculosis caused almost 25 per cent of all deaths in the United States. But advances in public health and the discovery of antibiotics brought many of those diseases under control. By 1990, pneumonia and tuberculosis caused less than 4 per cent of all US deaths.

Antibiotics were the wonder drugs of the 20th century. They cured children of meningitis, helped burn victims resist infections and reshaped the treatment of syphilis and gonorrhoea.

But as time crept closer to the 21st century, the tide began to turn. In 1987, antibiotic-resistant pneumococci − individual organisms of the species *Streptococcus pneumoniae* − had not been encountered. Just 10 years later, as many as 40 per cent of pneumococcus strains were resistant to penicillin and other commonly used antibiotics.

The cost of antibiotic resistance is high, both literally and from a health perspective. Literally, it costs fifteen times as much to treat a patient who has tuberculosis with a multidrug-resistant strain.

From a health perspective, the cost of antibiotic resistance is an increase in the seriousness of disease. For example, treating a person with tuberculosis caused by a strain that is killed by antibiotics is highly effective. In contrast, between 40 and 60 per cent of people who get antibiotic-resistant tuberculosis die.

The cost of misuse of antibiotics can be a weakened immune system. Researchers found that certain patients taking antibiotics had reduced levels of cytokines, the hormone messengers of the immune system. When your immune system is suppressed, you are more likely to develop resistant bacteria or to become ill in the future.

Here are steps to take to use antibiotics properly.

• Take antibiotics only for bacterial infections. Antibiotics work against bacterial infections, but colds and flu are caused by viruses. Doctors should know better than to prescribe them, but you can do your part by not insisting on an antibiotic for a cold or flu.

• Take antibiotics correctly. If you are prescribed an antibiotic, it's crucial that you take the entire course. Many people skip doses or stop taking the medication as they start feeling better, but that may help breed antibiotic-resistant pathogens. If you stop taking the drug early, the bacteria that are still alive can restart an infection.

• Don't use antibiotics to try to prevent infection. The drugs don't work that way. In addition, you're still likely to end up with an infection, but it could be a more dangerous, antibiotic-resistant one.

• Don't save or share antibiotics. A medical practitioner needs to evaluate each person every time they are ill.

• Avoid antibacterial hand soaps and lotions. One study from Tufts University School of Medicine in Boston found that an active ingredient in antibacterial soap, triclosan, can alter the genetic makeup of the *Escherichia coli* bacterium, producing resistant strains. By washing carefully with regular soap and water, you will get rid of as many germs as with any other product you can use. Soap loosens dirt and microbes, then water rinses them away.

10. Cheer Up
Use laughter to beat stress.

A child is said to laugh 400 times a day, while adults laugh only 15 times. Even though there may be no hard science to back up this statistic, it's pretty safe to say that children *do* laugh far more than adults. Just as the hands of time add wrinkles and rip out hair, they seem to make us more serious and less mirthful.

Life is too short to be so serious. Laughing boosts immune system function, says Dr Berndtson.

Researchers have found that the positive emotions associated with laughter decrease stress hormones and increase certain immune cells while activating others. In one study conducted at Loma Linda University

School of Medicine in California, 10 healthy men who watched a comedy video for an hour had significant increases in one particular hormone of the immune system that activates other components of the immune system.

To add humour to your life, simply find reasons to laugh. Rent a funny video; read a book of jokes. Have lunch with a friend known for her sense of humour. Taking things less seriously can boost your immune system, and it's a lot cheaper than going to the doctor.

PART

3

Preventing
and
Treating
Immune-Related
Diseases

Chapter

11

HOW TO CARE FOR YOURSELF AND YOUR FAMILY WITH IMMUNE-RELATED CONDITIONS

NOTHING MAKES A MEDICAL EXPERT OUT OF YOU FASTER THAN having a child with a health problem. For Susan Simmons of Olive Branch, Mississippi, that problem was her daughter's asthma. Over the years, Susan has learned many of the hard lessons immune-related disease has to offer, and she's become a strong, smart advocate for her daughter's health care.

'I didn't know a lot about asthma when Morgan was born,' Susan says, 'but now I can tell a kid who has it from across the room. I'm not an expert, but I've learned a lot over the years – most of it the hard way.'

That hard road included several hospitalisations for Morgan for respiratory ailments when she was just a baby, and more after she was diagnosed with asthma aged 2. But Susan and her husband, Gary, were determined that their daughter would have a healthy, normal life, and they took every possible step to provide it.

'The biggest things for us haven't been the medicines, the inhalers, or even the allergy shots,' Susan explains. 'They've been the things we've had to do at home.' Over the years, concerned paediatricians, allergists, immunologists and hospital staff gave the Simmonses advice on improving Morgan's health, and the family took it all to heart.

Among the 'prescriptions' they've followed are: daily swimming, year-round, to exercise Morgan's lungs; a curtain-, carpet-, stuffed-animal- and duvet-free world at home; plastic-wrapped pillows and mattresses for the whole family; vacuuming and damp dusting every single day; carefully monitoring Morgan's diet for highly allergenic foods; giving up an antique quilt collection; and, perhaps the hardest pill to swallow, moving out of their lovingly restored 100-year-old house into a newer one that harboured small amounts of dust mites, mould and other allergens.

Though the Simmonses' lifestyle changes have been significant, the benefits have been more than commensurate. The family's allergist once told Susan that Morgan had the worst case of asthma he'd seen in 35 years. You'd never know it, though, from the beautiful, healthy, outgoing 8-year-old who runs around the playground playing football and Barbies with her friends and rarely misses a day of school. 'She's down to just one medicine, too,' Susan reports, 'and we hope she'll be able to be weaned off that one very soon.'

A Combined Approach

Fortunately, not every family has to go to the extremes that the Simmons family did to ensure good immunological health. The main lesson they have to offer, though, is that promoting good immune health at home requires going far beyond just making a yearly trip to the doctor for a check-up. It's a complicated combination of self-care, traditional medicine and, in the best of worlds, at least a nod to the theories and practices of alternative and complementary medicine.

The Best Care Begins at Home

Any effort to deal with immune-related diseases and conditions starts at home with preventive self-care. Of course, when you're caring for a family, 'self-care' isn't just about you. It includes the care of children, a partner and perhaps an elderly parent or other family member. To prevent contagious diseases from striking the immune systems of your family, and to help manage immune conditions that already have, start by following these basic rules for good home health.

Wash your hands frequently. Good health at home starts right at the kitchen (or bathroom) sink. The majority of harmful organisms that cause contagious illnesses make their way into our bodies by way of our hands, says Susan Nelson, MD, a family physician at Cypress Family Care and Obstetrics in Memphis. Hand washing is one of the few factors within your control that can truly be effective in reducing the spread of disease in your home. Teach your children (and your partner, if you need to) to wash hands before every meal and after using the toilet, after playing or working in the garden, and after handling uncooked foods.

Children aren't likely to tolerate water hot enough to make a difference in how clean their hands get, so let them choose their water temperature as long as they'll consistently wash, says Dr Nelson. 'Soap increases their odds of avoiding the unhealthy germs, but even if you can only get them to rinse their hands, it'll make a big difference.'

An ideal wash is about 15 seconds with soap; try teaching children to recite the alphabet while they wash to encourage them to keep washing. To avoid killing off healthy bacteria on the skin, don't use antibacterial soap. A basic pump soap is fine, says Dr Nelson.

Keep things on schedule. Numerous studies suggest that stress is a factor in immune-related disease, so keeping it at a minimum in your household can affect your family's health. 'Day-to-day, one of the most important things you can do to reduce stress is make sure that your children have a schedule, and that that schedule isn't too taxing,' says Richard Glickman-Simon, MD, assistant professor of medicine at Tufts University School of Medicine in Boston and chairman of the Western biomedicine department at the New England School of Acupuncture in Watertown, Massachusetts. 'Children need to have a routine of sleeping, eating and

SUCCESS STORIES

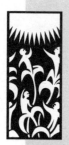

Natural Remedies Helped Her Overcome Crippling Arthritis

Nancy Etchemendy beat a devastating rheumatoid arthritis diagnosis with a vegan diet, acupuncture, regular exercise and relaxation therapies. Today, she's thoroughly enjoying life again.

When her illness struck, Nancy was in her early thirties and already had three children's novels in print with major publishers. She also ran a freelance graphics arts production business.

Mornings would find her leaning over a drawing board in her San Francisco Bay area home, lifting composites and overlays and wielding a razor blade, meticulously cutting around the edges of objects in photographs and aligning type elements. In the afternoons, she wrote. Then, one morning in 1986, her thumb wouldn't cooperate. It was sore and stiff.

'I thought I had strained it and it would go away,' she recalls. 'But it didn't.' Instead, the pain and stiffness spread. 'Before long, it was in my shoulders, and I was having trouble lifting my arms and doing my work.'

She saw doctors in her Stanford University community of Menlo Park, and within the year was diagnosed with rheumatoid arthritis. Then things got worse.

'Pretty soon it got to the point where I was having triggering in my fingers, and there was a lot of pain. Mostly it was in my upper body, elbows, neck, shoulders, wrists and hands. The doctor sent me to an occupational therapist because I couldn't hold my tools anymore. The therapist gave me some pointers about how to turn doorknobs, stuff like that. But it

times for work and play and family that they can predict.'

He also recommends making a regular interaction of sitting down with your children and asking them if they have anything they want to talk about. 'Even if they don't have any stresses they want to discuss,' he says, 'it's good for your family to know that that outlet is there, and that it's going to be there often, perhaps even daily.'

really was just a drop in the bucket. He also told me that I shouldn't lift any weight, not even my child.'

That was devastating. Her only child, Max, was just 3 years old.

And there were other disappointments and trials. 'I couldn't play the guitar or piano anymore, and I got to the point where I couldn't lift a glass without using both hands. Some days, I couldn't brush my teeth.'

At first, steroid injections helped, but then they worked for shorter and shorter periods. 'When they wore off, I would feel terrible,' she remembers. 'I got to the point where I just couldn't function anymore. I couldn't get through a day without bursting into tears. And I began to think continuously of suicide.'

The turnaround came when she realised that she needed a counsellor. She found a cognitive therapist, who helped her discover that despite the pain, she still was in control. He helped her learn to release anger and encouraged her to view her illness as an opportunity to grow and learn more about life. And he encouraged her to explore alternatives to caustic and often ineffective arthritis drugs. She started a vegan diet plus fish twice a week.

'Within a month of starting the vegan diet, I was getting normal blood work, normal sedimentation rates and less anaemia. I was feeling better,' Nancy says.

Then she saw a medical doctor who had studied Chinese medicine and treated her with acupuncture, and that helped a bit. After much research, she ultimately found a formula that works for her. It includes monthly counselling, acupuncture, daily meditation, qigong (slow-motion exercise that emphasises breath control), stress reduction techniques, nutritional supplements and daily walking.

Nancy still has occasional stiffness. 'But the difference is, I feel much more in control of the condition. And I'm totally enjoying life,' she notes.

She still can't pick up her son. But that's because he's grown up now. 'If he were a baby, I certainly could,' she says with pride.

Spend time outdoors. Making sure your family has time to get outside (even if that means sometimes giving them a push out of the door) is one of the best things you can do for their health, says Dr Glickman-Simon.

There are two main reasons: first, children (or adults) plus outside usually equals exercise, which benefits virtually all systems of the body.

Second, it's often the indoor environment that triggers immunological disorders – particularly, many allergies. 'The fact is that no matter how much you work on purifying your house, the air doesn't circulate as well there as it does outside,' Dr Glickman-Simon explains. In fact, the US Environmental Protection Agency has called poor indoor air quality one of the top five health threats of our time. Its studies suggest that indoor air is often 25 times more polluted than outdoor air – and sometimes as much as 100 times more polluted. Since most of us spend an estimated 90 per cent of our time indoors, experts say that getting out and breathing the fresh air may be one of the best things we can do for our health.

Remember that you're feeding your family's good health. As the caretaker for your family, the way you stock the shelves and the meals you put on the table affect much more than just you; they have a direct effect on everyone in your home. While family members dealing with immunological conditions may require very specialised diets, follow the suggestions in Activate Your Body's Immune Power with the MaxImmunity Diet, on page 51, for choosing the least allergenic, most healthy foods for your household.

'Of all the tools available to us in preventing and treating disease, the two areas I'd focus most on are nutrition and stress management,' says Russell Greenfield, MD, director of Carolinas Integrative Health in Charlotte, North Carolina, and co-author of *Healthy Child, Whole Child: Integrating the Best of Conventional and Alternative Medicine to Keep Your Kids Healthy.* 'You can't overestimate the importance of what you eat to your overall health and the health of your immune system.'

Good Health and Your Doctor

While many immune-related diseases remain a mystery to modern medicine, there are steps you can take with the help of your family doctor, your child's health visitor and medical specialists to help ensure the good health of your family.

Make sure that your family is vaccinated. Keeping up with the routine recommended vaccinations for your family is the simplest thing you can do to keep their immune systems well-equipped. Contact your doctor to be sure that the vaccinations you and your family need are up-to-date. Though there are some opponents to routine vaccination, compulsory immunisation is responsible for eradicating two devastating, once-rampant diseases (smallpox and polio) and for reducing the incidence of seven more diseases by 95 per cent or better. There are very rare health risks associated with vaccinations, but since we still do have outbreaks of some of the vaccine-preventable diseases, the benefits far outweigh the risks, says Dr Glickman-Simon.

Keep up with regular check-ups. 'Annual check-ups are very important in children and adults,' says Dr Nelson. 'They give the doctor and patient (or parent) time to review preventive health issues which may be overlooked when the patient comes for an illness.' In between yearly check-ups, stay on the alert for some of the symptoms of immune-related diseases: fatigue, muscle aches, or a persistent cold or cough, for example. 'If these symptoms linger for more than 2 weeks, see your doctor,' says Dr Nelson.

Work as a team. 'One of the most interesting developments in health care since the advent of the Internet is the number of patients who know more about their conditions than their doctors,' says Dr Glickman-Simon. 'A physician needs to know a lot about hundreds of diseases, but you can focus on your own.'

That change in the doctor/patient dynamic can be beneficial for everyone if you work together on your health care. 'Rely on your doctor to help you sort through what are evidence-based treatments (scientifically tested) and what are not,' Dr Glickman-Simon suggests. Working together, you can create a medical plan that combines your research and your doctor's medical knowledge, expertise and ability to make referrals to highly qualified specialists.

Note: It's especially important to work closely with your doctor whenever your child shows signs of any immune-related condition, since treatment recommendations and dosages for children can vary drastically from those for adults.

When Illness Strikes

No matter how cautious you are, there comes a time when the flu or a nasty cold makes its way into every family. Keeping it from spreading can seem an impossible task. Dr Nelson recommends that you start with the following strategies to contain the illness and get through it with a minimum of suffering.

Stop sharing. Teach your children that using one another's things – especially when someone in the family is ill – is an invitation to illness. Combs and brushes, hats, coats, pens and pencils, pillows, blankets and toys can all harbour illnesses, and keeping everyone with their own belongings during cold and flu season can help prevent the spread of germs. In particular, don't share food or take a taste from someone else's snack, and don't finish the leftovers from your child's plate.

Keep clean. Wiping down worktops, door handles and toys with a 10 per cent bleach solution from a spray bottle will keep surfaces virus-free, says Dr Nelson. Once the worst has passed, washing the ill person's bedding in hot water will help rid your house of germs that can spread through the family.

Watch for fever, but don't panic. Though conventional medicine often tells us that the first sign of fever should have us seeking urgent medical advice, that's not always true. Fever is one of the immune system's ways of mobilising against infection, and as long as it doesn't get too high (over 39°C/102°F in children or 38.5°C/101°F in adults) or last more than 2 days, Dr Nelson says there's no reason to be alarmed. 'Always bring your child to the doctor if you feel it is necessary,' she advises, 'but don't be afraid to settle your patient in at home and wait out a fever for a couple of days if you're comfortable with that.' More often than not, the results will be the same: a viral infection that passes of its own accord.

Don't expect a prescription. When you do decide to head for the doctor's surgery because you or your child is ill, keep in mind that a surgery visit shouldn't necessarily equal a prescription. Most colds and flu are caused by viruses, and viruses don't respond to antibiotics. Your doctor may be able to recommend medicines such as cough suppressants and fever reducers to help relieve your symptoms, but he or she will not have a cure.

If a bacterial infection is causing your symptoms, your doctor may prescribe an antibiotic. But if your illness is viral, do not ask for antibiotics 'just in case'. In the long run, unnecessary antibiotics can do more harm than good, says Dr Nelson.

Where Traditional Medicine Meets Alternative Care

For many patients with immune-related conditions, alternative treatments have a special allure. Alternative and complementary therapies focus on problems or imbalances that *cause or contribute to* symptoms, Dr Greenfield explains. When combined with conventional Western interventions, the alternative therapies might further relieve the symptoms to the point that the person feels cured.

The one thing alternative treatments should not do is replace the wisdom of conventional medicine. Always seek conventional medical advice before embarking on alternative treatments. Here are a few suggestions to help you combine complementary and conventional healthcare.

Consult your doctor. If you're going to pursue alternative treatments, you are going to be most effective with the advice of your doctor. 'Be sure you're working with a physician who meets you on your value system,' says Dr Greenfield. 'You don't necessarily need a doctor who is an expert in complementary practices, but you do need one who is open-minded.' A sceptical doctor, he points out, isn't always a bad thing. But one who doesn't want to discuss or look into alternative treatments probably isn't the best choice for a patient who wants to pursue those options.

The litmus test is to bring your doctor a few pages of literature about a treatment you'd like to pursue. See what kind of reaction you get. If your doctor wants to read about it and discuss it with you, you're probably in good hands. If your material is evaluated and you are counselled not to use the therapy in question because of potential dangers associated with your condition, or possible interactions with other medications, you are probably still in good hands. But if your curiosity is dismissed outright, you might want to start looking for a new doctor once your condition stabilises, suggests Dr Greenfield.

Be ready for the extra work. 'If you delve into the arena of alternative medicine, you'll have to do a lot of homework yourself,' Dr Greenfield explains. And that initial legwork in the library, on the Internet and on the phone is just the tip of the iceberg, he says. 'Alternative therapies are not about taking a different pill,' he explains. 'They're about making substantive changes in our daily lifestyles – and that takes a big commitment.'

Let the buyer beware. Because alternative treatments are so much less regulated by the government than traditional medicine is, the brunt of the responsibility for making sure that your acupuncturist, homoeopathic remedy, or herbal supplement is reputable falls to you. Here's a by-treatment guide to exploring alternative treatments.

Acupuncture. 'I've seen really, really good responses to acupuncture from people with immunological conditions,' says Dr Greenfield. Evidence suggests that acupuncture can help restore health to people with conditions as diverse as asthma, arthritis, migraine headaches, certain types of paralysis, sciatica and inflammatory bowel disease, including Crohn's disease. It can be especially helpful in alleviating chronic pain, fatigue and nausea.

Fortunately, the therapy involving the long, hair-thin needles inserted into strategic points on your body is better regulated than many other alternative therapies. Choose a practitioner recommended by the British Acupuncture Council (telephone 0208 964 0222). This organisation maintains a register of UK practitioners of acupuncture. You can write to them at Park House, 206–208 Latimer Road, London W10 6RE or email at *www.acupuncture.org.uk.*

Homoeopathy. Homoeopaths believe that a substance used at full strength can make a healthy person experience certain symptoms. That same substance, used in an extremely diluted form, can make a person with the same symptoms feel well. As with acupuncture, the goal of homoeopathy is to restore balance in the patient, and some patients find homoeopathic remedies helpful with disorders such as asthma and allergies, says Dr Greenfield.

Because the key ingredients in homoeopathic remedies are so diluted, there are few risks associated with using them. The one significant danger, Dr Greenfield points out, is that people sometimes skip their medically necessary traditional medications and decide to go the homoeopathic route alone. 'Homoeopathy can be used as an adjunct to traditional medicine, and it may be able to replace some treatments in the long run, but that kind of undertaking needs to be closely supervised with your medical doctor,' he explains.

In many cases homoeopathy is an area of specialisation for medical doctors, osteopaths, naturopaths and nurses, so your best bet for finding a reliable practitioner may be word-of-mouth recommendations. The British Homoeopathic Association (telephone 020 7935 2163) maintains a register of homoeopathic doctors and pharmacies. Members of the Society of Homoeopaths are not doctors but have completed a recognised course. Email them at *info@homeopathy-soh.org.*

Herbs and supplements. The range and variety of choices in herbal and other supplements are enough to overwhelm newcomers. Some herbs and supplements, though, may be well worth the trouble. Studies have suggested that glucosamine sulphate, for example, soothes arthritis pain as well as ibuprofen. Laboratory tests on animals suggest that green tea may even help to prevent arthritis in the first place.

As you choose herbal supplements, read labels carefully and beware of advertising gimmicks. Anything that claims to 'cure' an immune-related disease is probably a fraud, Dr Greenfield says.

Instead, look for bottles that are labelled as 'standardised' and that list the amount of the active ingredient they contain. Remember that bigger companies are more likely to be careful to protect their reputations. Make sure you understand the safety concerns, including interaction with medications, that are associated with some supplements. (See the Safe Use Guidelines, beginning on page 446, for those recommended in this book.)

To research which herbs might be helpful to you and learn about their possible benefits and side effects, there are several helpful websites to check out, says Dr Greenfield. Ask Dr Weil (*www.drweil.com*) is an excellent site, as is the site of the American Botanical Council (*www.herbalgram.org*). In addition, ConsumerLab.com (*www.consumerlabs.com*) appraises and rates supplements and vitamins and can be helpful for newcomers, says Dr Greenfield.

Stress reduction therapies. This broad group can include massage, yoga and hypnosis, and it might even extend to things like getting involved in your community or church. 'Over the years, we've seen that activities like massage and yoga really do impact people's stress levels, and so their overall health,' says Dr Greenfield. It may be a matter of the buttons a therapy is pushing on the body, but it's just as likely that the benefits of these types of therapies come from the quiet, peaceful contact they provide with other human beings.

Two very common stress reducers that you can do yourself at home and even teach to your children are relaxation and visualisation. 'The goal of relaxation techniques is to help alleviate the physical reactions our bodies experience when responding to chronic stress,' explains Dr Greenfield. The rush of adrenalin and quickening of your heart rate and respiration when you are under stress are your body's way of revving up for a fight or a flight, he explains, and in small doses, they're actually good for you.

'The problem is that sometimes we get to the point where our lives are so stressful that we are in that tense, emergency state all the time,' says Dr Greenfield. Though that response heightens our physical and mental capabilities in the short run, it weakens the immune system and physically wears us down if it's 'on' too much.

Different people find that different relaxation techniques work best for them. The core elements, though, are usually the same. First, set aside a time during which you will have no distractions, and sit or lie down in a comfortable position. Choose a setting that helps you feel relaxed. Second, breathe slowly and deeply from your abdomen. Just this basic breathing technique can help to pull your body and mind back to their resting condition and out of their keyed up response to stress, says Dr Greenfield.

To take relaxation one step further, try visualisation. Make a deliberate effort to picture a scene or a situation that calms you. For example, you might imagine yourself baking cakes with your children, or walking in the woods on a sunny day.

Even though those scenes are imaginary, your body relaxes when your mind is focused on things that don't stress you out, Dr Greenfield explains. You may even find success in visualising a positive outcome to stressful situations. For example, your child may be able to reduce stress about a difficult assignment by imagining bringing home a top grade. The idea is to keep your imagination from running wild and stimulating your adrenal response. Instead, visualisation can help keep your stress in check by helping you to feel in control of your situation.

'Everybody has stress in their lives,' says Dr Greenfield, 'but not everyone has enough tools in the toolbox to deal with it. These therapies, conventional and otherwise, give us more ways to cope with and rid ourselves of stress. And that, in turn, directly affects our health.'

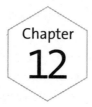

COLDS AND FLU

Some people come through even the nastiest cold and flu seasons unscathed. We'll give you a fighting chance to join their ranks.

Colds and flu are the most common illnesses people get. The average adult has one or two bouts a year, says Joseph Mercola, DO, osteopathic physician at the Optimal Wellness Center in Schaumburg, Illinois. Because colds and flu share many attributes and symptoms, sometimes it's hard to tell which is which. After all, both are respiratory tract infections, both are caused by viruses and both vary in intensity and duration. Most important, both can make us feel miserable and send us straight to bed.

Fortunately, there is a lot we can do to sidestep these conditions and to snuff them out quickly when we can't. This chapter will provide you with a virtual arsenal of strategies known to nip colds and flu in the bud. But before we get to that, it's important to understand the differences between a cold and a flu.

What Is a Cold?

Scientists haven't yet pinpointed which viruses cause up to half of the colds that afflict adults. According to the National Institute of Allergy and Infectious Diseases, researchers have identified more than 200 cold viruses, including more than 100 rhinoviruses and three strains of coronaviruses. To complicate things, viruses responsible for more serious illnesses, such as adenoviruses and Coxsackie viruses, cause 10 to 15 per cent of adult colds.

A cold, of course, is an infection of the upper respiratory tract – the nasal passages, throat and sinuses. To take hold, the virus must find its way into our noses. It begins multiplying once it latches on to our nasal cells. Then, within 12 to 24 hours, it takes effect. The first symptoms are a sore, scratchy throat; a runny nose and sneezing. During the first 2 days symptoms peak and we are most contagious.

Other common symptoms include headaches, chills, general malaise and hacking coughs. Sometimes, there is also a mild fever. Cold symptoms can be mild or severe and vary from cold to cold and from person to person, notes Jack M Gwaltney Jr, MD, head of the division of epidemiology and virology at the University of Virginia School of Medicine in Charlottesville.

Colds are most commonly passed hand-to-hand and then hand-to-nose or hand-to-eye (where the virus surfs down the tear ducts and on to the nasal membranes). You also can get the virus by breathing in droplets that someone has sneezed or coughed. In addition, because cold viruses can survive outside the body for a number of hours, you may get a cold if you touch an object contaminated with a cold virus and then rub your nose or eyes. Colds can last from 2 days to 2 weeks.

What Is Flu?

Flu, caused by a strain of influenza virus, is much more serious than a cold because it can be deadly. Particularly virulent strains can spread worldwide and cause millions of deaths. Major outbreaks (pandemics) in the 20th century included Spanish flu in 1918 and Hong Kong flu in 1968. While symptoms can be hard to distinguish from those of a severe cold, the flu virus doesn't lodge only in the nose, mouth and throat, but multiplies in the lungs as well and can lead to pneumonia.

Here are some of the things that distinguish the flu from a cold.

• A high fever (39°C to 40°C/102° to 104°F) for several days

- Prominent headache

- Severe general aches and pains

- Weakness and fatigue that can last 2 to 3 weeks

- Extreme exhaustion at onset

- Cough and chest discomfort that can become severe

Flu is passed via secretions from infected people and from coughing and sneezing.

Most people recover from the flu within 1 to 2 weeks.

Specific flu immunity is hard to develop, since flu viruses mutate. We are constantly confronted with altered viruses that are able to outwit our immune systems. Vaccine producers are forced to play an advance guessing game as to which mutations will arise in the next flu season.

Prevention Pointers

We cannot live in a glass bubble, breathing filtered, purified air and never touching contaminated surfaces. But we can make a conscious effort, especially during the cold and flu season (late summer through winter), to avoid close contact with people who have active colds or flu, says medical microbiologist Neal Rolfe Chamberlain, PhD, associate professor at Kirksville College of Osteopathic Medicine in Missouri. If you must be in contact with people who have the flu, stay out of the path of coughs and sneezes, he advises. Of course, once your family members get the flu, you cannot avoid proximity. In this case, you need to be particularly vigilant about washing your hands often and keeping them away from your nose, mouth and eyes. Since both the flu and colds are passed hand-to-hand, frequent, thorough washing with soap and water can wash away viruses.

While some holistic doctors and alternative practitioners question its widespread use, the annual flu vaccine is generally considered safe and is the top medical recommendation that doctors make for the elderly and those with compromised immune systems. If the strain in the vaccine is correct, these vaccines are 70 to 90 per cent effective in preventing flu in

NATURAL VACCINE BOOSTERS

One study has shown that taking a particular herb for a few weeks after getting the flu jab can significantly raise your body's flu-fighting antibodies and increase natural killer cell activity. Subjects received 100 mg of standardised ginseng extract Ginsana G115 daily for a period of 12 weeks after receiving a flu vaccine. There were only 15 cases of the flu or common cold afterwards in the study group; the placebo group reported 42 cases of flu or cold.

Another study in France looked at the efficacy of mineral and vitamin supplementation on immunity in elderly patients after flu vaccination over a 2-year period. The mineral group received a low dose of 100 mcg of selenium and 20 mg of zinc; the vitamin group received beta-carotene, ascorbic acid and vitamin E. Patients who received minerals alone showed a higher level of antibodies than those who took only vitamins.

Take the three – zinc, ginseng and selenium – 5 days before your flu jab and for at least 5 days after. Mark Stengler, ND, naturopathic physician at the La Jolla Whole Health Medical Clinic in California and author of *Nature's Virus Killers*, recommends 100 mg of Korean ginseng, 20 mg of zinc, and 200–400 mcg of selenium.

As an additional flu vaccine booster, Dr Stengler recommends taking 500 mg of echinacea and up to 2,000 mg of vitamin C daily. You can take 500–600 mg of vitamin C three times a day rather than 2,000 mg in one shot, as high doses of vitamin C may cause loose, runny stools in sensitive individuals.

healthy people under the age of 65, and they reduce the severity of symptoms for people who do contract it.

Mark Stengler, ND, naturopathic physician at the La Jolla Whole Health Medical Clinic in California and author of *Nature's Virus Killers*, agrees that immuno–compromised people should get the annual flu vaccine, and the elderly might want to consider it, too. For healthy people, however, he prefers a homoeopathic alternative, Influenzinum. He uses it himself. 'This is a homoeopathic preparation of flu virus,' explains Dr Stengler. 'I use it with patients, and most who take Influenzinum at the beginning of the flu season don't get the flu.'

Long-Term Protection

Washing your hands and staying out of the path of sneezes are good short-term ways to avoid coming down with a cold or flu, but they don't really do anything to boost your immune system over the long term. For that, you need to look at your lifestyle. According to Dr Stengler, the number one thing we can do to disease-proof ourselves against colds and flu is to practise positive ways of handling stress. 'Tons of studies have shown that mental and emotional stress does decrease the activity of the immune system,' he says. And it's not just the stresses that do the damage – it's how you perceive and react to them. Dr Stengler's first advice for people having trouble managing stress is to get more exercise, since exercise is a great stress reliever.

Which exercise is best? 'Whichever one you enjoy and will do regularly,' Dr Stengler says.

Beyond exercise, explore the vast variety of stress reduction techniques presented in Enhance Immunity with the Power of the Mind, on page 96. In addition, eating a healthy diet and maintaining good digestion and elimination are essential for long-term protection. These topics are discussed throughout this book. Finally, get plenty of rest, practise proper hygiene and see Booster 12, Celebrate Your Sensual Side, on page 123.

Conventional Treatment

Much of what conventional medicine has to offer cold and flu sufferers falls under the category of self-care: drink fluids, get bed rest, take over-the-counter medications. Here are some specific antiviral drugs available by prescription and some very effective remedies to buy over the counter.

• Doctors now have antiviral drugs that appear to have few or minimal side effects and can combat flu. They are available on prescription only, so ask your doctor about zanamivir (Relenza) and amantadine (Symmetrel) and rimantadine (Flumadine); they can shorten and lessen the severity of flu if taken soon after flu onset. Both, though, can have side effects such as nausea, light-headedness, nervousness and irritability. Other antiviral drugs are on the horizon.

• You can slow down a runny nose by taking a 'first-generation' antihistamine such as chlorpheniramine (Piriton, by prescription; also found in some over-the-counter products), brompheniramine (Dimotane, by prescription), or clemastine (Aller-eze, over-the-counter). These medications block a nervous system response that stimulates mucus flow. Unfortunately, first-generation antihistamines are the ones that cause drowsiness, and the non-drowsy formulas have not been shown to be effective for runny noses.

• Concurrent with taking the first-generation antihistamine, take an extended-release ibuprofen or naproxen tablet every 12 hours from the onset of your symptoms until they subside, Dr Gwaltney advises. 'Take the two together,' he says. The combination reduces most cold symptoms, including sneezing, runny nose, nasal obstruction, sore throat, cough and headache.

• For coughs that don't respond to the antihistamine/anti-inflammatory combination, use a dextromethorphan cough syrup or capsule, says Dr Gwaltney. Your doctor can prescribe something stronger if needed.

• If your nose is blocked up and you are uncomfortable, drink a litre (2 pints) of water for every 22.5 kg (50 lb) of body weight, and avoid sugar, grains and milk products. Chances are, they're making the problem worse, advises Dr Mercola.

• A prescription anticholinergic spray such as ipratropium bromide (Atrovent) can help dry up a runny nose if you experience drowsiness from antihistamines. Ask your doctor if it's suitable for you.

Alternative Treatment

While conventional medicine recommends using specific over-the-counter antihistamines and fever reducers and anti-inflammatories, many holistic doctors believe that these medications inhibit the immune system and slow healing while suppressing symptoms. Dr Mercola says that cold viruses reproduce less effectively at elevated body temperatures and that a mild fever can actually help speed recovery from a cold. (Doctors differ

THE RIGHT ZINC

Many studies have been carried out to demonstrate the effectiveness of zinc lozenges for fighting colds. About half show dramatic improvements, and about half show none at all.

This can be explained, says Guy Berthon, PhD, Directeur de Recherche at Equipe de Chimie Bioinorganique Medicale in Toulouse, France. He says that the type of zinc and the formulation used for the lozenges make all the difference.

Zinc lozenge studies that showed a significant improvement in the severity and length of colds used zinc acetate in a formulation that releases a potent dose of positively charged zinc ions at a specific pH. Zinc has not been shown to be effective in studies in which other forms of zinc were used, including those in which the zinc was mixed with sweeteners, citric acid, or vitamin C. These mixtures seem to eliminate the zinc's ionisation and deliver a different pH, Dr Berthon says.

In fact, as scientist George Eby, MA, and president of George Eby Research in Austin, Texas, reported in *Annals of Internal Medicine,* one study used zinc lozenges that released negatively charged zinc ions that actually *worsened* cold symptoms.

Eby, who discovered and first published the zinc ionisation theory, holds a patent on a positively charged zinc formulation, and he reports that many of the zinc lozenges on the market do not deliver an effective dose of zinc ions. He says that the following widely available zinc lozenges are effective.

- Cold-Eeze
- Cold-Free
- Cold Season Plus+
- Fast Dry

The way that the lozenge feels and acts in the mouth is a major tip-off, says Eby. Those with proper zinc ionisation have an astringent (puckering), drying effect.

on what constitutes 'mild', but most agree that any temperature over 39°C (102°F) should be taken seriously.) Drugs such as paracetamol and aspirin may actually prolong a cold.

Instead of turning to drugs, Dr Stengler uses herbs as his first weapon when a patient has the flu. In fact, he has developed what he calls his virus cocktail, which he recommends taking to boost the immune system. He advises keeping it and other herbal and homoeopathic remedies on hand. You can make the virus cocktail yourself using tinctures, which are also known as liquid extracts.

Add the following to 120 ml (4 fl oz) of warm water.

- 30 drops each of echinacea, astragalus, reishi and lomatium

- 10 drops of liquorice root

Drink this cocktail twice a day as a preventive measure when flu starts in your area and until the epidemic passes. If you are ill, take a cocktail every 2 to 3 waking hours until your illness is gone, which is usually 5 days, recommends Dr Stengler.

As an alternative to tinctures, take 500-mg capsules of one or two of echinacea, astragalus, reishi or lomatium every 2 to 3 waking hours when you're ill, Dr Stengler advises. You need not take all four to gain from these Immune Boosters.

In a small percentage of individuals, lomatium may cause a skin rash. It disappears once you stop taking the herb. Also take the liquorice root, but don't take more than about 1,500 mg per day (three 500-mg capsules) of this herb because high doses can cause some unwanted side effects, such as water retention and increased blood pressure.

In addition, drink ginger tea. You can make an infusion of the fresh root – cut off a 1.25 cm (½-inch) piece and steep it in 240 ml (8 fl oz) of hot water for 5 minutes. Or you can buy commercially prepared ginger tea in the supermarket. Drink three to four cups throughout the day.

Dr Stengler recommends picking either the virus cocktail or a couple of the aforementioned immune-enhancing herbs and using them consistently. Here are some other strong antiviral herbs that you may consider.

- Maitake mushroom: 3–7 g daily

- Olive leaf: 1,000–2,000 mg daily

- Elderberry extract: follow the label instructions.

For sore throats, Dr Stengler recommends propolis, a product of bees. 'Spray it right on your throat, or buy it as tincture and use drops. In my opinion, it has a tremendous antimicrobial effect as well as a natural anti-inflammatory effect. Some European doctors use it on wounds to keep them from getting infected.' Spray 1 ml three times daily.

Dr Stengler recommends seeing a qualified homoeopath for an individualised remedy specific to your condition. If that isn't possible, try following homoeopathic remedies when you have flu. He advises starting with one that most closely matches your symptoms, but he also says that you can take more than one homoeopathic remedy at a time; it usually speeds up the recovery time.

TAKE THE **FIRST STEP**

To increase your odds of getting through the cold and flu season unscathed even while everyone around you is ill, wash your hands – and do it often. Since both the flu and colds are passed hand-to-hand, thoroughly washing your hands with soap and water can flush away viruses. In addition, keep your hands away from your nose, mouth and eyes.

Homoeopathic medicines are completely non-toxic. Always check with your primary doctor to be sure that your condition does not require immediate medical attention. Take the remedies one at a time, and stop taking the remedy as soon as you see improvement because, in rare cases, taking too much of a remedy may make symptoms worse. If symptoms persist after self-treatment, see a professional homoeopath or your doctor. Finally, never treat chronic, serious conditions without professional supervision.

• Oscillococcinum. This remedy has been shown to stop flu quickly if taken early enough. It's a good one to start with, says Dr Stengler. Follow the label instructions.

• Gelsemium. 'This is very specific for the flu when you have tremendous muscle aching and feel chilled, dizzy, and tired,' Dr Stengler says.

• Arsenicum album. This is an appropriate remedy if you're 'experiencing very bad chills and have vomiting and diarrhoea at the same time, and if you feel a lot of anxiety with the flu,' notes Dr Stengler.

• For sinus congestion, you can take any homoeopathic combination remedy that says 'sinusitis' on it.

Self-Care

Much of what can be done for a cold or flu is self-care. You've no doubt heard numerous times before that you should get plenty of rest,

OLD-FASHIONED CHICKEN-VEGETABLE SOUP

There's nothing like homemade chicken soup when you're feeling miserable from a cold or the flu. And now, scientists have proved what mothers have known for years: chicken soup actually does have medicinal benefits. By helping to ease congestion, it can leave you feeling better in no time flat. And this version – loaded with nutrient-rich ingredients such as garlic, sweetcorn, green beans and courgettes – packs a powerful nutritional punch.

2	tablespoons olive oil
455 g (1 lb)	boneless, skinless chicken breasts, cut into 2 cm (¾ in) pieces
2	cloves garlic, finely chopped
1	onion, chopped
1 l (1¾ pt)	chicken stock
340 g (12 oz)	green beans, cut into 5 cm (2 in) lengths
230 g (8 oz)	fresh, tinned or frozen and thawed sweetcorn
1	red pepper, chopped
1	stick celery, chopped
1	small courgette, quartered lengthwise and sliced
4	sprigs thyme
¼	teaspoon salt
½	teaspoon freshly ground black pepper
15g (½ oz)	chopped celery leaves
2	tablespoons chopped fresh parsley

Heat the oil in a large saucepan over medium-high heat. Add the chicken and cook, stirring occasionally, for 10 minutes, or until lightly browned. Add the garlic and onion. Cook, stirring often, for 8 minutes, or until the onion is translucent.

Add the stock, beans, sweetcorn, pepper, celery, courgette, thyme, salt and black pepper. Bring to the boil. Reduce the heat to low, cover, and simmer for 10 minutes, or until the beans are tender. Remove and discard the thyme. Stir in the celery leaves and parsley.

MAKES 4 SERVINGS

Per serving: *310calories/1296 kJ, 31 g protein, 25 g carbohydrate (of which sugars 12 g), 11 g fat (of which saturates 2 g), 6 g dietary fibre, 599 mg sodium* drink plenty of fluids and monitor your condition. While flu is more likely to cause serious complications, colds, too, can get out of hand. Dr Mercola encourages you to be aggressive in self-treating colds and flu, but to see a doctor if you are uncomfortable about a symptom or response and if you are experiencing any of the following:

- Prolonged fever over 39.5°C/103°F

- Severe ear pain

- Green nasal discharge

- Wheezing and persistently coughing up green and yellow sputum

Here are some more steps you can take to limit flu and colds.

Take vitamin C. Some holistic doctors, like Dr Mercola, advise taking megadoses of 500–2,000 mg of vitamin C every few hours during a cold. As little as 1,000 mg a day has been shown to shorten the duration of colds. Dr Mercola cautions that if you develop loose or runny stools, you should stop taking vitamin C; some people have low bowel tolerance for it, as the vitamin can have a laxative effect.

Enjoy hot, steamy chicken soup. Homemade works best, in Dr Mercola's experience. The cysteine in chicken helps thin mucus and ease congestion. Dr Mercola suggests throwing in plenty of spicy peppers, which enhance the mucus-thinning effect. (See Old-Fashioned Chicken-Vegetable Soup on page 177 for a homemade chicken soup recipe.)

Take advantage of aromatherapy. You can use essential oils to create a refreshing and healing atmosphere. When you're feeling congested, mix 6 drops of eucalyptus essential oil in 30 g (1 oz) of skin cream or 12 drops in 30 ml (1 fl oz) of vegetable oil, and rub the mixture on to your chest. Or add 5 drops of lavender or clary sage to your hot bathwater, advises Kurt Schnaubelt, PhD, who is with the Pacific Institute of Aromatherapy in San Rafael, California. In his opinion, these herbs help boost the immune system. Please note that essential oils are not to be ingested; they are for external use only.

Avoid milk during the infection. Though this advice is controversial, it's commonly recommended by alternative medicine practitioners for treating colds and flu, as many people are sensitive to milk and milk tends to increase mucus production, says Dr Mercola.

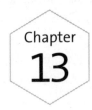

Chapter

13

ALLERGIES
AND ASTHMA

WHEN VIRUSES, BACTERIA, OR CANCER CELLS INVADE YOUR body, you *want* your immune system to haul out its heavy artillery. But when the invaders are harmless specks of pollen and mould, it's best if your immune system simply brings out its brooms.

And that's precisely what it does – if you *don't* have allergies. It quietly sweeps away pollen and mould with the rest of your bodily debris.

If you *do* have allergies, however, your immune system declares all-out war. Unfortunately, its primary target is *you*. So the next time you start sneezing and wheezing, don't blame pollen, mould, or other allergens. The true cause of your misery is your immune system's not-so-friendly fire.

'Allergy is really a failure of recognition,' says George Hinshaw, MD, of Wichita, Kansas, past president of the American Academy of Environmental Medicine. 'Our ability to distinguish friend from foe is out of kilter, and we start reacting to things that really bear no threat to us at all.'

What makes your immune system misbehave so badly? Part of the reason is genetic. If both of your parents have allergies, your odds of developing them are 75 per cent. If one of your parents has allergies, your odds are 30 to 40 per cent.

But lifestyle also plays a major role. An increasing body of evidence demonstrates that the Western lifestyle is associated with higher rates of allergies.

In one post–Cold War study, allergies were found to be much more common in materially rich West Germany than in materially poor East Germany. Since the two Germanys share a common genetic heritage, researchers concluded that the West Germans were choking on their own abundance.

Throughout the Western world, allergies and asthma are on the increase. In the United States, a recent poll shows that 38 per cent of Americans have some kind of allergy.

Fortunately, the picture isn't as bleak as it appears. 'You can't change an inherited predisposition to allergy,' says Andrew Weil, MD, director of the programme in integrative medicine and clinical professor of medicine at the University of Arizona College of Medicine in Tucson. 'But you can adjust your lifestyle and modify your environment to influence immunity in the right direction.'

That lesson applies whether you've battled allergies all your life or suddenly developed them in your forties or fifties. 'Many people in so-called midlife find that the cumulative effects of unbalanced diets, environmental toxins and stress can overstimulate and misdirect their immune systems,' Dr Weil says. 'Your goal should be to convince and reeducate your immune system to coexist peacefully with the common allergens you come into contact with.'

Common Allergy Triggers

When a national polling organisation asked people to name their worst allergy triggers, this is what topped the list.

- Trees, weeds, flowers, grasses: 27 per cent
- Drugs and medications: 19 per cent
- House dust and dust mites: 17 per cent

- Moulds: 15 per cent

- Indoor air pollution: 12 per cent

- Chemical fumes and gases: 12 per cent

- Perfumes: 12 per cent

- Pets: 11 per cent

- Personal care products: 11 per cent

- Insects and bees: 10 per cent

- Foods: 10 per cent

- Pesticides: 7 per cent

- Household cleaning products: 7 per cent

- Preservatives and food additives: 6 per cent

What Is an Allergic Reaction?

There is some confusion over what constitutes an allergy, with some people defining it as *any* adverse reaction to *any* substance. For the purposes of this book, however, we shall limit our discussion to allergic conditions with a strong, proven link to the immune system.

In most cases, the immune system's troublemaker is a tiny, Y-shaped antibody called immunoglobulin E, or IgE. Like the trigger on a bomb, these antibodies attach themselves to special cells called mast cells and basophils. Mast cells are found in your respiratory and gastrointestinal tracts as well as in your skin, while basophils are found in your blood. As many as 500,000 IgE antibodies can collect on a single cell.

When these IgE-loaded cells encounter an allergen, they explode, releasing a flood of inflammatory chemicals such as histamine. This prompts the formation of even more chemicals called prostaglandins and leukotrienes. People with allergies have 10 times as much IgE in their blood as people who are allergy-free.

Some experts believe that IgE's real purpose is to attack parasites. Since Western nations have largely eliminated parasites, it's thought that IgE has become a restless warrior that's turned its wrath on harmless allergens. This is the basis of the hygiene hypothesis, which suggests that we've become more susceptible to allergies because we've oversanitised ourselves.

Early exposure to antibiotics, in particular, is thought to deprive the immune system of the bacterial challenges it needs to develop normally.

'You want to have the right stimulus in your gut when you're an infant,' says Harold Nelson, MD, senior staff physician at National Jewish Medical and Research Center in Denver. As evidence, he points to a Swedish study showing that children who avoid antibiotics, eat lots of fermented food and have some contact with animals are half as likely as other children to be allergic.

Unfortunately, such measures cannot prevent allergies in older children and adults, whose immune systems are fully developed. Once you have allergies, you've usually got them for life.

TAKE THE **FIRST STEP**

If you suspect that you have an allergy, the first step you need to take is to go to your doctor for proper testing. After all, you can't limit your exposure to an allergen if you haven't properly identified it. Furthermore, allergens can travel through your bloodstream, so the cause of allergy symptoms is not always obvious, as when a food allergy causes hives or a rash.

The Main Types of Allergic Disease

The following conditions are commonly accepted as being of allergic origin.

Allergic rhinitis. Also known as hay fever, it affects the upper respiratory tract.

Asthma. A far more serious disease, it results in wheezing and shortness of breath due to a narrowing of the lungs' bronchial tubes.

Drug allergy. The most common drug allergy symptoms are hives (urticaria), rashes, stuffy nose, wheezing, dizziness and swelling of body parts. All reactions to drugs should be reported to your doctor immediately.

Dust mite allergy. Dust mites are tiny relatives of the spider that live on the dead skin cells we're constantly shedding from our bodies. They are common allergens that may affect millions of people each year.

Food allergy. Most common in children, it's usually caused by eggs, milk, nuts, wheat and shellfish.

Latex allergy. Most commonly triggered by latex gloves and condoms, this allergy has seen a rise in recent years. When people with this allergy come into contact with latex proteins, they may experience dry, crusted lesions on their skin; rash; hives; hay fever; or asthma. In severe cases, latex allergy can result in death.

Mould allergy. Reactions for people who are sensitive to mould can be even more severe than the reactions experienced by people who are sensitive to pollen. They include sneezing, runny nose and congestion. People with mould allergies can also develop asthma.

Pet allergy. Though many people with this type of allergy assume that it is their dogs' or cats' fur that causes their symptoms, the real culprit is a protein released with the animals' dander (dead skin cells) and saliva.

Stinging and biting insect allergies. Insects that sting, such as wasps, hornets and bees, are far more likely to cause allergies and potentially lethal reactions than insects that bite. Generally, people who are allergic to these stings are advised to carry an EpiPen, a hypodermic needle of adrenalin (epinephrine) they can administer themselves that will buy them time to get urgent medical attention.

Major Allergy Symptoms and Related Conditions

Because there are myriad allergy triggers, there are also myriad allergy symptoms. If you suspect that you have an allergy, you should consult your doctor. Following is a list of the major symptoms most commonly associated with allergic reactions.

Anaphylactic shock. The most severe of all allergic reactions, anaphylactic shock causes swelling of body tissues (including the throat), vomiting, cramp and a sudden drop in blood pressure. It often occurs in people who are especially sensitive to penicillin, stinging insects and shellfish or nuts. If not treated immediately, it can be fatal.

Eye reactions. Itchy, watery eyes whenever the pollen count goes up are a sign of seasonal allergic conjunctivitis; if this occurs year-round, it's a sign of perennial conjunctivitis. Much less common is vernal keratoconjunctivitis, which causes cobblestone-like bumps on the insides of the eyelids.

Skin reactions. These include the itchy rashes and oozing blisters of eczema; the swelling, redness and itching of hives (urticaria); and the rashes experienced after touching plants such as poison ivy or certain foods (known as contact dermatitis).

Upper respiratory symptoms. These include a runny or stuffed-up nose, sneezing, wheezing, congestion, coughing and postnasal drip.

Other conditions with a possible allergy link. Though more research needs to be done, scientists are currently investigating whether such conditions as otitis media (an acute or chronic inflammation of the middle ear) or rhinosinusitis (an inflammation of the paranasal sinuses) could be related to allergies.

How Are Allergies Diagnosed?

You might think that you know what you're allergic to. But because allergens can migrate via the bloodstream to any part of the body, they can fool you into making false assumptions. For example, a mother might blame her baby's rash on a soap. But the real cause could be a milk allergy.

The only way to be sure is to go to a doctor, describe a history of your reactions and get tested. Here are the tests most commonly used by conventional allergists.

Skin tests. Drops of suspected allergens are either placed on to or injected into your skin. If you're allergic to the substance, a round weal or flare will form on your skin after 15 to 20 minutes.

Blood tests. These tests measure either the total amount of IgE in your bloodstream or the IgE that's specific to certain allergens, such as ragweed pollen. As mentioned earlier, when IgE comes into contact with an allergen, it releases chemicals such as histamine, prostaglandins and leukotrienes. These chemicals cause the symptoms of allergies.

Pulmonary function tests. To measure airflow, a patient blows into a device called a spirometer and a reading is taken. If asthma is suspected, the patient is given a bronchodilator, then tested again. If airflow improves, it's a good indication that asthma is present.

Patch tests. A piece of blotting paper is soaked with the suspected allergen, then taped to the patient's skin for 24 to 48 hours. If a rash develops, it's a sign of allergic contact eczema.

Provocation tests. Generally performed by environmental medicine or alternative allergists rather than by conventional doctors, and usually done if specific allergy testing is not available, these tests require the patient to inhale or swallow a very small amount of the suspected allergen. Because of the risk of serious reactions, a provocation test must be done only under a doctor's supervision.

Environmental Control: The First Step in Managing Allergies

All allergy practitioners, from the most conservative to the most alternative, agree that environmental control should be your first 'treatment'. After all, it's natural, safe and extremely effective.

'The very best preventive measures are those that get the patient away from the cause of the problem,' says Betty Wray, MD, interim dean of the School of Medicine at the Medical College of Georgia in Augusta and a past president of the American College of Allergy, Asthma and Immunology. 'All the medications we give help blunt the response, but they don't do away with the problem.'

Environmental control isn't the same as 'running away' from your current environment. In most cases, moving to a new climate such as the mountains or beach is an exercise in futility. 'Some people even move to different parts of the world to "get away" from allergens,' Dr Weil says. 'For most, such moves are simply impractical, and often people find that in a short period of time they have developed new allergies to go with their new home.'

Fortunately, you can practise environmental control without packing your bags. If possible, avoid living near motorways, main roads and industrial parks. Environmental urban chemicals, such as ozone, carbon monoxide and nitrogen dioxide, can worsen asthma and allergies.

Next, focus on cleaning up your indoor environment. Because of improved home and office building insulation, indoor air can contain even more dust, lint, hair, smoke and pollen than outdoor air.

KEEP THE 'GREAT OUTDOORS' FROM GETTING IN

Creating an indoor oasis is hard work. Observe the following precautions to keep your sanctuary allergy-free.

• Keep the windows in your home and car closed to lower your exposure to mould, pollen and pollutants.
• To keep cool, use air conditioning instead of fans.
• Dry your clothes in a tumble dryer. If you hang them outside, they'll collect allergens that you will bring indoors.
• Be aware that allergens can be carried indoors by people and pets.

Here are strategies to minimise your household's exposure to common indoor allergens.

Insects and vermin

• Limit the spread of food around the house, and especially keep food out of bedrooms.

• Keep food and rubbish in sealed containers. Never leave food out in the kitchen.

• Mop the kitchen floor and wash worktops at least once a week.

• Eliminate water sources that might attract vermin, such as leaky taps and pipes.

• Plug crevices around the house through which insects and vermin can enter.

• Use bait stations and other environmentally safe pesticides to reduce infestation.

Dust Mites

• Encase your mattress and pillows in dustproof or allergen-impermeable covers.

• Wash all bedding and blankets once a week in hot water (at least 60°C/140°F) to kill dust mites.

HOW TO CREATE A DUST-FREE BEDROOM

Although you probably can't effectively control the amount of dust you inhale during waking hours at home and work, you can ensure a peaceful night's slumber by turning your bedroom into a dust-free zone. Here's how, starting with the most important steps.

Roll up the carpet. All carpets – especially the shagpile variety – trap dust. Some chemical treatments can even trigger allergic reactions. For maximum protection, replace the carpet with hardwood, tile or linoleum flooring.

Put your bed in a bubble. Encase pillows, duvets and mattresses in dustproof or allergen-proof covers. If you need to keep a second bed in the room, encase it, too.

Banish your furry and feathered friends. If you can't bear to part with your pets, at least shut them out of your bedroom.

Wash your bedclothes. Sheets, blankets and other bedclothes should be washed frequently in water that is at least 60°C/140°F. Lower temperatures will not kill dust mites.

Forgo unnecessary furnishings. Keep furniture and furnishings to a minimum. Instead of upholstered furniture, use wooden or metal chairs that can be easily scrubbed. Avoid venetian blinds, which can collect dust.

Clean dusty surfaces. Arrange for someone without an allergy to clean the dusty surfaces in your bedroom – floors, furniture, tops of doors, window frames, sills and so on – every week with a damp cloth or oil mop. He or she should air the room thoroughly, then close the doors and windows until you're ready to use the room.

Use an air filter. A high-efficiency particle arrestor (HEPA) filter can effectively remove many allergens. HEPA mechanical filters remove up to 90 per cent of home air pollutants. Place a freestanding HEPA unit (capable of purifying the air in a room several times per hour) in your bedroom. HEPA filters also are available for cars. Electrostatic filters are useful, too, but may emit asthma-inducing ozone if they're not functioning properly.

Lower the humidity. A room dehumidifier can turn dust mites into dried-up husks. Clean the unit frequently, however, to prevent mould growth.

Clear away clutter. Rid your bedroom of books, tapes, CDs and other dust collectors, or tuck them away in a closed cabinet. If a child sleeps in the bedroom, allow him or her to keep only washable toys made of finished wood, rubber, metal, or plastic in the room, and store them in a closed toy box or chest.

SUCCESS STORIES

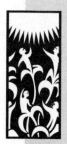

The Power of Positive Avoidance

George Miller, MD, knows what a difference avoiding food allergens can make: his pre-school son's bedsheets told the story clearly.

Like many parents, Dr Miller was perplexed by his pre-school son's habit of wetting the bed.

'In the middle of the night, his bladder would say, "Seth, we have to pee," but his brain would say, "Sorry, nobody home",' says Dr Miller, an environmental medicine specialist in Lewisburg, Pennsylvania, and president of the American Academy of Environmental Medicine.

When Seth was tested for allergies, it turned out that he was sensitive to two of his favourite foods: apples and chocolate. The chocolate, especially, left him spacey, glassy-eyed and unable to think clearly.

After Seth stopped drinking apple juice, his bedwetting ceased. 'It was just like turning off a faucet,' Dr Miller says. And after he stopped eating chocolate, his brain fog lifted.

Now in his twenties, Seth still practises positive avoidance. 'You couldn't pay this kid to eat a piece of chocolate today,' Dr Miller says. 'He's now in control, and that gives him a lot of power, self-esteem and good feelings about himself.'

• Replace wool or feathered bedding with synthetic materials and traditional stuffed animals with washable ones. Wash all bedding and toys frequently.

• If possible, replace wall-to-wall carpets in bedrooms with bare floors (linoleum, tile or wood).

• Use a damp mop or duster to remove dust. Never use a dry cloth, since it stirs up mite allergens.

• Use a vacuum cleaner with either a double-layered microfilter bag or a HEPA (high-efficiency particle arrestor) filter.

Food

• Designate a group of pots, pans and utensils specifically for the preparation of allergy-free meals. Even a trace of a food allergen, such as peanuts or milk, can cause a reaction.

• Prepare several allergy-free meals at a time and freeze them until they're ready to be consumed. This method will reduce the risk of cross-contamination that can happen when allergy-free and allergenic meals are prepared at the same time.

• Thoroughly clean your hands, utensils and kitchen surface areas before cooking allergy-free meals.

Most reactions occur when people eat food that they thought was safe. So it's equally important to master a few detective skills.

• Learn the scientific and technical terms of allergens (for example, casein is a milk product, and albumin usually comes from egg).

• Read every label on each product purchased, even if you buy the same product all the time. Manufacturers often change ingredients without warning.

• Avoid purchasing products without an ingredient listing.

• When dining out, inform the waiter about your food allergy, and clarify the ingredients used to prepare the selected meal.

• Emphasise to family and friends that food allergy is serious and that a reaction can be fatal.

Grass Pollen

• Get a non-allergic person to mow your lawn. If you must mow it yourself, wear a mask.

• Keep grass cut short.

• Be aware that pollen can also be transported indoors on people and pets.

House Dust

• Dust rooms thoroughly with a damp cloth at least once a week.

• Wear protective gloves and a dust mask while cleaning to reduce exposure to dust and cleaning irritants.

• Use electric and hot water radiators to provide a cleaner source of heat than blown air systems.

• Reduce the number of stuffed animals, wicker baskets, dried flowers and other dust collectors in your home.

• Replace carpets with washable rugs or bare floors.

• Instead of fabric curtains, cover windows with blinds made of material that you can wipe clean or remove and wash.

Mould

• Use a dehumidifier or air conditioner to maintain relative humidity below 50 per cent. In particular, you may need a dehumidifier in the basement. Remember to empty the container regularly and clean it often to prevent mildew formation.

• Air closed spaces such as cupboards and bathrooms.

• Vent bathrooms and tumble dryers to the outside.

• Check taps, pipes and ductwork for leaks.

• When first turning on the air conditioner in your car, drive with the windows open for several minutes to allow mould spores to disperse.

• Remove decaying debris from the garden, roof and gutters.

• Avoid raking leaves, mowing the lawn and working with peat, mulch, hay and dead wood. If you must do gardening, wear a mask and avoid working on hot, humid days.

Odours and Fumes

• Avoid perfumes, room deodorisers, cleaning chemicals, paint and talcum powder.

Pets

• Keep pets out of your home if possible.

• If keeping pets out of your home isn't possible, keep them out of bedrooms and confined to areas without carpets or upholstered furniture.

• If you keep a cat, wash it once a week with soap and warm water to reduce airborne dander. Keep it outside as much as possible.

• Wear a dust mask when you're near rodents such as mice and hamsters.

• After playing with your pet, wash your hands and clean your clothes to remove pet allergens.

• Avoid contact with soiled litter cages.

• Dust your home often with a damp cloth.

• Remember that pet allergens linger in house dust for months after the pet is gone. As a result, allergy and asthma symptoms may take some time to subside.

Pollen

• Save outside activities for late afternoon or after a heavy rain, when pollen levels are lower.

• If you buy trees for your garden, plant species that are less likely to aggravate allergies, such as dogwood, fig, fir, palm, pear and plum.

Tobacco Smoke

• Smoking should not be allowed in the homes or cars of people with asthma or allergies. Ask family members and friends to smoke outdoors.

• Seek smoke-free environments in restaurants, theatres and hotel rooms.

• If you smoke, find support to quit.

Wood Smoke

• Avoid woodstoves and fireplaces.

Drug-free Treatments

From immunotherapy to a modified diet to herbs and supplements, there are numerous things you can do to manage your allergies without

(continued on page 194)

THE PROS AND CONS OF ALLERGY DRUGS

There are numerous allergy drugs on the market that are effective at relieving symptoms. Unfortunately, as with most drugs, many of these allergy medications have side effects. Below is a list of the specific benefits and drawbacks to the most commonly used allergy drugs.

CLASS OF ALLERGY DRUG	BENEFITS	DRAWBACKS
Antihistamines	Relieve itching in the nose, throat and eyes and sneezing; reduce nasal swelling and drainage	Over-the-counter antihistamines cause drowsiness. So-called non-drowsy antihistamines may actually be sedating if taken with certain drugs. Be sure to tell your doctor about any medication you may be taking. Other common side effects of antihistamines include dry mouth, difficulty urinating and constipation. Children may experience nightmares, unusual jumpiness, or nervousness, restlessness and irritability.
Bronchodilators (theophylline)	Long-acting bronchodilators prevent asthma attacks; short-acting 'rescue' brochodilators relieve them by opening up the bronchial tubes so that more air can flow through.	Side effects include rapid heartbeat, anxiety, insomnia and headache. Elderly patients and children may be more sensitive to the side effects of bronchodilators.
Sodium cromoglicate, cromolyn (Intal), nedocromil sodium (Tilade)	Reduce inflammation in the airways	Almost none
Decongestants	Relieve nasal congestion by shrinking blood vessels, which decreases the amount of fluid that leaks out	Side effects include nervousness, sleeplessness and elevation in blood pressure. When used for a prolonged period, over-the-counter decongestants can cause 'rebound rhinitis', actually increasing nasal congestion. Prescription nasal sprays and drops don't have this effect and can be used for longer periods of time.

CLASS OF ALLERGY DRUG	BENEFITS	DRAWBACKS
Inhaled corticosteroids (AeroBec)	Decrease airway swelling in the bronchial tubes, reduce mucus production by the cells lining the bronchial tubes and decrease the chain of overreaction in the airways	Can cause hoarseness and thrush, a fungal infection of the mouth and throat. Such problems can be minimised by mouth rinsing and by using a spacer device that can reduce the amount of medication residue in the mouth and throat. Some studies show that these drugs may cause slower-than-normal growth in children. Several case reports suggest that psychiatric disturbances such as mania, depression and mood changes may occasionally occur.
Leukotriene modifiers (Accolate)	Leukotrienes are body chemicals that cause contraction of the smooth muscle in the airway, leakage of fluid from blood vessels in the lung and inflammation. Like antihistamines, antileukotriene medications neutralise these inflammatory chemicals.	Can make some drugs stay in the system longer, and the medication's actions are altered when it is taken with aspirin or theophylline (a bronchodilator). Side effects include headache, infection and nausea.
Oral corticosteroids (prednisone)	Relieve severe asthma that won't respond to any other treatment	Short-term use can cause slight weight gain, increased appetite, menstrual irregularities and cramps, and heartburn or indigestion. Withdrawal symptoms include loss of energy, poor appetite, severe muscle aches and joint pains. Long-term use can cause ulcers, weight gain, cataracts, weakened bones and skin, high blood pressure, elevated blood sugar, easy bruising, decreased growth in children, depression, mania and mood disturbances.
Topical nasal steroids	Relieve hay fever by reducing the number of mast cells in the nose, mucus secretion and nasal swelling (often used in combination with antihistamines)	Mostly the same as for inhaled corticosteroids, as well as an increased risk of nasal irritation and bleeding

the use of drugs. Always work with your doctor to find the plan that allows you to best regulate your allergy symptoms. (Bear in mind that for serious conditions such as asthma, your plan will probably need to include both drug and drug-free strategies.)

Conventional Immunotherapy

Immunotherapy, or desensitisation therapy, is a century-old therapy that is based on the theory that a little 'hair of the dog that bit you' can relieve your allergies. Commonly known as allergy injections, it is the closest thing to a cure for hay fever, asthma caused by allergy to pollens and dust mites, and stinging-insect allergy.

After testing positive for certain allergens, patients begin receiving injections containing weak concentrations of those allergens. Over a period of weeks or months, the concentration is gradually increased so that patients build up a tolerance to the allergens in their environment.

'The only way you can really alter your allergic response is to get allergy shots, which can create blocking antibodies that compete with allergic antibodies,' says Robert Nathan, MD, an allergist in private practice in Colorado Springs. 'After a number of years, you also get an actual decrease in the allergic antibodies.'

Allergists have long believed that immunotherapy is effective, but until recently, there was little scientific proof. Today, Dr Nathan notices that allergy injections relieve hay fever in up to 90 per cent of his cases.

Don't be surprised, though, if your doctor refers to this therapy as 'vaccination'. It seems that allergists have battled public confusion over the term *immunotherapy* for decades. 'When you tell people they can be vaccinated against allergies, they understand,' says Dr Wray. 'But when you say "immunotherapy", they think you're talking about a cancer treatment.'

In addition to some PR problems with terminology, there are also some medical drawbacks that you should be aware of before beginning immunotherapy.

• Risk of adverse reactions. Some patients develop swelling at the site of the injections. This reaction can be resolved by taking oral antihistamines, using ice packs and adjusting the dose or vaccine. Rarely, a person may experience asthma symptoms or anaphylaxis.

• Inconvenience. Immunotherapy requires patience and a substantial time commitment. After each injection, you must remain in the clinic for at least 20 minutes so that staff can monitor you for adverse reactions.

• Limited applications. Immunotherapy won't work for non-allergic hay fever. In addition, researchers have yet to develop safe and effective immunotherapies for food and latex allergies.

Environmental Medicine Forms of Immunotherapy

Conventional immunotherapy isn't the only desensitisation process available to people with allergies and asthma. Since the mid-1960s, clinical ecologists or environmental medicine doctors have promoted their own forms of immunotherapy.

'The standard allergist would begin treatment with a very weak dose,' Dr Hinshaw says. 'An environmental medicine doctor can start with a dose that is many times stronger, but still will not produce symptoms, and will give symptom relief, sometimes with the very first treatment.' Unlike conventional allergists, environmental medicine doctors also use allergy injections to treat food and chemical sensitivities.

Although conventional doctors do not claim that these higher concentrations are necessarily harmful, they believe that allergy injections are primarily useful for inhalant allergies – pollens and mould – and that such injections can be dangerous when used to treat food allergies.

Here are two of the forms of immunotherapy used by environmental medicine doctors.

Optimal-dose immunotherapy. The 'optimal' dose is just short of the dose that produces symptoms. By starting with higher doses, environmental medicine doctors have shown that patients can complete a course of immunotherapy in as little as 2 years.

Enzyme-potentiated desensitisation. This form is used to desensitise patients to an entire category of allergens. For example, the aeroallergens category would include pollens, moulds and animal dander. The patient is given a series of tiny injections of these allergens several weeks apart. Since doses are much weaker than other allergy injections, an enzyme called beta-glucuronidase is added to increase, or 'potentiate', the effect.

Diet

Since people with allergies and asthma already have pro-inflammatory immune systems, eating a pro-inflammatory diet is like throwing fuel on the fire. Diets that are very rich in inflammatory materials, such as saturated fat, are going to make people worse.

Eat natural products, avoid processed foods and avoid preservatives. choose fruits, juices, whole grains and vegetables.

It is well known that foods such as broccoli, spinach and strawberries are good for you, but they can also help to relieve your asthma and allergies. The following is a list of allergy 'superfoods'. For better health, try to increase your consumption of them.

Apples. A British study of 2,512 middle-aged men showed that those who ate five apples a week had significantly better lung function than those who ate no apples. Experts believe that apples contain numerous healthy compounds, including antioxidants that improve lung health.

Borage oil, blackcurrant seed oil and evening primrose oil. These three oils are all rich sources of gamma linolenic acid (GLA), which has anti-inflammatory properties. In fact, borage oil is the subject of ongoing research at the Center for Complementary and Alternative Medicine Research in Asthma, Allergy and Immunology at the University of California, Davis.

Cold-water fish. In addition to plant sources, the following fish are rich sources of omega-3 fatty acids: mackerel, anchovies, herring, salmon, sardines, trout and tuna. To get the most benefit, either bake or poach the fish. Eat two or three servings per week.

Fruits and vegetables. Any richly coloured fruit or vegetable is loaded with antioxidants, vitamins and bioflavonoids. Eat more blueberries, raspberries, strawberries, cranberries, sweet potatoes, peppers and tomatoes.

Magnesium-rich foods. Some studies have demonstrated that people with asthma are magnesium deficient. Magnesium-rich foods include spinach, haricot beans, pinto beans, sunflower seeds, tofu, halibut, cashews, artichokes and black-eyed beans.

Olive oil. Since it's monounsaturated, consider using extra-virgin olive oil as your main source of fat.

Spices. Eat ginger and turmeric regularly for their anti-inflammatory effects.

Spirulina. This is bioflavonoid-rich algae, available in tablet and powder form. *Caution:* To avoid possible heavy-metal contamination, buy spirulina only from reputable sources. Check the label for an indication that it has been analysed for heavy-metal content.

Walnuts and walnut oil. These are a great source of allergy-fighting omega-3 fatty acids. Other plant sources include soya oil, flaxseed and flaxseed oil and wheat germ.

Yoghurt. A study at the University of California, Davis, showed that people who ate 230 g (8 oz) a day of yoghurt with active cultures had one-tenth as many allergies.

Zinc-rich foods. Some studies have demonstrated that people with asthma are zinc deficient. Zinc-rich foods include plain yogurt, tofu, lean beef, lean ham, oysters, crab, the dark meat of turkey and chicken, lentils and other pulses, and ricotta cheese.

Dietary Supplements

'Nutritional supplements such as antioxidants, essential fatty acids and anti-inflammatory herbs can quell symptoms before they start,' says Robert Rountree, MD, a holistic physician and co-founder of the Helios Health Center in Boulder, Colorado, who has used dietary supplements to treat allergies and asthma for 20 years. 'And, best of all, a holistic allergy programme can soothe your problems at their source – an imbalanced immune system.'

Based on scientific research and clinical observation, Dr Rountree has devised the following supplementation schedule for people with allergies and asthma. Number one on his list is quercetin, a bioflavonoid.

With the exception of liquorice root, all of the supplements listed below can be used with conventional medications. So, depending on the severity of your condition, Dr Rountree recommends experimenting with various combinations until you find the one that's right for you.

Dr Rountree's recommendations for nutrients are:

- Tocopherol (vitamin E) complex (d-alpha tocopherol): 125–250 mg

- Selenium: 200 mcg
- Zinc: 20–40 mg
- Vitamin C: 2,000 mg
- Quercetin: 500–3,000 mg
- Proanthocyanidin (grape seed extract): 50–150 mg
- GLA (from borage or blackcurrant seed oil): 300 mg

In addition to the above, consider a daily supplement of one or more of the following herbs, all of which are rich in antioxidants and anti-inflammatory phytochemicals, or plant chemicals.

- Green tea: 3 cups daily or one 250-mg capsule, three times daily
- Ginger: 500 mg, three times daily
- Curcumin (from turmeric): 500 mg, two times daily
- Liquorice root: 500 mg, three or four times daily

Supplements for Leaky Gut Syndrome

According to proponents of this controversial theory, many allergic woes are caused by large food molecules that 'leak' from inflamed small intestines into the bloodstream. Once the molecules pass into general circulation, they affect numerous body systems, causing symptoms ranging from headaches, fatigue and bloating to skin rashes and autoimmunity.

'With small children, the number one cause of leaky gut is food allergy – more often than not to cow's milk,' Dr Weil says. 'In adults, gastrointestinal inflammation often results from the use of nonsteroidal anti-inflammatory drugs such as aspirin and ibuprofen.' Other troublemakers include excessive amounts of alcohol (distilled spirits, not a daily glass of wine), sugar, caffeine (more than one cup of a caffeinated beverage a day), antacids, food additives and prescription drugs, including antibiotics.

Once you've eliminated the causes of leaky gut syndrome, Dr Weil recommends these supplements to promote healing of the gastrointestinal tract.

- Glutamine. Take 2–3 g of this amino acid per day.

- Vitamin A. Do not exceed 3,000 mcg daily.
- Folic acid (400 mcg), B_{12} (1,000 mcg), and zinc (30 mg)
- Aloe vera juice. Look for a preservative-free brand. Follow dosage recommendations on the product label.
- Acidophilus, lactobacillus GG strain. Take one or two capsules a day. Supplements can restore normal bowel flora.

First Steps: Natural Quick-Relief Strategies

So far, most of the advice in this chapter has addressed the long-term *prevention* of allergies and asthma. If you need immediate relief, however, the following home remedies can calm down your overactive immune system.

Nettle. Also called stinging nettle, this herb will relieve allergy symptoms readily in most people, and it has no toxicity. Instead of side effects, you get bonus trace minerals. The best form to buy is a freeze-dried extract of the leaves, sold in capsules. Take one or two 300-mg capsules every 2 to 4 hours as needed. Some experts advise that allergy symptoms may worsen initially when trying nettle, so you may want to take only one dose a day for the first few days.

Nasal rinsing. Flushing your sinuses with salt water removes allergens, reduces congestion and soothes irritated mucous membranes. Mix approximately ¼ teaspoon of salt and ⅛ teaspoon of baking soda in 120 ml (4 fl oz) of warm water. Using a bulb syringe or a neti pot (a porcelain container that resembles Aladdin's lamp), rinse your sinuses twice a day.

Aromatherapy. Essential oils have long been used to relieve sinus and chest congestion. Eucalyptus oil, for instance, works as an antiseptic, antispasmodic and expectorant. It can be massaged on to the chest or back during an asthma or allergy attack, or it can be inhaled to help clear the sinuses and free congestion in the chest. Other useful oils include hyssop, lavender, frankincense, rosemary and cajeput. Mix 12 drops of essential oil with 30 ml (1 fl oz) of vegetable oil to use for massage. To inhale, place 1 drop on a handkerchief.

Caution: Since essential oils can trigger allergic reactions, start with only a tiny amount and stop if you experience any symptoms. Never take these essential oils internally.

To counter mild to moderate reactions to food, try these remedies, recommended by Dr Hinshaw and other experts. Do not, however, use these remedies for serious food reactions, such as anaphylaxis. These are medical emergencies and should be treated with injectable epinephrine (adrenalin), such as an EpiPen.

Buffered vitamin C. Mix 1 teaspoon of the powder in a glass of water and drink it. If there is no improvement in 15 minutes, try the following remedy.

Epsom salt. Mix 1 teaspoon in a glass of water. Drink.

A Special Action Plan for People with Asthma

So far, no alternative asthma regimen has proven as efficacious as conventional treatment. In fact, one study shows that adults who manage their asthma with either herbs or black coffee or tea are up to three times as likely as adults using conventional treatments to end up in a hospital.

Still, you can combine conventional and alternative approaches – including dietary changes, exercise and stress reduction – to achieve better results than if you use conventional treatments alone.

To ensure that you get the best possible care, work with your doctor to develop a written action plan. Such a plan should include detailed instructions for taking maintenance medications, managing acute attacks and knowing when to get urgent care.

Here are two essential self-care skills.

Monitor your breathing. You may recognise your own signs of an impending attack (slight coughing, wheezing, or shortness of breath at night, after laughing, or following minimal exertion). But many people do not. To accurately measure your lung function, use a home peak-flow meter. Depending on the severity of your asthma, you may need to measure airflow once or twice daily or only a few times a week. Your doctor can give you detailed instructions on using peak-flow meters and interpreting the results.

Treat attacks early. The earlier you know that an attack is on the way, and the sooner you intervene, the less medication you will need to control your symptoms. If your action plan fails to provide relief, seek immediate medical attention.

Prevent Exercise-Induced Asthma

Although exercise improves lung function, reduces stress and improves immunity, many people with asthma experience wheezing from strenuous workouts. Still, doctors say that it's the one allergy trigger you *shouldn't* avoid.

To prevent exercise-induced asthma (EIA), conventional doctors recommend using a short-acting bronchodilator such as salbutamol (Ventolin) 15 to 30 minutes before exercise. If this doesn't prevent symptoms, your doctor may recommend adding sodium cromoglicate (Intal) or nedocromil sodium (Tilade).

To stay symptom-free during sustained exercise, some doctors recommend using a long-acting bronchodilator such as salmeterol (Serevent) or ipratropium bromide (Atrovent) beforehand.

If you prefer a drug-free approach, try these natural prevention strategies.

Warm up and cool down. Since sudden changes in activity can trigger symptoms, buffer your workouts with at least 10 minutes of warm-ups and cool-downs.

Drink up. Dehydration impairs breathing, so drink plenty of water before, during and after exercise.

Reduce salt intake. One study showed that a low-sodium diet – no more than 2,000 mg per day – improves breathing and prevents exercise-induced asthma.

Take more vitamin C. One study showed that taking 2,000 mg of vitamin C before exercise eliminated symptoms in 80 per cent of participants with EIA.

Bundle up. Wear a scarf over your mouth and nose during winter to humidify the cold, dry air.

Get wet. Swimming and water aerobics are excellent exercise choices because the warm air above the water enhances breathing, allowing you to work out for longer.

Avoid unnecessary exposures. Exercise indoors during peak allergy seasons, extreme heat or cold, or when outdoor air quality is poor.

Exercise with a friend. It's best to exercise with a partner in case you have a serious attack.

Keep medication handy. Use your quick-relief inhaler at the first sign of symptoms.

Chapter

14

AUTOIMMUNE
DISORDERS

I F YOU WERE TO HIRE A SECURITY GUARD FOR YOUR HOME, YOU'D make sure that he or she knew just what to protect. You'd want your guard to instantly recognise you and your family, be able to tell your pets from any strays in the neighbourhood and have a clear idea of which visitors to let in and which to turn away.

But what if your security guard turned out to be more than a little bit confused? What if he or she blocked invited guests as they tried to enter your house, or worse yet, what if your guard became violent and actually injured a family member instead of protecting him or her?

This imaginary scenario is not entirely unlike what happens when your body's security guard – your immune system – mistakes cells that it should protect (body cells) for invaders that it should attack (for example, bacteria or viruses). When you have an autoimmune (literally, 'self-immune') disorder, your immune system directs its powerful defensive abilities against your own tissues. Seeing enemies within, the immune system produces autoantibodies, cells that target and destroy the body's own tissues. This inner battle leads to a variety of symptoms, depending on which cells the autoantibodies choose to target – they may be cartilage, nerve, intestine, or just about any other kind.

The Gene Connection:
Only a Partial Explanation

Medical experts believe that most people who have autoimmune disorders probably have a genetic tendency toward getting the disease: that is, they may possess a gene (a tiny unit of cellular information) making them more susceptible to a certain disorder than someone without that gene. But not everyone with these tendencies goes on to actually develop the disease.

For example, there are cases where one identical twin develops type 1 diabetes, an autoimmune disorder, and the other twin does not. Because twins share identical genes, if type 1 diabetes were purely genetic, whenever one twin develops the disease, the other should too – but they don't. 'Actually, most people who have the gene don't go on to develop the disease,' says Denise Faustman, MD, PhD, a diabetes researcher and associate professor of medicine at Harvard Medical School. The gene sets the stage, but something else is needed to get the self-destructive process started.

Another outside factor, most likely a virus, is believed to be the crucial, additional trigger that turns the immune system against itself. Currently, many researchers are focusing on trying to discover the virus or viruses involved, with the hope of locating the causes of, and possible cures for, the variety of autoimmune disorders.

Understanding the Most Common
Autoimmune Disorders

All autoimmune problems have a common basis in an overactive immune system. Although quite a few autoimmune disorders overlap (people with one often have another as well) each disease manifests its own set of troubling symptoms, and each disease must be treated with a tailored approach.

Read on for an overview of the most prevalent autoimmune disorders.

You'll learn what happens in the body as these diseases develop, as well as the warning signs you shouldn't ignore. You'll also get a sampling of the steps you can take to prevent complications and treat symptoms.

Insulin-Dependent (Type 1) Diabetes

Type 1 diabetes used to be called juvenile diabetes because it frequently makes its first appearance in childhood. Now, however, so many adults are being diagnosed with this disease that it is more often called by the name of the problem it leads to: becoming insulin-dependent, or having to rely on injections of insulin in drug form. (Type 2 diabetes, also known as non-insulin-dependent diabetes, is a metabolic disorder rather than an autoimmune disease.)

Insulin is a hormone that is produced in the pancreas and used throughout the body. In the right amounts, insulin performs the important job of allowing glucose (sugar circulating in the blood) to enter your body's cells and provide energy.

In the case of type 1 diabetes, however, there's an insulin shortage, because cells in the pancreas (called beta cells) that normally produce insulin in response to foods, activity level and other cues become the targets of an immune system gone awry. Antibodies in the blood attack the beta cells, hindering and eventually halting insulin production altogether. By the time symptoms of type 1 diabetes arise, most of the beta cells have been destroyed.

This is no small matter. Without enough insulin available to them, cells cannot take in the glucose they need to carry out vital functions. 'Type 1 diabetes is basically a disease of starvation,' explains Dr Faustman. This means that regardless of how much food a person with type 1 diabetes eats, the body goes hungry at the cellular level.

In addition to the serious problem of starving cells, glucose that can't be put to work builds up. While you need *some* glucose in the blood (more on this later), unchecked high amounts of blood sugar will cause a host of problems that most people are lucky enough not to have to worry about until they've reached old age: stroke, heart disease, kidney failure, blindness and amputations.

Early Warning Signs of Type 1 Diabetes

Unlike the symptoms of the more common type 2 diabetes, which may be noticeable for years before a person is diagnosed, the symptoms of type 1 come on relatively quickly, developing over only weeks or months. Here are the most common signs that indicate type 1 diabetes.

• The need to urinate frequently. When blood sugar soars, so does sugar in your urine. Your body will naturally pull extra water out of the blood and into the bladder to help thin out the concentrated urine; this makes your bladder fill up faster.

• Increased thirst. As water gets diverted from your blood to your bladder, you get dehydrated and end up feeling constantly parched.

• Increased hunger combined with weight loss. These symptoms seem contradictory, but they're actually related. You're always hungry because without insulin, your cells can't absorb the glucose they need for energy. In a search for another source of energy, your body begins to break down muscle and fat, causing you to lose weight.

• Weakness. Without energy from glucose, muscle cells lose strength and power, leaving you weak.

Prevention and Treatment of Type 1 Diabetes

Primary prevention – preventing diabetes before it can ever start – is still a scientist's dream, according to Dr Faustman. Lots of work is being done on potential approaches, including tests to identify people at risk for type 1 who haven't actually developed any symptoms yet (a daunting enough task in itself), as well as the creation of a vaccination that someday may help such people sidestep the disease. Research is also being done on ways to prevent transplanted beta cells from being rejected by the person who receives them. Until prevention becomes a reality, however, people with type 1 diabetes need to focus on effective treatment.

The more common form of diabetes, called type 2, may be treated with nothing more invasive than lifestyle changes, such as getting more exercise and cutting back on dietary fats and sugars. While these steps make good sense for anyone (with or without diabetes), an important difference between the two types of disease is that people with type 1 must control their blood sugar by taking insulin, usually by injection. If you have type 1 diabetes, you need insulin to survive.

Relying on injections may make you feel as if you have no control over the treatment of your diabetes. Nothing could be further from the truth: in fact, there are two crucial ways that you can get involved to make your diabetes treatment simpler and more effective.

Practise tight control. Until fairly recently, if you were diagnosed with type 1 diabetes, you were advised to test your blood sugar levels and inject yourself with insulin once or twice a day. Now, doctors are more likely to recommend that you monitor your blood glucose level more often and use several measured doses of insulin throughout the day. The approach is called tight control. Research shows that using this method to keep glucose levels as close to normal as possible can minimise diabetes-related health problems.

One study in Stockholm, Sweden, showed that tight control helped people with type 1 prevent worsening of autonomic neuropathy, a potentially deadly diabetes complication involving the heart, lungs and nervous system. After 11 years, participants in the study who failed to use tight control developed more heart rate, breathing and balance problems related to nerve damage than those who kept their blood sugar levels closely in check.

Consider a pump. A small electronic device that automatically delivers a measured dose of insulin through a needle inserted into the skin (usually around the abdomen) can help make tight control much easier, says Dr Faustman. Currently available pumps are worn externally, strapped to your waist or leg; internal, surgically implanted devices are currently being tested.

Using a pump takes some motivation. You will have to learn how to clean and maintain the equipment as well as the needle site, and you will still have to test your blood glucose level many times a day and stay alert for the possibility of hypoglycaemia, or low blood sugar. But for people willing to make the effort, the health benefits of better control are worth it. 'If I had diabetes, I would do it,' says Dr Faustman.

SUCCESS STORIES

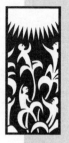

Single Mother Fights Back against Diabetes

Diabetes and heart disease dealt Charlotte Libater a double blow, but she fought back with her diet and exercise. Today, her will to win is keeping her active, involved and cheerful against all odds.

When Charlotte was diagnosed 40 years ago with type 2 diabetes, she was a struggling single mother of a 10-year-old boy. Her husband had died suddenly several years earlier, leaving her as her son's sole support in Charleston, South Carolina, the city Charlotte had moved to when she was first married.

She was scared.

What would happen without her good health? Her son had already lost his father, who had had a heart attack.

Charlotte knew that she had some control over type 2 diabetes, which could be managed with a nutritious diet and exercise. She began steaming vegetables and turned to fish, chicken and turkey for her protein. Her office was not even a mile away, so she walked every day. 'The best part is that I felt so much better,' she says.

Even with the most vigilant care, however, diabetes can be an insidious

Natural Approaches for Treating Type 1 Diabetes

At this time, type 1 diabetes requires treatment with insulin. There is presently no herb, vitamin, or other supplement pill that can substitute for your body's own insulin the way prescription medication can. But that's not to say that natural or alternative approaches have no place in treatment. Natural remedies can help you avoid complications and provide support for your tight-control programme. Here are just two to try.

Consider chromium. The trace mineral chromium is often recommended for type 2 diabetes because of its insulin-boosting effects. At the cellular level, chromium improves the way our bodies use insulin in two ways. First, it makes the attachment spots on cells, called receptors, more disease. Within 20 years, she became insulin-dependent and had to learn how to give herself insulin shots every day. Then – Charlotte remembers it as if it were yesterday – on February 10, 1991, she had a heart attack.

She was scared, again.

This time, something her surgeon told her gave Charlotte the courage to bounce back. She had survived because she had taken such good care of herself. Her immune system was strong, and she needed to continue to keep it that way.

Charlotte joined a hospital cardiac rehabilitation programme. To this day, she goes 3 days a week to work out on the treadmill and the stationary and recumbent bicycles. 'I still watch my diet, and I check my blood sugar levels twice a day,' she says.

While she attributes her renewed good health to her healthy lifestyle, Charlotte contends that she would not feel as good about herself were she not involved in so many activities in the community and her synagogue. She does voluntary work for the Charleston chapter of the Mended Hearts, a non-profit, volunteer support group for heart disease patients and their families; she sings in choirs, including the Jewish Choral Society; and she is a volunteer usher at the Charleston Symphony and at the Dock Street Theatre.

'I now force myself to rest every afternoon, to sit quietly and read. I haven't much energy or time left for housework, so I do as little as I can,' she says happily. 'I realise that it's possible to take care of your health, no matter what the obstacles.'

sensitive to insulin, meaning that they react more strongly. Second, chromium increases the actual number of insulin receptors, providing more doorways for insulin to enter cells.

Enhanced sensitivity to insulin is particularly important for people with type 2 diabetes, where the problem is trouble using available insulin (not a shortage of it). But chromium might benefit people with type 1 as well, according to Kathi Head, ND, author of *Natural Treatments for Diabetes*, senior editor of *Alternative Medicine Review*, and a naturopathic physician in private practice in Dover, Idaho. Chromium may improve the effectiveness of insulin, 'whether it is produced in the body (as in type 2) or injected (as in type 1),' says Dr Head.

There is no RDA for chromium, but a dose of 50–200 mcg is considered safe and adequate. Diabetes researchers have used levels both lower and higher than that. If you decide to try chromium, it's important that you get your doctor to supervise. Chromium may reduce your need for insulin; if you don't adjust your insulin dose accordingly, you could end up with blood sugar levels that dip too low (hypoglycaemia). Low blood sugar can be just as dangerous as high blood sugar.

Look after your feet. One serious complication of diabetes seems entirely unrelated to blood sugar: foot amputations. Diabetes is the leading cause of foot amputations because of the nerve damage caused over time by high glucose levels, which leads to loss of feeling in the feet.

Gradual loss of sensation can leave you totally unaware of the small cuts and blisters that we all get on our feet from time to time. If they are left untreated long enough, even minor foot injuries can become dangerously infected. People with type 1 diabetes can prevent this tragic and crippling situation, which is unfortunately currently on the rise, by paying extra attention to their feet.

A daily footbath laced with lavender essential oil is more than just a way to relax, says Kathleen Duffy, LPN, CCA, a certified clinical aromatherapist and owner of the Herbarium in Chicopee, Massachusetts. Soaking your feet daily gives you a chance to carefully examine them, and the warm water and healing herbal oil can soften hangnails and dry skin that could otherwise snag and tear, preventing future problems. Use a basin of water big enough for both feet, and test the water with your elbow before stepping in to prevent an accidental burn, recommends Duffy. Add 4 to 6 drops of essential oil of true lavender and soak until the water cools.

Rheumatoid Arthritis

Like age-related osteoarthritis, rheumatoid arthritis (RA) causes joint pain, swelling and stiffness. But that's where the similarities end between the two different diseases. RA is unique in that it usually happens symmetrically: affecting the same joints on each side of the body, mirror-like.

While RA most often targets the wrist and finger joints, it can also cause pain elsewhere in the body as well as fever, fatigue and a general feeling of illness.

Though some question that the condition even exists, leaky gut syndrome (also known by its more formal name, intestinal hyperpermeability) is one explanation given by some doctors for the autoimmune activity seen in RA. These doctors believe that, in certain situations, proteins from food are able to 'leak', in their whole, undigested form, from the intestine into the bloodstream. 'The lining of the gut is similar to the lining of the mouth,' explains John McDougall, MD, founder of the McDougall Wellness Center in Santa Rosa, California. 'If the cell layer lining the intestine is damaged, it becomes permeable.' Damage to the intestines can be caused by many things, including medication (such as aspirin and nonsteroidal anti-inflammatory drugs), bacteria, food allergy, or a genetic tendency toward inflammation.

Proteins from animal-based foods, such as pork, beef, chicken, eggs and dairy products, are the culprits to worry about here. In their undigested state, these proteins prompt the body to react as if a foreign invader had entered the bloodstream by producing antibodies. The catch here, says Dr McDougall, is that animal proteins are extremely similar to human proteins (after all, we *are* animals) and the antibodies produced to attack a milk or pork protein work just as eagerly to target and destroy the similar-enough proteins in your wrist or finger joints.

When the immune system attacks, white blood cells flood the tissue that lines the joint, creating heat and swelling. As the inflammation continues, the lining begins to grow abnormally, invading nearby cartilage and bone and affecting muscles and tendons in the area. Eventually, the joint becomes painful, deformed and weak.

Early Warning Signs of Rheumatoid Arthritis

There is no single test that can detect rheumatoid arthritis. A doctor's diagnosis will be made after considering any symptoms and ruling out other possible causes. The following are some of the common symptoms of RA.

- Tender, warm and swollen joints, especially in the wrists and fingers, but also in the neck, shoulders, elbows, hips, knees, ankles and feet

- A symmetrical pattern to the problem; if one wrist is affected, so is the other

- Fatigue or weakness

- Low-grade fevers

- Stiffness, especially if it gradually improves with movement

- Rheumatoid nodules, lumps of inflamed tissue under the skin

Treatment for Rheumatoid Arthritis

Lifestyle-related steps are essential in RA treatment. Rest and exercise are both vital: rest is important during periods of active inflammation; exercise maintains strength and flexibility during less painful times. Splinting a swollen joint and using self-help tools around the house (such as zip pullers and jar openers) can reduce pain and prevent overuse of affected joints. Stress reduction techniques are also very useful: while stress may not cause RA, it can increase pain levels.

Most people with RA will also have to take medication. While no drug offers a cure, some are effective for pain and inflammation, and others seem to slow the progression of the disease.

- Nonsteroidal anti-inflammatory drugs (NSAIDs), including aspirin and ibuprofen, are often the first drugs used by people with RA to help relieve pain and inflammation. These drugs work, but they may cause stomach irritation, contributing to leaky gut syndrome. Plus, some NSAIDs – especially ibuprofen (Motrin), naproxen (Naprosyn), and indometacin (Indoci) – may actually encourage damage to other joint tissues. The newest members of the NSAID family are known as COX-2 inhibitors: celecoxib (Celebrex) and rofecoxib (Vioxx). The great benefit of these drugs is that they can alleviate pain while causing fewer cases of gastrointestinal problems, such as ulcers.

- Disease-modifying antirheumatic drugs (DMARDs) may slow the development of rheumatoid arthritis. This group of medications includes injectable gold (Myochrisin), penicillamine (Distamine), anti-malarial drugs and sulfasalazine (Salazopyrin). Up to two-thirds of people who take DMARDs will show improvement; unfortunately, these drugs also have some serious possible side effects.

• Immunosuppressive drugs, including methotrexate (Maxtrex) and the newer drug cyclosporin (Neoral), work more quickly than DMARDs but have worse side effects.

• Relatively new medications known as TNF blockers may be prescribed for people who have not seen significant improvement with other drugs, such as DMARDs. These medications work by targeting tumour necrosis factor (TNF). Scientists have discovered a dramatic increase in the level of this protein circulating in the bloodstreams of people with rheumatoid arthritis. This increase contributes to making joints swollen and painful. Two TNF blockers for treating rheumatoid arthritis are etanercept (Enbrel) and infliximab (Remicade).

Surgery can help people with severe RA by reducing pain and improving the look and function of the damaged joint. Joint replacement is the most common procedure; younger people considering this surgery should be aware that artificial joints may eventually need to be replaced, entailing more surgery.

Natural Approaches for Treating Rheumatoid Arthritis

The Internet is swamped with remedies claiming to be effective natural treatments for rheumatoid arthritis. Unfortunately, the science is lacking for most, if not all, of the alternative options out there. However, some approaches are safe enough – and show enough anecdotal evidence – that experts are willing to recommend them. Talk to your doctor if you'd like to try one of the approaches given here.

Eat an animal-protein-free diet. To address the possible effects of leaky gut syndrome, Dr McDougall recommends eliminating the animal proteins that may be encouraging an autoimmune attack. While the idea is to follow an animal-free diet for life, for some people who try it, symptoms respond right away – in about 4 to 7 days, according to Dr McDougall. 'It surprises people to see how quickly they get better,' he says.

To test this approach, you will need to avoid all animal foods, including meat, fish, eggs and dairy products. Eat whole grains, seeds, pulses, nuts and vegetables such as broccoli, sweetcorn, potatoes and peas for protein. Use soya milk fortified with calcium or vegetables such as kale, cauliflower and brussels sprouts as calcium sources. 'If it takes more than 4 months,' says Dr McDougall, 'you should try something else.'

Try the 'mushroom of immortality'. Chinese medicine often relies on plant-based remedies. The reishi mushroom is a safe and effective natural anti-inflammatory, according to Janet Zand, LAc, OMD, a licensed acupuncturist and oriental medicine doctor in Austin, Texas. Look for reishi at your local health food shop; following the dosage instruction on the label, try this tonic food supplement for 2 months to see if it helps ease your pain.

Lupus

The full name is systemic lupus erythematosus (SLE), but this is more commonly known simply as lupus, which means 'wolf' in Latin. The disease was named to describe the appearance of one of its most common symptoms, a red facial rash that resembles a wolfish snout.

Unfortunately, the effects of lupus are more than skin-deep. The destructive autoimmune processes involved in lupus are widespread: besides the skin, they will also attack the joints, the central nervous system and the kidneys, heart and lungs. The body seemingly becomes allergic to itself.

There are two forms of SLE. One group of people with lupus have *non-organ-threatening lupus:* they will have aches, fatigue, fever and swollen glands or rashes, but they will not show any signs of internal organ involvement. About the same number of people with lupus will have *organ-threatening lupus*, a more serious form of the disease that involves the heart, lungs and kidneys. Without treatment, organ-threatening lupus can be fatal.

Lupus affects up to two million people in the United States, making it more common than multiple sclerosis, cystic fibrosis, cerebral palsy, sickle-cell anaemia and AIDS *combined*. The vast majority of people with lupus are women of childbearing age.

Early Warning Signs of Lupus

Like many of the other autoimmune disorders discussed in this chapter, lupus can be difficult to diagnose. Part of the problem is that the older a person is, the longer it seems to take to establish the cause of illness. Children generally show more obvious symptoms and can be diagnosed quickly; people over 60 may feel ill for years, visiting doctor after doctor before finally getting a definitive diagnosis of lupus. Lupus can also occur in combination with other autoimmune diseases, confusing the diagnosis process further, according to Daniel Wallace, MD, clinical professor of medicine at UCLA, past president of the Lupus Foundation of America and author of *The Lupus Book*.

The most important thing to consider is that early signs of lupus look very much like a number of other illnesses. If you suspect lupus, getting a reliable diagnosis requires a thorough medical examination – preferably by a rheumatologist (an arthritis specialist) – who will examine you from head to toe and most likely order blood tests for more information, says Dr Wallace.

The most common symptoms that can point to lupus include:

- Joint pain and swelling (seen in 50 per cent of people with lupus)
- Facial rashes (in 20 per cent)
- Malaise (generally feeling unwell) and fatigue (in 70 per cent)

This trio may go hand in hand with other, more general symptoms, such as low-grade fever and loss of appetite that leads to weight loss.

Prevention of Lupus

Preventing lupus is a complicated proposition. The disease may be genetic (although a lupus-specific gene has yet to be discovered), which would make prevention harder to control. Other likely candidates for causing lupus are factors that are also known to bring on flare-ups for those already diagnosed.

The following possible triggers may induce lupus in those who are already susceptible to the disease. Bear in mind, though, that there are

GENE THERAPY FOR LUPUS?

Autoimmune disorders are difficult to treat at best. For those who have the most extreme form of the autoimmune disorder lupus, the sad fact is that lack of a cure can ultimately be deadly.

Researchers seeking a cure for lupus (as well as for other autoimmune diseases) have focused their hunt on genes: tiny units of information located on the chromosomes within every cell. They already know that a particular section of chromosome referred to as the human leucocyte antigen (HLA) region contains a group of genetic markers that – singly or in various combinations – may give a person a tendency to develop lupus, as well as many other related diseases. Learning more about these markers and what they mean to the people who possess them may be the key to a new kind of treatment.

Gene therapy may be able to help both people at risk for lupus and those who already have the disease. 'We hope to someday take people at risk for lupus – say, children (of parents with the disease) – and potentially vaccinate them against it with an injection,' says Daniel Wallace, MD, clinical professor of medicine at UCLA, past president of the Lupus Foundation of America, and author of *The Lupus Book*. For people who are already experiencing the effects of lupus, gene therapy may be able to repair and replace a defective gene or set of genes and effectively 'turn off' the disease process.

Researchers are hopeful that gene therapy for lupus will become a reality in time for readers of this book to benefit. 'I'd say useful therapy is 10 to 20 years away,' says Dr Wallace.

many uncontrollable factors – genetics and viruses included – that may put people at risk of autoimmune disorders. Avoiding potential lupus triggers might be a good idea, but not to the point where it seriously affects your everyday lifestyle.

Eat less alfalfa. In 1989, the amino acid L-tryptophan was linked to an autoimmune-like illness. While that scare may have been due to manufacturing impurities, another amino acid called L-canavanine has been proved to cause or worsen inflammation in people with various autoimmune diseases, including lupus, says Dr Wallace. Alfalfa sprouts contain high amounts of this amino acid.

Be aware of the sun's effect. Two of the three types of ultraviolet radiation, UVA and UVB, are known to aggravate lupus, causing rashes and fatigue, and may be involved in initiating the disease process, according to Dr Wallace. Using sunscreen that blocks both UVA and UVB can help, and so can staying out of the sun during the peak hours of 10 a.m.–3 p.m.

Avoid aromatic amines. Chemicals called aromatic amines may play a role in causing or aggravating lupus and other arthritis-like diseases in certain people. These chemicals are found in hair dyes (paraphenylenediamine), tobacco smoke and some food colourings and drug preservatives (tartrazines). By law, all cosmetics sold in shops must carry ingredient labels. However, because those sold in salons are not covered by this rule, you might want to avoid them altogether. Tartrazine is a common name for E102 which is required by law to be listed as an ingredient on packages containing it. Normally, these chemicals are broken down in the body by a process called acetylation. However, approximately half of the population is 'slow acetylators,' meaning that they break down these chemicals more slowly and may have an immune-related response to them.

Be aware of the risk from medication. Prescription drugs are thought to cause up to 20,000 new cases of lupus each year. More than 70 different troublemaking medications have been identified, but 90 per cent of the cases can be linked to three drugs that are now rarely used: hydralazine (Apresoline) and methyldopa (Aldomet) for hypertension, and procainamide (Pronestyl) for heart problems. If you take any prescription drug and notice a rash, fever, or swollen joints, seek urgent medical advice. Once you stop taking the drug, symptoms should reverse.

Treatment for Lupus

More than 90 per cent of people with lupus need to take medication. The most highly prescribed drugs for lupus are the anti-inflammatories, including aspirin as well as NSAIDs.

Aspirin inhibits prostaglandin, a chemical that boosts inflammation and pain. Research has shown that aspirin is helpful for lupus because it can lower fever, help headache, ease muscle aches and pains and reduce malaise. Aspirin cannot, however, cure lupus or help treat any internal organ problems. In addition, aspirin can cause stomach, liver and kidney problems in some people. Too much aspirin can also cause ringing in the ears.

NSAIDs (including ibuprofen) have been available since the mid-1960s. These drugs are stronger than aspirin (meaning that you can take fewer pills to get the same pain-relieving effect) but most have more side effects to worry about. Like aspirin, NSAIDs inhibit prostaglandins and so reduce inflammation. Unlike aspirin, NSAIDs have not been studied for use specifically against lupus. Despite the lack of scientific evidence, many people with lupus take NSAIDs regularly, even daily. But as helpful as NSAIDs can be for people with lupus, they can also be very dangerous: all NSAIDs have the potential to cause liver or kidney failure in up to half of all patients using them long-term. The COX-2 inhibitor class of NSAIDs, however, which we mentioned earlier for rheumatoid arthritis, seems to pose less risk to the liver and kidneys. These drugs will be discussed in greater length shortly.

If lupus affects your kidneys or liver (which can happen in up to half of cases), you should avoid aspirin as well as oral NSAIDs. Fortunately, there are two other options to relieve pain and inflammation without risking serious side effects.

Consider topical pain relief. You don't have to swallow an NSAID to get the prostaglandin-inhibiting benefits. Certain NSAIDs (usually ketoprofen, the generic form of Orudis, and diclofenac, the generic form of Voltarol) can be added to gels that you rub into sore joints twice a day, going straight to the source of pain and bypassing the liver and kidneys. 'Topical NSAIDs are a good option,' says Dr Wallace. Talk to your doctor about getting a prescription for them.

Find out about a new type of NSAID. The next generation of prostaglandin-inhibiting NSAIDs, called COX-2 inhibitors, came on the scene in 1999. This relatively new group of drugs includes celecoxib (Celebrex) and rofecoxib (Vioxx). As mentioned earlier, COX-2 inhibitors appear to be safer for the kidneys and liver than standard NSAIDs. These medications are available only on prescription; ask your doctor whether you should give one a try.

Other prescription drugs may also be used for lupus, sometimes for mild cases, but especially for the more severe, organ-threatening form of the disease. These stronger drugs are referred to as disease modifiers, and they do more than just ease inflammation. Disease-modifying drugs can actually change the course of the disease. The three general types of disease-modifying drugs used against lupus are antimalarials, steroids and immunosuppressants.

• Antimalarial drugs were accidentally discovered to have an effect on lupus and rheumatoid arthritis in 1951. Doctors have been prescribing them – usually hydroxychloroquine (Plaquenil) and chloroquine (Avloclor) – for early-stage lupus ever since. Though antimalarials are generally safe to take, chloroquine is associated with permanent eye damage if taken in high dosages or taken over a long period of time.

• Steroids (a common one is prednisone) work by blocking chemical pathways in the body and decreasing immune activity, and can be used as creams, injections, or intravenous treatments. Steroids save the lives of many people with severe lupus; unfortunately, the drugs also cause a list of potentially serious side effects, including easy bruising and skin thinning, obesity, diabetes, high blood pressure, mood changes, ulcers and increased risk of infection. Lowering the dose or combining steroids with other drugs can reduce some side effects.

• Immunosuppressants are used against severe lupus that does not respond to steroids. Similar to chemotherapy for cancer (in fact, some of the medications are used for both), immunosuppressants are powerful and very toxic drugs, but they may slow the progress of lupus and allow people to reduce their steroid doses.

After years without any new options for treating lupus, a unique prescription alternative to steroids and immunosuppressants is on the horizon. If the FDA approves it, a patented form of the hormone DHEA (dehydroepiandrosterone) will be marketed for lupus in the US under the name Aslera (the generic name is prasterone).

In the past, over-the-counter DHEA has been touted as a cure for just about everything, lupus included. While experts have held that DHEA *does* show promise for lupus, taking it without a doctor's supervision could be useless at best – or quite dangerous at worst. 'Over-the-counter versions are very unreliable,' cautions Dr Wallace. 'You don't know what you are getting in each pill.' In high amounts, the hormone may cause endocrine-related side effects, including acne and facial hair growth, and it could even have a stimulating effect on some tumours. That said, a reliably pure form of DHEA like Aslera, if approved by the authorities, may prove to be the best treatment in the future.

Natural Treatment for Lupus

No natural or alternative therapies have been studied specifically for use against lupus. But certain herbs have been shown to help counter two common side effects, depression and mental and physical fatigue.

Deal with depression. Depression is the most common day-to-day problem associated with lupus. Fortunately, it's a good candidate for natural treatment, according to Dr Wallace. St John's wort has been used medically for years in Europe and is now becoming just as popular worldwide. The herb offers a way to address lupus-related depression without side effects though it should not be taken with antidepressants. 'It's really similar to Prozac,' says Dr Wallace. If you'd like to try St John's wort, discuss it with your doctor first. Then, look for tincture or capsules standardised to 0.3 per cent hypericin (the active ingredient in the plant). A typical dose is 300 mg, three times a day.

Try ginkgo for mental and physical fatigue. Another herbal medicine may help counter the debilitating malaise and mental fog that people with lupus often find themselves pushing through. 'Ginkgo seems to have positive cognitive effects,' says Dr Wallace. As with any natural medicine, let your doctor know if you decide to start taking ginkgo. Tea made from ginkgo leaves won't be strong enough; you should look for tablets concentrated to 24 per cent ginkgoflavoglycosides and 6 per cent terpenes lactones. A standard daily dose is 120 mg, taken in the form of one 40-mg tablet three times a day.

Multiple Sclerosis

Picture an electrical cord that has been targeted as a cat's favourite toy. Imagine the telltale teeth marks where the protective covering has been worn away, exposing the delicate inner wires. Then imagine what will happen when you try to turn on the lamp attached to that cord: Flicker, flicker, spark, then nothing.

In multiple sclerosis (MS), the immune system does the 'chewing'. For unknown reasons, the body creates autoantibodies that randomly wear away the protective coverings (made of a protein called myelin) that insulate nerve cells throughout the body and normally allow electrical messages to be sent at lightning speed.

When myelin gets destroyed, nerve messages are delayed. If the part of the nerve cell normally protected by myelin (called the axon) is itself destroyed, messages are stopped completely. Because the damage is random, and because nerve conduction can be affected by other factors as well, the disease commonly waxes and wanes: onsets of symptoms are called relapses; their spontaneous disappearance is called remission.

There are different stages, or phases, of MS. People commonly start out in the *relapsing-remitting* phase. People with this form of the disease first show symptoms between the ages of 20 and 40. These people tend to recover fully after their first attack; weeks or years can pass before the second attack. After each attack that follows, recovery is not as complete. Many people with relapsing–remitting MS stay at this point in their disease, having one attack every year or two, and never progress to the next phase.

After up to 20 years, a small percentage of people in the first phase of MS enter the *secondary progressive* phase. At this point, the damage caused by attacks is pretty much constant, and periods of remission disappear. A third, smaller group of people will develop MS symptoms that slowly get worse over time and never go into remission; this is called *primary progressive*.

Early Warning Signs of MS

Some symptoms of MS call attention to themselves, letting you know that something is wrong. But they can also be so subtle and mild that you might not even decide to see a doctor – or the symptoms may be gone by the time you do. Because damage to nerve coverings can happen anywhere in the body, symptoms can be different in each person affected.

Here are some of the most common early signs.

- Weakness in the arms and legs
- Numbness or tingling anywhere, including the head and face
- Eye pain
- Dimmed or blurred vision, usually in one eye

In later stages, MS can also cause dizziness, bladder and bowel problems and memory loss, among a list of possible symptoms.

Treatment for MS

Modern medical treatment for MS takes two approaches: one is to prevent relapses and stop the disease from progressing, and the other is to deal with symptoms.

'Until 1993, there were no true treatments for MS,' says Patricia K Coyle, MD, professor of neurology and director of the MS Comprehensive Care Center at the State University of New York at Stony Brook. Medications had been tested, of course, but none were proved to slow the disease process until a large clinical trial showed that a substance called interferon beta 1b (also known as Betaferon) could reduce the number of MS flare-ups by about one-third. Since then, another drug, involving interferon beta 1a, has been approved for use for MS – Avonex – and a third, Rebif, has been submitted to the FDA in the US for approval. Mitoxantrone (Novantrone), a chemotherapy drug, has also been used successfully for MS, says Dr Coyle.

Interferon is a protein normally made by white blood cells. Scientists believe that interferon regulates immune activity in healthy people. Interferon beta 1a (Avonex) is identical to the interferon produced in our bodies; interferon beta 1b (Betaferon) is slightly different.

Interferon beta 1a is known to help people who already have a definite case of MS. A study at the State University of New York at Buffalo has shown that treating people with interferon at the first signs of the disease may prevent them from going on to develop full-blown MS. Researchers gave weekly injections of interferon beta 1a to 193 people who had one MS-related symptom as well as an MRI test showing nerve sheath damage and a high risk for MS. Another group of 190 people received placebo injections. The study ended when any of the participants developed definite MS. Three years after the study, researchers found that people who received interferon treatment were significantly less likely to go on to develop MS.

Another non-interferon drug has also been shown to reduce the number of relapses in people diagnosed with MS. Glatiramer acetate (Copaxone) resembles a small part of the protein of which nerve sheaths are made. Its exact mechanism is unclear, but Copaxone may work by shutting down destructive immune activity. Of all the MS drugs, Copaxone seems to have the fewest side effects.

Treatment for active attacks generally calls for steroids, according to Nancy Holland, RN, EdD, vice president of clinical programmes for the US National Multiple Sclerosis Society. Injected or oral steroids (such as methylprednisolone, cortisone, or prednisone) can speed recovery from an attack and are the best treatments that doctors have to offer right now, says Dr Holland. But frequent or long-term steroid use puts you at risk for a list of side effects. You can minimise side effects by using the drugs only when necessary and by taking the lowest effective dose for the shortest length of time.

Individual problems associated with MS, such as fatigue, nerve pain in the face or limbs and bladder infections, can be treated with prescription drugs specific to each symptom.

Natural and Self-Help Treatments for MS

Though there doesn't seem to be any sure way to reduce the severity of MS relapses, certain self-help approaches have been shown to help many people avoid 'pseudo-exacerbation', a temporary worsening of symptoms that does not reflect new disease activity. Here are five to try.

Keep cool. Heat temporarily makes symptoms worse for some people. 'MS actually used to be diagnosed with a "hot bath test" to see if symptoms got worse in hot water,' says Dr Holland. If heat causes flare-ups for you, avoid overly hot showers or baths and stay out of direct sun. In warm weather, drink plenty of cool liquids and 'stay cool'. Air conditioning is considered a medical necessity for MS in some locations.

Take control over your bladder. Serious bladder problems can be dramatically improved by medication, or in some cases by learning to self-catheterise, says Dr Holland. 'Urine sitting in the bladder is an ideal place for infection to grow,' she warns. Learning to handle the simple equipment can prevent a trip to the hospital and also relieve worries related to loss of bladder control or 'emergency' situations when a lavatory isn't available. Doing it yourself is much easier than you think, says Dr Holland. Ask your doctor to teach you how to self-catheterise, or for any help with your bladder problems.

Try tai chi. A small study shows that the gentle Asian exercise known as tai chi can make physical activity easier for people with MS. Nineteen people with the disease took part in an 8-week tai chi class. At the end of the programme, researchers saw a 21 per cent increase in walking speed and a 28 per cent improvement of flexibility in the back of the leg (hamstring). Mental and social abilities also improved, suggesting that tai chi offers all-round help for those with MS.

Healthy eating may help. MS tends to flare up and calm down with no apparent cause, making it difficult to pinpoint foods that may trigger trouble. While no one diet has been proved to help, experts agree that a low-fat approach rich in fruits, vegetables and whole grains certainly cannot hurt. Avoiding alcohol and caffeine may also relieve MS symptoms.

Add some special fats. Along with an overall healthy low-fat diet, increasing the amount of certain essential fats, called omega-3 fatty acids, is worth a try for people with MS. Omega-3 fatty acids are found in oily fish such as salmon and mackerel, as well as in rapeseed oil and soya beans. Modern eating doesn't provide enough of these healthy fats; increasing the intake of omega-3s balances out other fats (known as omega-6s) that promote inflammation. 'Basically, omega-3s favour health,' says Robert Wildman, RD, PhD, associate professor in the nutrition programme at the University of Louisiana at Lafayette. Eating fish at least twice a week or grinding 60 g (2 oz) of flaxseed on to your morning cereal could result in less pain and inflammation, says Dr Wildman.

Crohn's Disease

People with Crohn's disease suffer from deep and ongoing inflammation of the lining of the intestine, leading to all manner of digestive problems that are very difficult to treat.

Crohn's disease is considered an inflammatory bowel disease (IBD). Unlike other IBDs, though, Crohn's is generally thought to be caused by an autoimmune reaction, most likely to a bacterium or virus. It has also been linked with the measles vaccination and diet. There is probably a genetic connection as well: Crohn's tends to run in families.

Chronic inflammation changes the walls of the intestine, eventually leaving them scarred and thickened and prone to blockage, the most common complication of this disease. Inflammation can also lead to sores that fail to heal and instead grow into tunnels that affect nearby areas such as the bladder, anus, or vagina. These tunnel-shaped sores are called fistulas and often become infected, requiring medication or surgery.

Early Warning Signs of Crohn's Disease

Symptoms of Crohn's are very similar to those of other intestinal illnesses such as irritable bowel syndrome and ulcerative colitis. If you notice any of the following early signs persisting for more than a few weeks, see your doctor for a proper diagnosis.

- Abdominal pain, especially in the lower right area
- Diarrhoea
- Rectal bleeding (see your doctor immediately)
- Weight loss
- Fever

Prevention of Crohn's Disease

No steps have yet been found to prevent Crohn's, but some controllable factors are known to increase your risk of developing the disease.

Avoiding the two potential triggers here will benefit your health in other ways as well.

Keep away from cigarette smoke. Cigarette smoke – either first-or secondhand – can double your odds of developing Crohn's disease, according to Eugene May, MD, retired gastroenterologist and honorary staff member at Riverside Methodist Hospital in Columbus, Ohio. If you really need convincing, consider that smoking adds to other digestive problems as well, including ulcers and heartburn, and can increase your risk of gallstones and liver disease.

Try to manage stress. 'Stress can make anything worse, and certainly, some people feel that stressful events precipitated the onset of their Crohn's,' says Dr May. 'We already have proof that stressful events can flare ulcerative colitis.' While no one can avoid stress completely, you can stay aware of your level of stress and take action to relieve it through methods such as meditation, prayer and guided imagery before it affects your health.

Treatment for Crohn's Disease

Steroids used to be a mainstay of treatment for Crohn's relapses, says Dr May. But, he says, 'They have so many bad side effects long-term on the emotions and the body that they are used now in the major centres more for acute disease complications only.' Instead, people with Crohn's are being urged to consider immunosuppressants to keep their condition in remission. That appears to be good advice, says Dr May.

A double-blind study from the London Clinical Trials Research Group in Ontario showed that the immunosuppressive drug methotrexate, an effective treatment to shorten relapses, can also keep Crohn's in remission when taken over the long term. Forty out of 76 people whose disease was currently in remission were chosen to get 15-mg injections of the drug once a week. The remaining 36 received placebo injections. After 40 weeks, 65 per cent of the people receiving methotrexate were still in remission, compared with only 14 per cent of the people in the placebo group. Furthermore, only one person taking methotrexate had side effects severe enough to withdraw from the study.

There is now another option available for people whose symptoms do not respond to immunosuppressive medicine. Infliximab (Remicade), the first drug approved specifically for use in Crohn's, targets TNF, a protein that is produced by the immune system and that may be responsible for the inflammation caused by Crohn's. Infliximab removes TNF from blood before it gets to the intestines, preventing inflammation. This new drug is available, and some studies have shown a substantial improvement in patients who are treated with it, but researchers are continuing to study people who are taking the drug to monitor its long-term safety and effectiveness. (As mentioned earlier in this chapter, it is also being prescribed to help ease the swollen and painful joints of people with rheumatoid arthritis.)

Drugs such as antibiotics and antidiarrhoeals may also be prescribed to deal with Crohn's symptoms. Severe Crohn's may also be treated with surgery to remove the affected part of the intestine, but the inflammation tends to return to the area adjacent to that which was removed. Many people with Crohn's have other surgeries to repair complications such as intestinal blockages or abscesses.

Natural Treatments for Crohn's Disease

Since Crohn's is a disease of the digestive tract and people with the disease are often malnourished because of it, natural remedies focus on foods. The two approaches mentioned here may help, but they are not meant to substitute for medical treatment. Try them in conjunction with your doctor's recommendations.

Try a Chinese approach. Traditional Chinese medicine (TCM) takes a unique dietary approach to Crohn's disease that differs from the traditional Western view. 'It's considered an acid condition,' says Dr Zand. To counter the tendency, TCM practitioners recommend a diet low in extremely acidic foods such as lemons. A licensed practitioner can determine whether TCM remedies are suitable for you.

Add some yoghurt to your diet. Some experts believe that Crohn's disease may be initiated by a lack of beneficial bacteria. 'Today's better hygiene and more sanitary water supply may prevent our guts from being exposed to certain bacteria that would otherwise protect us from other bacteria that may damage the intestine,' says Dr May. Adding yoghurt to your daily diet is a way to deliver some healthy, and possibly protective, bacteria directly into the digestive tract.

Scleroderma

If you studied any Greek at school, then you know what scleroderma does to nearly everyone diagnosed with it. This autoimmune disorder leads to hardening *(sclero-)* of the skin *(-derma),* most often on the fingers, hands, forearms and face.

As with the other conditions discussed in this chapter, we don't know for certain what causes scleroderma (though there are some interesting possibilities: see 'Prevention of Scleroderma' on page 230). Once someone develops the disease, however, his or her symptoms can be traced back to an autoimmune response that leads to the overproduction of collagen, a protein that's a major component of what is called connective tissue, which includes the skin, the oesophagus and digestive tract and the lungs, kidneys, heart and other internal organs.

In people without scleroderma, the immune system normally sparks cells to make collagen and create a scar as part of healing after an injury or infection. In people with scleroderma, the immune system sends mistaken signals, telling connective tissue cells to produce collagen when it's not needed. Scar tissue then randomly builds up, causing thickness, tightness and pain in the skin and other areas.

Scleroderma can appear in different forms, depending on the type and extent of symptoms. The following are the two main groups, or classifications, of scleroderma.

Localised scleroderma. The localised form affects children more frequently than adults, and shows up as patches or lines of thickened skin. Linear scarring to the forehead and scalp resembling a knife slash is referred to as *un coup de sabre,* 'a cut of the sabre'. Localised scleroderma usually doesn't involve internal organs, and it generally will not progress to the systemic form.

Systemic scleroderma. Also called systemic sclerosis, systemic scleroderma affects the skin as well as the internal organs and the small blood vessels. This form is further divided into two smaller subgroups – limited and diffuse – depending on the amount of skin affected.

Early Warning Signs of Scleroderma

The early stages of both localised and systemic scleroderma generally look the same. Unfortunately, many symptoms can be vague and may overlap with other health problems, making it difficult to recognise the disease and get a proper diagnosis the first time. If your doctor suspects scleroderma, you should be referred to an arthritis specialist (a rheumatologist) and possibly a dermatologist as well.

The following early symptoms of scleroderma show up in nearly everyone who has the disease.

- Thickening or hardening of the skin of the fingers affects 98 per cent of people with scleroderma.

- Raynaud's disease (abnormal sensitivity to cold, especially in the hands and feet) affects 95 per cent of people with scleroderma.

- When they are tested for, antinuclear antibodies (antibodies that attack the nuclei of other cells in the body) show up in the blood of more than 95 per cent of people with scleroderma.

Other signs occur less frequently and may include the following:

- Joint pain and stiffness

- Digestive problems, such as heartburn and a feeling that food is 'sticking' on the way down

- Weakness and fatigue

- Sjögren's syndrome (dry mouth and eyes)

- Lung and heart problems (such as shortness of breath on climbing a flight or two of stairs, a chronic cough, or high blood pressure) and, rarely, kidney failure

Prevention of Scleroderma

Since it isn't known what causes scleroderma, current prevention is limited to avoiding possible environmental triggers that make the disease more likely to develop. Two substances have been linked to scleroderma, one falsely.

Silicone does not play a role, according to research done so far. After a number of women with silicone breast implants complained of scleroderma-like symptoms that disappeared when the implants were removed, researchers became curious. Since then, there have been at least five studies done showing no connection between the implants and development of the disease, according to Daniel E Furst, MD, director of arthritis clinical research at the Virginia Mason Research Center in Seattle.

Dr Furst notes, however, that there are a couple of caveats to consider. 'There is a reasonable amount of data to show that, in test tubes, silicone can cause immune hyperreactivity,' he says. Plus, increased levels of antinuclear antibodies (a marker for increased immune reactivity) can occur in women with implants who otherwise show no signs of the disease. 'It's hard to know which came first,' says Dr Furst. Regardless, if you are concerned about developing scleroderma, it's probably a good idea to avoid augmenting your figure with silicone.

While the evidence for silicone may be unclear, there is no argument that another similar-sounding but unrelated substance – silica – *is* associated with an increased risk of scleroderma, says Dr Furst. Silica, also called silicon dioxide, is a hard mineral used in dental materials, among other things – although there is no evidence that dental materials are associated with scleroderma, he says. People whose jobs expose them to very high amounts of silica – in particular, coal miners, sandblasters, rock drillers and roofers – develop scleroderma in above-average numbers.

Treatment for Scleroderma

Since each person with scleroderma can have a unique set of symptoms, treatment needs to be tailored to the individual. In general, treatment for localised scleroderma will focus on relieving symptoms that are limited to the skin, while treatment for the more severe systemic form aims to prevent potentially life-threatening complications.

Localised skin thickenings have been treated with steroids, in either injection or cream form. Mild skin symptoms can be left alone, but trying treatment may be a better option. 'We like to treat early, in the hopes that we can prevent the body from producing even more collagen,' says Dr Furst.

In serious cases of systemic scleroderma, small blood vessels can be damaged by collagen growth, leading to an emergency kidney condition called renal crisis. There was no effective treatment for this until recently, when it was discovered that drugs called angiotensin-converting enzyme (ACE) inhibitors (usually prescribed for high blood pressure) can work miracles. 'This complication used to kill people within 6 weeks,' says Dr Furst, 'but medication now makes a huge difference.'

Potent immunosuppressive drugs, such as methotrexate and cyclophosphamide (Endoxana), which are most commonly used against cancer, are also being enlisted to treat systemic scleroderma. 'We are trying many things, but it's all still experimental. Some of these drugs seem to help a number of people, but they can also be very dangerous,' Dr Furst explains.

An advanced medical technique called stem cell transplantation shows promise for the people seriously ill with scleroderma. In this risky procedure, specialised cells that produce blood and bone marrow are removed from the blood. High doses of medication and radiation are then used to destroy the cells responsible for the overproduction of collagen. The stem cells are then replaced and, hopefully, go on to produce new blood and bone marrow that will be normal and healthy. According to Dr Furst, this is a very hopeful treatment for those with the worst prognosis. Ask your doctor if you'd like to be involved in an early study (called a clinical trial) of stem cell transplantation for scleroderma.

Natural Approaches to Scleroderma

Unfortunately, there is little evidence that natural remedies can affect the root cause of scleroderma: the overproduction of collagen. One supplement, an amino acid called N-acetyl-cysteine (NAC), has been studied because of its powerful antioxidant effects and the hope that it could help break down collagen. Dr Furst was involved in NAC research in 1972.

While NAC is considered relatively safe, the researchers had to use huge amounts to see any effect, and the results weren't particularly relevant to people with scleroderma. 'Antioxidants worked very well in test tubes, but the effect doesn't translate to humans,' Dr Furst says. 'It's unlikely that antioxidants are going to be effective against this disease.'

Sjögren's Syndrome

If you've ever had a stuffed-up nose and woken up sandy-eyed and parched after a full night's sleep of mouth-only breathing, you have a vague sense of what it's like for someone with Sjögren's (pronounced 'show-grens') syndrome. This uncomfortable autoimmune disorder is the result of overreactive white blood cells attacking the body's moisture-making glands. Sjögren's causes problems most frequently in the eyes and mouth, but sometimes it can also affect the vagina, skin and lungs. It affects up to 1 per cent of the population, mostly middle-aged women.

In about one-third of cases, the disease can also become systemic, involving more parts of the body and causing additional symptoms, including pain, fatigue and possible kidney trouble. People already diagnosed with another autoimmune disorder, such as rheumatoid arthritis or scleroderma, may also develop Sjögren's as a secondary problem.

Early Warning Signs of Sjögren's Syndrome

We've all experienced bouts of dryness on occasion: think of the last time you had a head cold, overindulged in salty food, or spent time in windy or arid weather. That's why symptoms of Sjögren's are often overlooked or labelled as being caused by something else. In particular, postmenopausal women complaining of vaginal dryness who are actually showing signs of Sjögren's often go undiagnosed, says Stuart S Kassan, MD, past chair of the medical advisory board for the Sjögren's Syndrome Foundation and clinical professor of medicine at the University of Colorado Health Sciences Center in Denver.

When the most common signs of Sjögren's *are* recognised, it may be your optometrist or dentist who identifies it. Constantly dry eyes (the medical term is *sicca*), especially when accompanied by a gritty or sandy feeling and sticky debris that builds up in the inner corners, is one warning sign. Another is dry mouth (called *xerostomia*), which can lead to difficulty in speaking and swallowing and can spur cavities and other dental problems. A person with Sjögren's may also notice dry skin; women may suffer from dry vaginal tissues, leading to painful intercourse.

Treatment for Sjögren's Syndrome

As with other autoimmune disorders, there is no proven way to prevent or cure Sjögren's syndrome. Medical treatment can offer relief from symptoms and may stop the disease from getting worse.

There is a prescription drug to target mouth symptoms effectively, says Dr Kassan. Pilocarpine (Salagen, taken in pill form) stimulates the branches of the peripheral nervous system that include the salivary glands and encourage them to be more productive. Side effects are minimal, and the necessary dose is relatively small. You should see relief within a few days of starting the drug; ask your doctor if it would be right for you.

Most of the time, Sjögren's starts out mildly and progresses very slowly. In about one-third of cases, however, people with the disease will have other symptoms in addition to dryness. For fatigue, low-grade fever and achiness, antimalarial drugs such as hydroxychloroquine (Plaquenil) can be taken long-term. Severe lung, kidney and blood vessel involvement may call for stronger drugs, including immunosuppressive medicines or steroids.

Self-Help for Sjögren's Syndrome

If your symptoms are mild, or if medical treatment isn't enough, self-help strategies can make you more comfortable. Try these basic tips to ease chronic dryness and prevent complications.

Sip water often. Keeping a cool drink of water on hand at all times will make speaking and eating less awkward. More important, developing the habit of drinking plenty of liquids during your meals can prevent accidental choking.

Mend a parched mouth. Specialised mouthwashes, generally available over-the-counter, can be used as often as needed to soothe and soften dry mouth and throat tissues, says Dr Kassan.

Protect your teeth. Since saliva normally helps to protect your teeth from plaque build-up, the saliva-sapping effects of Sjögren's can cause an increase in cavities and other tooth trouble. See your dentist and hygienist twice a year for check-ups and cleanings, brush and floss after every meal and avoid sticky, sugary snacks. You can also ask your dentist about prescription-strength fluoride gel treatment that can help prevent cavities, says Dr Kassan.

Try using eyedrops. Like saliva, tears normally serve a protective function. Without their lubricating moisture, eyes feel itchy. With extreme dryness, sores called corneal ulcers can form on the surface of the eye. Artificial tears, in the form of eyedrops, offer relief from that scratchy feeling and make blinking smoother. Try over-the-counter brands, or ask your doctor for a prescription for Liquifilm Tears.

Graves' Disease and Hashimoto's Thyroiditis

Think of your thyroid – a butterfly-shaped gland that smoothly (and normally, invisibly) wraps around the front of your throat – as your metabolic thermostat. Turned up, you get warm. Turned down, you cool off.

The thyroid produces thyroid hormone, a chemical that has important regulatory effects on other parts of the body. In healthy people, the right levels of thyroid hormone smoothly control metabolism (the rate of calorie burning) without inadvertent heat surges or unexpected cool-downs. When the thyroid is attacked by autoantibodies, however, over- or underproduction of thyroid hormone will sway the balance one way or the other and show up as ripple effects throughout the body.

In Hashimoto's thyroiditis (also called autoimmune thyroiditis), antibodies target and gradually destroy the thyroid gland, leaving the body with a lack of thyroid hormone. In Graves' disease, abnormal antibodies fool the thyroid into continuously releasing thyroid hormone. Too much thyroid hormone overstimulates metabolism. Other symptoms, including serious eye problems, may actually be related diseases rather than side effects of thyroid trouble, according to H Jack Baskin, MD, past president of the American Association of Clinical Endocrinologists and director of the Florida Thyroid and Endocrine Clinic in Orlando.

In some cases, Graves' disease will evolve into Hashimoto's as the thyroid slowly burns itself out, says Dr Baskin. It's also possible that some people will show signs of both disorders at the same time.

Early Warning Signs of Autoimmune Thyroid Trouble

Both Graves' disease and Hashimoto's thyroiditis are frequently misdiagnosed. The people Dr Baskin sees with these conditions have often had numerous tests done and have visited an average of four doctors before coming to him.

In addition, doctors may miss signs of thyroid problems in menopausal women because many of the symptoms, such as vaginal dryness, thinning hair and weight gain, are also associated with ageing. Knowing the signs of a hyper- or hypoactive thyroid can help you seek medical advice or get a second opinion sooner rather than later.

Because of the regulating effect that the thyroid has on metabolism as a whole, symptoms of a thyroid gone wrong will affect various body parts as well as behaviours such as sleep and appetite. Symptoms of thyroid diseases, including Graves' disease and Hashimoto's thyroiditis, mirror each other because an overstimulated metabolism will have the opposite effect of a sluggish one.

Symptoms of Graves' disease include:

- A tendency to feel warm
- A fast or irregular heartbeat
- Fatigue
- Difficulty sleeping
- Feelings of anxiety
- Increased sweating
- Diarrhoea
- Weight loss (especially in later stages or in elderly people)

WOMEN AND AUTOIMMUNE DISORDERS: A HORMONE CONNECTION?

It's a fact (but a mysterious one) that autoimmune disorders strike far more women than men. Almost three out of four people with autoimmune trouble are women; most of them are in their childbearing years.

Why the imbalance? When you consider that certain autoimmune disorders show up more frequently during postmenopause, others occur or flare up with pregnancy and still others actually improve when a woman is with child, the evidence seems to point to a role for female hormones, which also wax and wane at those key times.

A number of female sex hormones have been shown to have complex actions on the immune system, says Patricia K Coyle, MD, professor of neurology and director of the MS Comprehensive Care Center at the State University of New York at Stony Brook. The major ones are progesterone (a hormone that fosters pregnancy), prolactin (a hormone associated with breastfeeding), androgens ('male' hormones that are also present in women) and a variety of oestrogens (a class of 'female' hormones), says Dr Coyle.

Of course, every woman's body produces hormones, but not all women will develop autoimmune trouble. There are other possible factors behind the gender-slanted phenomenon: for example, the genes related to autoimmune disorders may occur more often or in greater numbers on the X chromosome, of which women have two. Women may also be somehow more susceptible to environmental triggers, such as viruses, that are suspected to contribute to the development of autoimmune problems.

The uneven distribution of these disorders may also relate to the possibility that women simply have more robust immune systems than men. 'There is good data that the female immune response is more potent,' says Dr Coyle.

Symptoms of Hashimoto's thyroiditis include:

- A tendency to feel cold

- Fatigue

- An urge to sleep more than usual

- Constipation

- Decreased appetite

• Weight gain (especially in later stages)

Both types of thyroid disease will cause fatigue. A person with Hashimoto's thyroiditis will have the urge to sleep more, and may even fall asleep inappropriately, for example, during a film. A person with Graves' disease will feel energetic due to the alerting effects of thyroid hormone, but will tire easily. That's because the stimulating effect of Graves' disease prevents deep sleep and hinders night-time energy storage.

Treatment for Graves' Disease and Hashimoto's Thyroiditis

Surgery used to be the main medical treatment for the hyperactive thyroid seen in Graves' disease. Removing part or all of the thyroid gland was a sure way to bring metabolism under control and prevent complications. After the procedure, thyroid hormone would be replaced with a synthetic supplement in just the right amount.

Today, doctors use a modified approach to quell an out-of-control thyroid, says Dr Baskin. 'Radioactive iodine has been used for more than 50 years and doesn't show any side effects,' he says, 'and usually, one dose does it.' Iodine from foods and other sources is absorbed only by thyroid tissues, where it is normally used to make thyroid hormone. In the form of a radioactive pill, iodine selectively destroys just the thyroid gland, eliminating the need for surgery. Afterward, synthetic thyroid replacement medication needs to be taken daily.

Treatment for Hashimoto's underactive symptoms boosts thyroid function using the same synthetic thyroid hormone. Levels of hormone must be carefully calculated for each individual.

People taking replacement thyroid hormone for either condition generally take the same specialised dose for the rest of their lives, although hormone needs may change at times. During pregnancy, for example, a woman will probably need to increase her dose, says Dr Baskin. 'We may have to increase her dose once or twice during pregnancy,' he notes, 'possibly because of the weight gain or an increase in metabolism.' Pregnant women taking thyroid replacement should have their thyroid function tested every 6 weeks.

Natural Treatment for Thyroid Disease

Naturopathic physician Dr Head recommends a special type of replacement thyroid hormone, a blend called Armour Thyroid, which is a natural preparation containing several thyroid hormones. 'Synthroid (generic name, levothyroxine) is a synthetic drug – one of the most commonly prescribed by conventional doctors – and contains only one of the hormones that is missing if your thyroid is no longer working,' she says. 'Armour Thyroid is a prescription item, but it's more natural and, in my experience, it's more effective.' Ask your doctor about trying this alternative form of thyroid hormone.

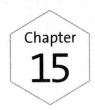

CANCER

If you don't have cancer and you don't want to get it, you're too late: You've almost certainly already had it. In fact, you've probably had cancer several times in your life without knowing about it.

The reason you didn't know it is that your immune system intervened and annihilated the cancer before it had a chance to take hold and spread. Cells that were on their way to becoming malignant were discovered and destroyed. A cancer that might have put you in an early grave was flushed out of your system, and you went about your business never knowing that a cellular catastrophe had been avoided.

In this chapter, you'll learn how to help your immune system keep winning its war against cancer.

On Guard against Cancer

You are not the same person you were a year ago. The 10 trillion cells in your body are constantly giving birth to new cells and then dying off. At that rate of replication, the odds that something might go genetically wrong aren't high; they're *certain*. Cells that should die can mistakenly keep on reproducing, growing out of control until they start to threaten the tissues and organs around them. Sometimes, cells become chronically irritated – by persistent heartburn, perhaps, or a chronic bowel disease, or after too much exposure to the sun – and after a while, they can begin to mutate. Viruses and bacteria can attack cells, too, causing internal damage that turns them malignant. Or you may have a genetic predisposition that gives you higher-than-usual odds of developing a certain type of cancer.

Whatever the reason, cancer cells are twisted traitors in your body. Somehow, their DNA gets damaged, and they begin to grow out of control. It's the immune system's job to clean up those mistakes before they get out of control. It does this by producing cells that recognise abnormalities in other cells. Once a cancer cell is recognised, immunity cells attack. They can kill off cancer cells in one of two ways, according to Ronald B Herberman, MD, director of the University of Pittsburgh Cancer Institute. They can release a substance that punches holes in the outer membranes of the cancer cells, causing them to leak and then explode. Or they can send a chemical signal that rewrites the cancer cell's DNA with a new set of instructions: instructions that tell its nucleus to disintegrate. Dr Herberman agrees that there's a sense of poetic justice in the latter case, because the immune system is using cancer's own DNA-corrupting strategy to defeat it. If our immune systems have such effective anti-cancer weapons at their disposal, how do some cancer cells manage to evade those weapons and grow? One answer to that question, Dr Herberman says, is that the cancer cells have their own defence mechanisms that can kill or at least impair the functioning of the attacking immune cells. Other times, cancer cells disguise their presence (how they manage this is not completely understood) so that the immune system doesn't recognise them. If they get away with this deception long enough, the cancer can become too advanced to overcome.

One of the most insidious problems with cancer is that, as it grows, it gradually weakens the immune system's ability to resist it. That can lead to a vicious cycle: a weakened immune system lowers your body's ability to fight off the development and progression of cancer. That's why people who have acquired immunodeficiency syndrome (AIDS) often develop multiple malignancies.

The bottom line is this: the stronger your immune system, the more

A VACCINE FOR CANCER?

What if you could get an injection that would protect you against cancer the same way you get a vaccination against tetanus? Scientists are working on it, and some are optimistic that cancer vaccines could be a fact of life by the middle of this century. Given the spectacular potential for healing that a cancer vaccine would have (and the spectacular profits that such a vaccine would bring), it's not surprising that this is one of the hottest areas in medical research today.

At this early stage, most cancer vaccine research is focusing on curing people with cancer, rather than on preventing it. The immune system is a key player in many of these studies. Normally, the immune system will detect abnormal cells and destroy them before they spread into malignancies. But sometimes, mutating cells avoid detection. If that goes on long enough, a tumour can form; then it may be too late for the immune system to successfully overwhelm it.

Scientists are trying to develop vaccines that would help the immune system notice those renegade cells before they get out of control. One way of doing this is to extract some cells from a patient's tumour and insert into them genetic material that is known to produce certain proteins in the body. When these altered cells are then reintroduced into the patient's system, the proteins they produce will cause the immune system to notice the tumour cells – it's like programming the tumour cells to flash an electric sign.

Much of the research so far has focused on melanoma, a form of skin cancer, and on kidney cancer. These cancers have relatively high rates of spontaneous remission, which suggests that the immune system can reverse them once it is alerted to their presence. Other potential vaccines are being aimed at pancreatic, colon, breast, prostate and lung cancer, among others.

A few tests of cancer vaccines on small groups of patients have shown dramatic results. In a few cases, tumours almost 'melted away,' says Ronald B Herberman, MD, director of the University of Pittsburgh Cancer Institute. But Dr Herberman and others are cautious about predicting that vaccines will produce a cancer cure any time soon. Even in successful trials, patients whose malignancies disappeared were limited – in the 10 to 20 per cent range, he says – and studies involving far larger groups of patients are needed. Meanwhile, early predictions of a vaccine breakthrough have not been realised as quickly as expected.

Still, the sheer numbers of scientists at work on the challenge and the progress they've made so far suggest that, sooner or later, the elusive breakthrough will occur. Then, hopes will likely shift to the next frontier: vaccines that could actually prevent cancer from developing at all.

likely it is that your body's inevitable cellular mistakes will be killed in their infancy. Here's how to make sure that that happens.

Cellular Self-Defence

'Well people don't get cancer.'

That's how herbalist Douglas Schar, DipPhyt, MCPP, who practises in London and Washington, DC, sums up his philosophy on defeating everyone's most feared disease. What exactly does it mean?

It means that you can lower your risk of getting cancer by keeping yourself healthy, because healthy people have healthy immune systems. Holistic healers believe that the body's natural state is one of health. We compromise that basic state of health by doing things that interfere with our various natural body functions, says Keith Berndtson, MD, medical director at Integrative Care Centers in Chicago and Glenview, Illinois. Bad health habits are like weights, dragging our bodies down, Dr Berndtson believes. The goal, therefore, is to eliminate that excess weight by taking care of ourselves. 'Less drag means more thrust,' he says.

Take sleep, for example. When we sleep, our bodies embark on what Dr Berndtson describes as a restoration phenomenon, during which growth hormones are pumped throughout the system. These growth hormones help maintain and restore our organs, our tissues, our cells and all our 'metabolic pathways,' as Dr Berndtson puts it, including our immune systems.

Our immune systems face especially weighty challenges today because we live in an especially stressful world. 'Modern life compromises our vitality in a thousand ways,' says Schar, 'and when your vitality is compromised, you're vulnerable to all sorts of health problems — whether it's the athlete's foot fungus you're exposed to at the gym, or cancer. If our vitality is decreased, then whatever we can do to increase it is good.'

One way to avoid compromises to your body's natural vitality is to

TAKE THE **FIRST STEP**

Tonight, try going to bed a little earlier. Scientists have found that as we sleep, growth hormones coursing through our bodies actually work to restore our organs, tissues and other cells. By making sure that you get plenty of rest, you're actually helping your body to mend itself – and that can lower your risk of cancer.

avoid the forms of bodily stress that have been shown to lead to cancer. Don't smoke cigarettes, don't drink too much alcohol, don't indulge in unsafe sex that can lead to AIDS, don't spend too much time in the sun and don't expose yourself to too much pollution.

Beyond all that, there are some simple measures that experts say will minimise bodily wear and tear and keep your immune system at its cancer-fighting best, day after day, year after year. Here are the basic building blocks they recommend.

Defy Cancer with Your Diet

When it comes to beating cancer, diet counts. It's been estimated that as many as 40 to 70 per cent of all cancers are related to what we eat – either because we don't eat the foods our bodies need or because we eat foods that actively contribute to disease, or both, according to James S Gordon, MD, director of the Center for Mind-Body Medicine in Washington, DC, and co-author of *Comprehensive Cancer Care*.

To be sure that your diet is healthy, keep the following points in mind.

Stock up on fruits and vegetables. Nature has built cancer-fighting elixirs into fruits and vegetables. These are called phytonutrients, and some of them seem to be part of a plant's own immune system, developed to help it ward off assaults from germs and disease. The wonderful thing is that plants pass the protective capabilities of their phytonutrients on to us when we eat them.

One of the primary ways that phytonutrients help to maintain our immune systems is through their antioxidant power. Antioxidants protect the body from attack by free radicals. These are oxygen molecules that somewhere along the way – because of various sorts of wear and tear, normal and otherwise – have lost an electron. As they attempt to regain their missing electrons, they sweep through your body, stealing electrons wherever they can. The molecular victims of these raids are damaged in the process and become free radicals themselves. This is a chain reaction that over time may result in cancer, among other diseases.

Phytonutrients step between the marauding free radicals and your body's cells, offering up their own electrons. Free radicals take them, become stable again and stop doing their damage.

Phytonutrients also help fight cancer in several other ways. Some help the body flush out toxic chemicals, including carcinogens, before they have time to make us ill. Others help keep the level of hormones in the body in balance, which helps prevent hormone-related cancers, including breast cancer and ovarian cancer. Still others prevent the growth of tumours by keeping blood vessels from growing nearby. The whole package adds up to an anti-cancer powerhouse, which is why a number of studies show that people who eat lots of fruits and vegetables appear to be at less risk of cancer than people who eat less of these foods. For an overview of specific phytochemicals, what they do and what foods have them, see Activate Your Body's Immune Power with the MaxImmunity Diet, starting on page 51.

Buy natural foods. One idea to keep in mind as you shop for groceries is that, in general, less processed is better. 'Every machine that comes in contact with your food is likely to strip out nutrients,' says Dr Berndtson. Besides taking healthy things away from your foods, processing often puts unhealthy things in: preservatives, colourings, sugar, sugar substitutes and trans fatty acids, to name a few. Such additives can not only weaken a food's cancer-fighting capabilities, Dr Berndtson points out, but they may also promote cancer themselves.

Insist on whole grains. If you want evidence that less is more when it comes to food processing, look no farther than the bakery aisle of your local supermarket. When it comes to carbohydrates, most of us tend to fill up on refined grains: white bread, cakes, biscuits and the like. They taste good but the refining process removes virtually everything that was nutritious in the grain and throws it in the dustbin.

Whole grains, by contrast, are packed with nutrients, including plenty of ones that fight cancer, such as fibre, which may lower your risk of colon cancer; antioxidants, which keep free radical damage in check; lignans, natural compounds that are linked to lower rates of breast cancer; and trace minerals such as zinc and selenium, which strengthen the immune system. To find foods that are a good source of whole grains, look for a nutrition label with those words on.

Follow a low-fat diet. The evidence is in, says Dr Gordon, and it's irrefutable: eating fatty foods increases your chances of getting cancer. One major reason for that is the direct impact that high–fat diets have on immune function: they decrease it. On the other hand, people who limit fats to 25 per cent of their total calories or less have significantly higher levels of cancer-killing immune cells in their systems.

There are several reasons why fat and cancer tend to go together, Dr Gordon says. One is that carcinogenic substances tend to accumulate in saturated fat, particularly animal fat, which prevents them from being flushed safely out of the system. Fat also retains sex hormones, which can lead to cancer. In addition, fats make cell walls less flexible and therefore more apt to break down.

That can set the stage for mutation. Finally, eating fat makes you fat. Studies have shown that overweight people have an increased risk of getting cancer, and a lower chance of recovering if they do get the disease.

Perhaps the easiest way to reduce fat consumption is to cut back on meat, dairy products, and processed foods, all of which tend to be packed with saturated or trans fats, a particularly unhealthy kind of fat. The

BYPASS THE BAKERY

There's a disturbing mystery afoot in the land concerning lymphoma: cancer of the immune system. Levels of the disease in the United States have about doubled over the past 25-plus years, according to William Ralph Vogler, MD, scientific programme director of the American Cancer Society, and no one knows exactly why. People with AIDS often contract lymphoma, and that's part of the reason for the increase, but that doesn't account for it all.

Another piece of the puzzle may have fallen into place recently after a study was conducted by the Harvard School of Public Health. The study looked at the diets of some 88,410 women. It found that those who ate the most trans fatty acids (the type of fats found in most shop-bought pies, cakes and biscuits) had twice the risk of developing lymphoma as those who ate the least trans fatty acids. 'Cutting out trans fats may be one of the best ways to avoid lymphoma,' says researcher Shumin Zhang, MD

To do this, simply watch out for products that list 'partially hydrogenated oil' as an ingredient, which is where trans fats come from.

benefits of cutting back on high-fat foods in your diet are cumulative: eating fewer high-fat foods automatically means that you'll start eating more low-fat foods – exactly the foods that help lower your risk of cancer. Aim for foods with no trans fats, and eat foods with saturated fats only if that type of fat makes up less than 10 per cent of the total food calories, adds Dr Berndtson.

Remember that not all fats are created equal. There's good news for the fat lovers among us (a category that includes just about everyone): some fats actually help prevent cancer. Among these, according to Dr Gordon, are the monounsaturated fats found in olive oil and the omega-3 fatty acids found in fish.

In a study of people in 24 European countries, British researchers found that those who regularly included fish in their diets were much less likely to get cancer. Indeed, they estimated that having small servings of fish three times a week, in addition to limiting the amount of animal fats in the diet, would reduce the death rate from colon cancer in men by nearly one-third.

Flaxseed oil is another excellent source of omega-3 fatty acids. Flaxseed itself is nature's richest reservoir of lignans, which have powerful antioxidant properties.

Lignans can also help subdue cancerous tumours after they've begun to develop, making it less likely that they'll turn into full-blown cancer.

Anti-Cancer All-Stars

Nature's gifts are bountiful, and the list of excellent cancer-fighting foods is a long one.

Some of the best ones are listed below. Bear in mind as you read that all of these foods are likely to be helpful in preventing many types of cancer (as well as other diseases), although research studies often home in on a specific type of malignancy. Add these foods to your diet, and you'll help your immune system in its daily battle against cancer.

Blueberries. Holly McCord, RD, nutrition editor at *Prevention* magazine, recently named blueberries as 'nature's number one source of antioxidants'. She backs up that claim with a study from Tufts University in

Boston, which showed that blueberries beat 39 other common fruits and vegetables in antioxidant power.

Other excellent antioxidant foods (also chosen by researchers at Tufts) include kale, strawberries, spinach, broccoli, brussels sprouts, butternut squash, cantaloupe melon, kiwi fruit, navel oranges, papayas, sweet potatoes (baked), red peppers and watermelon.

Mushrooms. Because mushrooms grow in places where they have to fend off lots of potential predators – bacteria, viruses, other fungi – evolution has provided them with an arsenal of natural immune enhancers with which to defend themselves. They also have compounds that inhibit the growth of tumours. Virtually all mushrooms have these properties, but natural healers recommend maitake and shiitake mushrooms for their anticancer properties.

Soya. Soyabean products contain high levels of genistein, an oestrogen-like compound shown to inhibit cancer cell development and division. We don't yet have all the proof we need of soya's anti-cancer effects, but we do know that Japanese women, whose daily diet contains soya products such as tofu, have only one-quarter as much breast cancer as American and European women. There is also evidence that eating soya lowers a man's risk of developing prostate cancer, or of dying of it when it does develop.

Tomatoes. What a blessing that one of the most widely used and delicious foods happens to be one of our most potent weapons against cancer. Tomatoes, which turn up in everything from pizza sauce and ketchup to salsa and soup, are one of nature's best sources of a red pigment called lycopene. Researchers think that lycopene is the reason why frequent tomato consumption is linked to reduced risks of all sorts of malignancies, including cancers of the prostate, lung, stomach, breast, colon and cervix.

Tomatoes are one case where processed foods still have excellent nutritional value: tomato purée, for example, is basically concentrated tomatoes, and thus a great source of lycopene. Lycopene is also present in tomato sauce and ketchup, where it is easily accessible to the body because it has been processed into small pieces. Other sources of lycopene include

DR DUKE'S SALAD

The idea that you can prevent cancer by eating the right foods is nothing new for James Duke, PhD, author of the hugely popular herbal handbook *The Green Pharmacy*. For years, Dr Duke has enjoyed making his Cancer Prevention Herbal Salad.

The recipe is easy. Simply throw together the following in a bowl: garlic, onions, red peppers, tomatoes, red clover flowers, chopped cooked beetroot, fresh marigold flowers, celery, fresh chicory flowers, chives, cucumbers, cumin, peanuts, purslane and sage. Dr Duke tops his salad off with an anti-cancer dressing that includes flaxseed oil, evening primrose oil, garlic, rosemary, a dash of lemon juice and – for a little spice – hot peppers. *Bon appétit!*

pink or red grapefruit, guava and watermelon.

Pomegranates. Cancer cells forget how to die, and then run out of control. A chemical called ellagic acid can remind these wayward cells that they are supposed to lie down and die. A pomegranate is one of the best sources of ellagic acid. Other rich sources are raspberries and strawberries.

Green tea. Green tea is packed with enzymes that help flush toxins out of the body, and is an excellent source of antioxidants. In fact, the main antioxidant in green tea is 200 times more potent than vitamin E and 500 times more potent than vitamin C. Various studies suggest that green tea can help fight skin cancer, breast cancer and prostate cancer. More research needs to be done to confirm these findings. But Andrew Weil, MD, director of the programme in integrative medicine and clinical professor of medicine at the University of Arizona College of Medicine in Tucson – among other physicians – is convinced enough to recommend drinking green tea regularly. One cup a day should be sufficient.

Garlic. A recent 'meta-analysis' of 22 studies regarding the impact of garlic on cancer found that people who consumed six or more cloves of garlic per week had a 30 per cent lower rate of colorectal cancer than did those who ate one clove of garlic or less per week. The garlic lovers also had a 50 per cent lower rate of stomach cancer. The analysis found some evidence that garlic also has a protective effect against prostate, breast and laryngeal cancers. Garlic's role in strengthening the immune system is important for fighting cancer.

Salmon. Fish that swim in cold water, such as tuna, rainbow trout, and mackerel, as well as salmon, keep warm by producing a type of fat called omega-3 fatty acids. People who eat lots of those types of fish generally have lower rates of cancer, and researchers believe that's because omega-3s block certain compounds that promote the growth of tumours. You can enjoy this protective effect by eating three small servings of fish a week, and salmon is one of the more succulent ways to fill that prescription. For those with a taste for luxury, a small, 30-g (1-oz) serving of caviar will also do.

Water. Staying hydrated with plenty of water helps reduce your risk of bladder cancer. In a 10-year study of nearly 48,000 men (men run a much higher risk of bladder cancer than women), those who drank six 240 ml (8 fl oz) glasses of water daily were half as likely to develop bladder cancer as those who drank just a glass a day. Those who drank 10 or more glasses of water lowered their risk even more.

Herbal Immunity

If you're looking for ways to fortify your immune system against cancer, take a look at any herb garden. 'In my work, I've studied a minimum of 500 plants with immune-stimulating capacity, and that's just the tip of the iceberg,' says herbalist Schar, who is in the process of adding a PhD in immune-boosting plants to the herbal medical degree he has already earned.

Based on his research, Schar recommends a two-pronged herbal approach to cancer prevention, an approach that includes a general immune-boosting regimen in addition to herbs that have been shown to fight specific cancers. If that sounds too complicated, Schar stresses that you should use only what fits comfortably into your schedule and your lifestyle. 'Common sense must prevail,' he says.

For the same reason, Schar is not fussy about the form in which these herbs are used. If you like drinking tea, he says, drink a herbal tea; if you find taking a pill in the morning more convenient, then take your herbal medicine in capsule form, following dosage instructions.

The one exception is that he recommends avoiding standardised extracts of these herbs, because he believes that we don't yet know exactly which molecular components of the herb actually have the immune-boosting effects. In fact, he says, the herb's medicinal effect may well be derived from the combined action of many of the herb's molecular components. Ask for products that contain the whole herb.

Immune-Boosting Herbs

In order to keep your immune system in peak condition for cancer prevention, take an immunity-boosting herb for about half of the year, Schar says. Try taking the herb 2 weeks on, 2 weeks off, or every other month. Why the intermittent schedule? Because it's easy to overdo herbs to the point where their effectiveness is compromised, notes Schar. Nonetheless, he adds, if you're going through a particularly stressful time, or anticipating a stressful time, go ahead and stay on your immunity regimen until you get through it.

There are five herbs that Schar recommends as choices for this basic immunity regimen. Which is best for you is really a matter of personal taste. Just as some people prefer paracetamol to aspirin, some will find astragalus more to their liking than echinacea. Try one for a month or so and see if you feel that it works for you. (Bear in mind that herbs are slower-acting in general than conventional medications.) If it doesn't work for you, try another.

Echinacea. Schar calls echinacea 'the immune system rocket fuel,' but he quickly adds that its very effectiveness means that many people tend to overuse it. The herb builds immunity in several ways, including boosting the body's production of interferon, a virus and cancer killer.

Maitake. Research has shown that the maitake mushroom stimulates the production of immune cells in the body, Schar says. Although maitake mushrooms were once rare (and have been considered a delicacy since Roman times), they are now cultivated commercially and are widely available.

Yarrow. This herb has been used to heal wounds since ancient times;

it is said that it helped mend Achilles' famous heel. Besides being an effective antibacterial and antiviral agent, yarrow also stimulates the immune system.

Turmeric. One of the elements of turmeric, curcumin, has been shown in the test tube to prevent DNA damage in cells, which means that it may stop the mutations that lead to cancer.

Astragalus. Evidence indicates that astragalus stimulates the bone marrow to produce more immune cells. It also stimulates those immune cells to be more active.

Herbs to Target Specific Cancers

Once you have your immune system running along efficiently overall, you can build in some extra protection against specific cancers. That's a reasonable precaution to take, Schar says, if you have a family history of a certain type of malignancy, or if you have some other risk factor you're concerned about (smokers who want to hedge their bets against lung cancer, for example).

Schar lists the following six herbs, each of which addresses the health of a basic body system in which cancers commonly occur. The philosophy underlying all of these herbal recommendations is that if you can keep a particular organic system healthy over time, it is less likely to develop a malignancy.

Chasteberry (also known as vitex) for female reproductive cancers. This herb is known for its ability to regulate hormone imbalances during the menstrual cycle, which makes it an ideal preventive agent for women concerned about breast, uterine and cervical cancers, Schar says. As with many herbs, you should not take chasteberry if you are pregnant.

Saw palmetto for male reproductive cancers. This herb keeps male hormones in balance much as chasteberry keeps female hormones in balance, Schar says. For men, the main issue is prostate cancer, and saw palmetto has been shown to be a tonic that helps maintain good prostate health.

Schar does recommend a standardised brand for saw palmetto, in contrast to many other herbs. Look for extracts of saw palmetto berry standardised to contain 85 to 95 per cent fatty acids and sterols.

Milk thistle for liver cancer. The active ingredient in milk thistle, silymarin, binds to the membranes of liver cells, preventing toxins from damaging them. It also helps speed healing of liver tissues that have already been harmed. 'In a world filled with liver-damaging pollutants,' Schar says, 'milk thistle is a powerful herbal ally.'

Liquorice for respiratory cancers. Herbalists have long used liquorice both as an anti-inflammatory agent and for its ability to clear congestion. The combination of those properties makes it the herb of choice for soothing irritated lungs and throat tissues. Because chronic cellular irritation can lead to mutation, soothing irritation can help stop cancer before it begins.

Aloe for skin cancer. Schar recommends aloe for its ability to help irritated tissues heal themselves. Look for a pure aloe gel to rub on your skin after exposure to the sun.

Camomile for cancers of the digestive tract. Camomile is a soothing herb, and Schar recommends it as a preventive agent for stomach and intestinal cancers for the same reason that he recommends milk thistle for the liver, liquorice for the lungs and aloe for the skin: prolonged irritation can lead to cancer, and camomile is helpful for soothing and healing irritated tissues.

Saving Supplements

Is it absolutely necessary to take vitamin supplements in order to avoid cancer? No, says Dr Gordon. If you're feeling great, you don't need to worry about taking anything at all. If, on the other hand, you're feeling out of sorts, run down, or stressed, taking vitamin supplements may be called for. That's true for health reasons in general, and specifically to help support your immune system in its ongoing fight against the sorts of cellular breakdown that cause malignancies. Here's how supplements can help.

Antioxidant vitamins. Antioxidant vitamins such as vitamins C and E are important in fighting the ongoing cellular damage from free radicals that can lead to mutation and ultimately to cancer. Antioxidants are also immune system stimulants, helping to ward off the bacterial and viral infections that can lead to cancerous mutations as well as cancer itself.

Co-enzyme Q_{10}, a vitamin-like substance that is present in the cells of all mammals, is a powerful antioxidant that has shown promise as an antitumour agent. It has mainly been used for treating patients who already have cancer, according to Dr Gordon, rather than for cancer prevention, but it does enhance immunity. 'I would certainly take it if I had cancer in my family,' he says. 'The only downside I can think of is that it's expensive.'

B vitamins. The B vitamins help cells reproduce safely and repair DNA damage. They also help flush potentially cancerous toxins from the body. The B vitamin folic acid in particular has been found in two major studies to help prevent cervical cancer and colon cancer in women.

Minerals. Calcium may help protect against colon cancer, while chromium and magnesium promote the body's effective management of glucose, which may help control cancer cell growth. Selenium is an antioxidant mineral that has been shown to have particularly potent anticancer properties. In one study, those who took a 200-mcg selenium supplement daily for 10 years cut their risk of lung, prostate and colorectal cancer in half. Zinc has been shown to enhance immunity and to enhance the effectiveness of antioxidants.

For the supplement regimen recommended by Dr Gordon, see 'A Basic Supplement Plan' on page 254.

Mind-Body Cancer Prevention

Anyone who doesn't feel stressed at times in today's world probably isn't thinking clearly. But that tension can undermine our immune systems, and even lead to cancer. 'As every year goes by, more data accumulates showing that our emotional, psychological and spiritual states have a definite impact on our immune systems,' says Dr Berndtson.

The good thing about knowing that the mind and body are interrelated is that it gives us a whole range of new opportunities to practise cancer prevention. The trick is cultivating what one researcher described

A BASIC SUPPLEMENT PLAN

One way to prevent cancer is to make sure that your immune system has all the vitamin support it needs to do its job. Here is the basic supplement regimen for adults recommended by James S. Gordon, MD, director of the Center for Mind-Body Medicine in Washington, DC, and co-author of *Comprehensive Cancer Care*.

Twice a day, take 1,000 mg of vitamin C and 250 mg of vitamin E, and once a day (at breakfast), take 200 mcg of selenium. In addition, he says, most people need a B-complex vitamin, which contains more than the usually recommended amounts of folic acid, B_6 and B_{12}. Dr Gordon also suggests taking a multimineral – one with iron for women who are menstruating, one without iron for post-menopausal women and for men – once a day with food.

as stress hardiness. Stress hardiness is, in essence, an attitude that enables you to weather life's vicissitudes cheerfully and confidently, without being overwhelmed.

Stress hardiness means more than just being well-defended, Dr Gordon points out. It also means being engaged. Several landmark research studies found that people who have cancer do better medically if they feel in control of their lives and passionate about living. Dr Gordon believes that the benefits of this sort of involvement extend to healthy people as well. Developing a sense of engagement with one's life, he says, can help strengthen your resistance to cancer.

Dr Berndtson agrees. 'The idea is to orchestrate your life so that you feel that you have a reason for living,' he says. 'That communicates a message from your head to the rest of your body, including your immune system, that says, "Hey, we're worth fighting for!"'

How exactly that advice translates into your life is up to you, but in general, the idea is to take positive steps to avoid feeling victimised, passive, detached or trapped. However, stress hardiness is an attitude that can be learned. 'It's really about living a fuller, more engaged life generally,' Dr Gordon says. 'The simple act of taking a look at how you're dealing with your life is the beginning of making the shift from passivity to engagement. It can be done, and I see people doing it all the time.'

Here are some fundamental steps toward developing stress hardiness, suggested by Dr Gordon and Dr Berndtson specifically with cancer prevention in mind.

Make time for meditation. You don't have to sit in a lotus position with sitar music playing in the background to meditate, Dr Gordon points out. 'Meditation is nothing fancy,' he says. 'It's simply using one of many different techniques to slow down, to be present in the moment, to become aware of one's thinking and sensing and feeling, to both relax and become aware. And that's the beginning of becoming engaged in one's life.'

One of the simplest ways of practising meditation, Dr Gordon notes, is to simply go for a walk for 20 minutes or so. Pay attention to the thoughts in your head, the sights you see, the smells around you and the feeling of your body as you walk. You'll find that the more you practise this sort of observation, the less tense and preoccupied you'll feel and the more you'll enjoy being alive. That can translate into better mental and physical health.

(For more on meditation, see Enhance Immunity with the Power of the Mind, on page 96, and Facet 4: The MaxImmunity Stress Relief and Sleep Plan, on page 347.)

Practise guided imagery. A further step toward getting in touch with yourself is the use of imagery. This is basically a form of intentional daydreaming, where you close your eyes and let images – sounds, tastes and feelings as well as sights – come into your mind. Your imagination is a powerful tool, and imagery lets you use it to evoke a peaceful, relaxing state of mind.

For example, the spiritual teacher and writer Marianne Williamson often begins her lectures by asking members of her audience to close their eyes and envision themselves walking into a beautiful temple, surrounded by flowing fountains and filled with golden light. Other people might picture nature scenes: a favourite mountain meadow, perhaps, or a beach at sunset. Using such images can help you centre and calm yourself, creating an atmosphere of inner tranquillity.

Imagery can also be used in more directed ways, Dr Gordon says. Visualising scenes from your life, for example, can allow repressed feelings

Success Stories

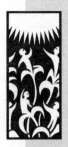

She Took Charge When Confronted with Breast Cancer

The following account was written by Suzanne Wymelenberg, a health writer in Cambridge, Massachusetts, and a contributor to this book. As you will see, Suzanne played an active role in her treatment – and her recovery.

I'm not an optimist. I can worry with the best of them. When I was told that my mammogram showed a lump, what kept me from panic was the fact that, at the time, my desk was covered with information on breast cancer. I'm a medical writer, and I was getting ready to do a special report on breast cancer for Harvard Health Publications. I was becoming familiar with types of biopsies, the different forms of breast cancer and how they behave and the various surgeries available.

Not that I'd ever had any doubt about the operation I would prefer: if my cancer wasn't aggressive and wasn't large, I wanted a lumpectomy. As a reporter covering national breast cancer conferences, I'd learned many years ago that, for many cancers, a lumpectomy is as effective as a mastectomy. Cancers detected by mammography tend to be found before they can be felt, and they're often good candidates for lumpectomy.

to surface from the subconscious. Solutions to various problems can similarly bubble up from within if you peacefully picture the situation or person involved. This is a common prayer technique: many people imagine themselves bringing their troubles to a beloved religious figure – Jesus, for example – to ask for comfort and counsel. Imagery also can focus the body's energy on healing: cancer patients often imagine that their immune systems are attacking and killing their tumours.

Write your story. Keeping a personal diary or journal is another way of paying attention to what's really happening inside yourself. Don't worry

When my doctors had all the lab findings about my cancer, the only surgery we discussed was a lumpectomy. My lump wasn't tiny – it was about an inch and a half in diameter – and it was an invasive but not aggressive type of cancer. A lumpectomy would provide the same medical results as a mastectomy but leave me my breast.

When the tumour was removed, no signs of spread were found, so chemotherapy didn't seem necessary. To kill any stray cells that couldn't be detected, however, I had radiation therapy.

From my doctors and from my reading, I learned that I, like many people, probably carried cancer cells in my body for years. What triggered them into forming a tumour may simply have been ageing. Today, in all likelihood, my body still has some cancer cells; hopefully, my immune system can deal with them.

Fortunately, I'm a healthy person. My work may be sedentary, but when I'm not at my computer, I garden, walk the dogs several times a day and work side by side with my husband on many house projects. I avoid fad diets, regardless of their promises. I try to have a lot of variety in my diet, with lots of fruits and vegetables. I take some vitamin supplements and seldom have an alcoholic drink. I've never smoked.

Today, it's almost impossible to discern which of my breasts was operated on. I feel well. I try to take care of my immune system. Even when I don't feel like it, I exercise. My biggest struggle is to eat fruit or vegetables instead of chocolate when I want to relax and snack. Fortunately, I know that chocolate has recently been found to be a powerful antioxidant!

about how elegant your prose style is, Dr Gordon says. The important thing is to get the feelings out. If you're going to change your attitudes and your approach to life for the better, the place to start is where you are right now. Keeping a journal can reveal emotional and mental patterns that are holding you back. At the same time, the very act of writing your feelings down is a positive step in self-care – Dr Gordon calls it 'a manifestation of the fighting spirit'. As such, keeping a journal can be instrumental in helping you develop the sort of stress hardiness that preserves good health.

Stay connected. The therapeutic value of being connected with a supportive, loving community has been documented in many studies. In one, a group of patients with melanoma (a potentially deadly form of skin cancer) met with a leader in small support groups once a week for an hour and a half. Months later, blood tests revealed that these patients had significantly higher levels of immune cell activity than patients who had received only conventional medical treatment. In the long run, it turned out that their survival rate was also significantly higher.

Dr Berndtson believes that one of the reasons social support is so critical to health is that it gives you an opportunity to share your troubles with other people. 'A problem shared is a problem halved,' he says. 'You've cleaned yourself out. You're not investing energy in either denying or in covering up.'

Stay active. When you exercise regularly, you begin to feel out of

DIARY BASICS

There is no 'right' way or 'wrong' way to keep a diary, says Mike Heller, PhD, professor of English at Roanoke College in Salem, Virginia, who has taught journal writing at Pendle Hill, a Quaker centre for study and contemplation near Philadelphia. In fact, that's one of the things Heller likes best about diary writing: the directions and contents are entirely yours. You may wish to choose a special notebook or folder for your diary; this helps bestow a sense of ritual to the time you spend with it, he says. When you write is up to you. Some teachers recommend that you spend half an hour a day, 5 days a week. Many people like to write first thing in the morning or last thing at night. Heller carries his diary with him so that he can jot down a few lines whenever he has a few idle minutes, or whenever inspiration strikes. Some days, he'll make five entries; other days, he'll make none.

Heller finds it useful to begin his diary sessions by spending a few quiet moments contemplating the open page; he finds that it helps him still the surface noise in his mind and turn his attention inward. A few moments of calm reflection when you've finished your writing can likewise help make what you've written sink in.

sorts if, for some reason, your exercise routine is interrupted. That's evidence of the mind-body connection at work, and of the fact that some form of exercise – whether it be walking, lifting weights, playing tennis, practising yoga, or any other form of movement – is essential for overall well-being.

An extensive body of research has documented that you not only *feel* healthier when you exercise, you *are* healthier. Laboratory studies have found that exercise helps prevent cancer by stimulating the immune system's ability to fight the formation of tumours. Studies of actual humans bear these findings out. For example, when researchers followed 1,806 women for 11 years, they found that those who were moderately active – walking, gardening, or even simply doing housework several times a week – had a 50 per cent lower risk of breast cancer compared with sedentary women. Women in the study who did vigorous activity – swimming, running or playing tennis at least once a week – were *80 per cent* less likely to develop the disease.

Exercise also helps prevent cancer by keeping your weight under control. A 1999 study by the US Centers for Disease Control and Prevention tracked rates of colon cancer in a group of 13,420 men and women over some 20 years. The leanest people – both male and female – had the fewest malignancies. The heavier people became, the more their risk of cancer increased.

How much exercise do you need? The standard recommendation is to do some form of exercise for 30 minutes a day, 5 days a week.

However, this need not be an exhausting gym class. Even moderate exercise, such as walking, can be just as effective.

Visit an acupuncturist. Most of us who live in the West think of getting acupuncture (if we think of it at all) as a potential remedy for some physical problem. In China, however, a visit to the acupuncturist at the change of each season is seen as a step one routinely takes in order to *maintain* good health. The idea is that acupuncture helps keep the body's vital energies in balance. Dr Gordon believes, and some research demonstrates, that the immune system definitely benefits from such regular acupuncture sessions.

Have fun. If it's true that we live in a stressful world, then we should take steps occasionally to cheer up. Constantly living in 'vigilance mode', as Dr Berndtson puts it, wears you down and sucks vital energy away from your body, your immune system included. His prescription for all of us: take time for a little rest and relaxation, and don't take yourself so seriously.

Chapter 16

HIV AND AIDS

Imagine that you're the commander of an army, and your troops have settled into camp for the night. As they sleep, a secret army of spies steals into the camp, quietly killing all your soldiers and then dressing in their clothes and moving throughout your ranks. You now have an idea of the way that HIV operates in the body.

The human immunodeficiency virus directly targets and disables the immune system, leaving you highly vulnerable to other severe infections and tumours. HIV often leads to a characteristic cluster of complications that have been labelled the acquired immunodeficiency syndrome, or AIDS.

Approximately half of HIV-infected adults will develop AIDS within 8 to 10 years of HIV infection; for others, it will be longer. While most people who are infected will develop AIDS, why a small minority of HIV-infected people remain healthy for many years is unknown. The difference between those who do and those who do not become extremely ill is still being studied, but it appears that it may depend upon the amount of virus the person is exposed to, as well as the state of the person's immune system.

Experts say that as experience with the disease grows, it seems that good nutrition can boost the immune system and may help slow the progression of the disease. A healthy way of life also may ease the side effects of the strong drugs used to treat it.

How the AIDS Virus Works

The road to AIDS starts when the HIV virus enters the body, where it targets the white blood cells called CD4 cells, which direct and buttress our immune defences.

HIV enters the CD4 cells and uses the cells' own reproducing mechanisms to make thousands of HIV copies. In the process, the CD4 cells are killed. The newly made viruses spread throughout the bloodstream, infect and kill even more CD4 cells as they go, and make additional thousands of copies of themselves.

Day after day, long before any symptoms appear, a person with HIV produces thousands of new, uninfected CD4 cells to fight the thousands and thousands of new copies of HIV now living in the bloodstream. Eventually, the body's ability to generate CD4 cells weakens, their number diminishes and the person's resistance to tumour growth and infections falters. Often at this point the diagnosis becomes AIDS.

How Does HIV Enter the Body?

HIV is a virus that is carried chiefly by blood, semen and breast milk. It is less potent in anal or vaginal secretions, and weakest in tears, saliva and urine.

The virus travels readily via certain body pathways.

- By way of the vagina, anus and mouth, in semen

- Into the bloodstream via a transfusion of blood from a person who has the virus (Donor blood is screened for HIV antibodies, which signal the presence of the virus.)

- On an intravenous needle or syringe that has already been used by a person carrying the virus

- By means of accidental pricks, cuts, or punctures with HIV-

A PREVENTION PRIMER

Though great progress has been made in the treatment of AIDS, there is still no cure. Therefore, prevention is as important as ever. Here are the best ways to keep yourself safe, spelled out in black and white.

• Unless both you and your partner have been tested and are HIV-free, use a male or female latex or polyurethane condom for oral and vaginal sex. For anal sex, use a male condom. Do not use natural membrane condoms, which are made from lamb's intestine – they do not act as a barrier against this virus.
• Have sex only within a mutually monogamous relationship, which means that you and your partner have sex only with each other.
• Keep in mind that even with condom use, the risk of HIV increases with the number of sexual partners you have.
• Before beginning a sexual relationship, you and your partner should both be tested for sexually transmitted diseases, particularly HIV.
• Don't share intravenous needles or syringes. The person you might be sharing with might not even know if he or she has HIV.
• For the same reason, don't share razors, earrings for pierced ears, toothbrushes, or anything that might have come into contact with another person's blood.
• If you are pregnant or thinking about getting pregnant and don't know the HIV status of your partner, get tested. Treatments exist for protecting your baby.

contaminated needles or other medical instruments

• Through an unprotected scrape or cut or an open sore that comes into contact with infected blood, semen, or vaginal secretions

• From a mother's bloodstream to her baby before birth, because they share a blood system

• In breast milk when the mother has HIV

• By artificial insemination with sperm from a man with the virus

- Through receiving transplanted tissue or an organ from a donor who is carrying HIV

Unlike some other viruses, HIV cannot be transmitted by kissing, shaking hands or hugging. You cannot catch it when someone with the virus coughs or sneezes near you, or by sharing eating utensils or telephones or swimming pools. You shouldn't, however, share earrings for pierced ears, razors and toothbrushes, since these items may have touched blood and that blood could be contaminated.

Because it can take many years for HIV to manifest itself, many men and women unknowingly may be carrying the virus, and can inadvertently spread it. Unfortunately, it is especially infectious during its early days.

Symptoms of HIV and AIDS

When an HIV infection is just getting under way, it may produce no symptoms at all or the symptoms could easily seem to be something else

WOMEN AND HIV

Although men still make up the majority of people with HIV/AIDS in the West, that proportion is changing. Today, the number of women with this infection is climbing, and sexual intercourse now is ahead of intravenous drug use as the most common way of acquiring the disease.

Research shows that HIV is passed more readily from a man to a woman. Women need to be vigilant about the use of condoms: their lives may depend on it.

Some women aren't diagnosed with HIV/AIDS until they develop obvious symptoms or give birth to a baby who is ill with HIV. Such a late diagnosis has a negative effect on the length of time a woman can survive with the disease, because treatment starts so late in the course of the infection. If diagnosed and treated early, a woman will live the same length of time as a man.

All women who are sexually active or using intravenous drugs are at risk for HIV infection and should be tested for the virus. In addition, having a sexually transmitted disease can make a woman more vulnerable to the virus.

altogether. They include fatigue, headaches, muscle pain, fever and swollen lymph nodes.

On the other hand, when the immune system has been extensively weakened by the virus, the body becomes vulnerable to all sorts of illnesses. A yeast infection in the mouth, called oral thrush, is often the first. Persistent vaginal yeast infections also may be a sign of HIV/AIDS.

In addition, a person whose infection has worsened might experience:

- Persistent diarrhoea (lasting more than 1 week)
- Heavy night sweats
- Shortness of breath
- Swollen lymph nodes
- Profound tiredness without a cause
- Recurring fever
- Dry cough
- Rapid weight loss

Sometimes, the purple markings of the cancer called Kaposi's sarcoma will appear on the skin or in the mouth.

If the person's brain has become infected, there might be signs of memory loss, depression, or a personality change.

Testing For HIV

If you have symptoms that suggest HIV infection, you need to be tested – for your own health and to protect others. You can be tested at your doctor's surgery or at a health centre. A blood test will check for antibodies against the virus. If your test result is negative, you may be advised to have another test in 3 months' time because antibodies can take that long to develop.

Counselling is given before and after the test to discuss the implications of a positive result.

If it's determined that you have HIV, you will need to get regular blood tests to monitor the severity of the infection and the effectiveness of your treatment. With the new drugs available today in the developed world, many people with the infection are living longer lives.

Medical Therapy for HIV

HIV is what's known as a retrovirus: a type of virus that is capable of altering a cell's DNA to make copies of itself. The medications used against it are called antiretroviral drugs. A combination of these drugs is used to stop HIV from multiplying, limiting the body's viral load and allowing its CD4 cells to increase.

If your CD4 count remains low, you may need medicine to treat infections such as oral thrush. Such opportunistic infections can take advantage of your weak immune system. To ward off as many of these infections as possible, your doctor may suggest vaccinations against the most common troublemakers: hepatitis B, pneumonia and flu.

Because many of these drugs, particularly the antivirals, cause side effects, you should be monitored frequently by your doctor.

Nutritional Therapy for HIV

Poor nutrition and its side effects complicate this illness even further. Not only does it make the infected person even more vulnerable to other illnesses, it can also diminish an effective response to drug therapies.

Poor nutrition is only part of the problem, however. A body affected by HIV undergoes a host of changes: tissue wasting, body fat accumulations, increased levels of blood fats and changes in metabolism, all of which can have a marked effect on the outcome of this disease.

If you have been diagnosed with HIV/AIDS, one of your primary goals should be to keep yourself well-nourished, says Cade Fields-Gardner, RD, director of services at The Cutting Edge, a caregiving and research company in Cary, Illinois, that specialises in HIV nutrition issues. This may be hard at times, since you may have little or no appetite or may be too tired to prepare food or shop for groceries. Although it's not very common any more, you may also be dealing with opportunistic infections that may affect your mouth or throat and make eating difficult, and, since the medicines you've been prescribed can cause nausea or diarrhoea, you may not want to eat.

In addition, it's particularly common for people who have HIV/AIDS to have problems absorbing nutrients. 'Taking vitamins and antioxidants doesn't mean the body is able to use them,' observes Fields–Gardner.

Yet 'there is a suggestion that good nutrition supports the body to better withstand the progression of this disease,' says Fields–Gardner. 'We

CHOOSING YOUR CAREGIVERS

As with other complex diseases, people who seek the care and advice of specialists in HIV/AIDS will have more information available to them than people who consult generalists. In addition, Marcy Fenton, MS, RD, a nutritionist at AIDS Project Los Angeles, advises people living with HIV/AIDS to look for caregivers 'who are up to date. Look for a doctor and a dietitian who follow the latest evidence-based professional literature and attend professional meetings. And make sure that your dietitian and doctor communicate and coordinate with each other.'

It's important for physicians and dietitians to keep up-to-date on HIV/AIDS because changes are occurring all the time, points out Jenna Bell-Wilson, MS, RD, consulting dietitian at South West CARE Center, which specialises in HIV/AIDS services, in Santa Fe, New Mexico. 'We're facing new issues all the time because life spans are being extended, different drugs are being used and the needs of those living with HIV are ever-changing.'

Specifically, choose a nutritionist or dietitian who is knowledgeable about what happens during the infection process and who can tailor nutrition care and recommendations to the individual's needs, suggests Cade Fields-Gardner, RD, director of services at The Cutting Edge, a caregiving and research company in Cary, Illinois, that specialises in HIV nutrition issues.

You can contact a state-registered dietitian via your GP or local hospital . For details of private dietitians in your area, send a stamped addressed envelope marked 'Private Practice' to the British Dietetic Association, 5th Floor, Charles House, 148/9 Great Charles Street, Birmingham B3 3HT (*www.bda.uk.com*).

know that if a person's nutritional status is compromised, she or he can get ill more often and may die earlier.' She cautions, however, that 'we must remember that nutrition is just a support, not a treatment. It's not reasonable to think that nutrition will cure the HIV infection.'

Nutritional status is important, agrees Marcy Fenton, MS, RD, a nutritionist at AIDS Project Los Angeles. 'At every visit, you should remind your doctor what supplements you're taking and if you're having any digestive problems such as diarrhoea and nausea.'

In addition, people living with HIV/AIDS need to advocate for themselves, Fenton says. 'Don't be afraid to tell your doctor about what's going on with your body every time you see him. Every person with HIV infection requires an individualised nutrition care assessment and plan. There is no longer one natural progression of this disease, and the nutritional aspects of it are complex,' she points out.

Nutrition experts consider that nutrition care and drug therapy work together to preserve the body's important protein stores. Having normal protein stores is vital to body function and survival, and maintaining it is the target of much nutrition-related therapy.

Experts point out that drug therapy is lifelong with this disease, presenting the possibility that there will be all sorts of interactions between side effects, food and body metabolism. You may be able to reduce the number of side effects, however, by managing your symptoms skillfully and keeping your body well-nourished.

Although you may be eager to try every new vitamin and herbal supplement you hear about, your first priority should be to make sure that your basic nutritional needs are being covered, says Fields-Gardner. This includes making sure that you take in enough fluids, calories, proteins and nutrients in foods. There is so much we don't know about how supplements interact with HIV infection and treatments that it's difficult to make general recommendations, says Fields-Gardner.

Special Nutritional Concerns

By eating a wide range of vitamin-rich foods, most healthy people are able to derive enough vitamins and minerals from their diets. If diarrhoea becomes a problem in people who have HIV/AIDS, however, their nutritional status may deteriorate and they may need more of these nutrients to help repair damaged cells.

People with HIV/AIDS who are not getting enough nutrients will begin to lose weight. If the loss is lean muscle instead of fat, the phenomenon is termed *wasting syndrome* or *cachexia*. If it is left untreated and it continues, wasting syndrome can be deadly. The key is to have body composition measurements done every 3 months, advises Joanne Maurice, MS, RD, CD, a dietitian at the Madison Clinic of Harborview Medical Center in Seattle, which specialises in HIV/AIDS services. Bioelectrical impedance analysis (BIA) is one type of measurement that is a quick and easy way to check muscle and fat. You should also keep an eye on your weight: if you lose more than 5 per cent of your usual body weight, see both your doctor and your nutritionist.

Another danger signal for people with HIV is the development of extremely high levels of fat in the blood, particularly triglyceride and cholesterol levels. Over time, excessive levels of these lipids can contribute to heart disease, stroke and pancreatitis. 'Abnormal triglyceride levels may be the result of the effect of certain drugs on the liver,' reports Maurice. Other factors might be a diet that's high in fat and the inability to absorb some nutrients.

Whatever the cause, Maurice says, high levels of blood lipids are unhealthy and need to be lowered. Often, they can be brought down through changes in diet. To help lower your cholesterol, you need to reduce the amount of saturated fats and eat more monounsaturated fats and soluble fibre. 'Adding more fish and reducing the total amount of high-fat meat in your diet can help,' she says.

When you want to eat meat, choose lean types, such as loin cuts, advises Jenna Bell-Wilson, MS, RD, consulting dietitian at South West CARE Center, which specialises in HIV/AIDS services in Santa Fe, New Mexico. Reading package labels will help you find meat that is lower in saturated fat.

To lower elevated triglyceride levels, it's important to reduce the amount of sugar and alcohol in your diet, notes Bell-Wilson. Simple sugars in the form of sweets, desserts, carbonated drinks, and lots of sugar

WATCH OUT FOR FOOD POISONING

Even when a person is in the best of health, food poisoning is miserable and can be dangerous. When you have HIV, it's especially so. HIV weakens your immune system, so you are much more at risk for a serious reaction to the microorganisms in contaminated food.

If you have HIV, be extra careful about refrigerated food. Eat leftovers within 3 days or throw them out. Avoid eating rare meat, chicken and fish, as well as barely cooked eggs.

Take extra precautions when you're handling food, too. Always wash your hands before preparing food; in fact, get into the habit of washing them every time you enter the kitchen. And tell anyone who cooks for you about the necessity of hand washing.

When it comes to cleaning up, use plenty of soap and hot water on worktops and sinks. If you need to clean up meat juices, use paper towels first, followed by hot, soapy water.

Be aware that people with AIDS are especially vulnerable to salmonella poisoning. To reduce your risk of salmonella and other bacterial poisoning, thoroughly scrub cutting boards and knives used for meat, especially chicken, immediately after use. Wash your hands again after working with raw meats. Finally, don't taste uncooked pastry or sauces that contain raw eggs.

As you work in the kitchen, be careful to avoid cross-contamination. Keep raw meat, eggs and fish away from green salad, fruits and vegetables. Use different utensils and cutting boards for salads and other raw vegetables.

Finally, use sponges, rather than dishcloths, in the kitchen. You can wash your sponges in the dishwasher whenever you do a load of dishes. And remember that a towel used for drying hands should not be used for drying dishes.

in your tea or coffee should be avoided. Because alcohol is a form of sugar, its consumption also should be cut back or eliminated.

Conventional medicines for high cholesterol, such as simvastatin (Zocor), are a last resort if you have HIV/AIDS because they can stress the liver, Bell-Wilson notes. In healthy people, this is not often a problem, but if you are already taking HIV medications, altering your diet and adding exercise is the first approach.

Tips for Good Nutrition

Getting enough vitamins and minerals is essential if you've been diagnosed with HIV/AIDS. Bell-Wilson suggests the following practical tips.

• As soon as you've been diagnosed, start eating more protein and complex carbohydrates with moderate amounts of fat. Also, a moderate exercise programme, such as walking and weight training, will help to develop and maintain good muscle mass.

• Make sure your diet includes lean meat, fish, pulses, seeds and nuts, whole-grain breads and cereals and plenty of fruits and vegetables every day. This helps to supply your body with enough fuel for exercise and well-being.

• Include small amounts of fat for energy and calories, but instead of chips and crisps, try nuts, avocado dip, peanut butter or seeds for a snack.

• If nausea or poor appetite is an issue, try smaller portions and try six smaller meals a day instead of three regular-size meals.

• Fluid is essential throughout the day, but avoid drinking a lot of liquids at mealtime, because they can make you feel full and reduce your appetite.

If you don't have much of an appetite, you might want to follow some advice that nutritionist Phyll Ribakoff, RD, and her team at Nutrition Works in Boston give to their clients with HIV/AIDS. They suggest setting a timer to remind you periodically to have a high-protein snack or to eat a small meal. Nutrition Works is a joint programme of the AIDS Action Committee, the American Red Cross of Massachusetts Bay and the Boston Living Center. 'It's important for persons with HIV/AIDS to try to get 100 g of protein each day,' Ribakoff notes.

A milkshake is a tasty, easy-to-swallow way to get needed nutrients. 'Invest in a blender and invent some homemade recipes for milkshakes,' Bell-Wilson suggests. 'You don't need expensive ingredients; in fact, I usually tell my clients to use common items from their grocery store.'

According to Bell-Wilson, the basics for milkshakes made at home can be ice cream (low-sugar ice cream if triglycerides are creeping up),

HIGH-PROTEIN, LOW-COST SNACK IDEAS

If you've been diagnosed with HIV/AIDS, it's important that you maintain good muscle mass. In order to do this, you'll need to exercise and make sure that your diet includes foods that are good sources of protein. Fortunately, a lot of ordinary, inexpensive foods make excellent high-protein snacks. Eat them between meals or instead of a regular meal. Here are a few options.

FOOD	PROTEIN (g)
Chopped egg sandwich (2 boiled eggs)	20
Tuna (90 g/3 oz can)	20
Milkshake made with ice cream (240 ml/8 fl oz milk)	16
Peanut butter sandwich (2 tbsp)	13
Hot dog with cheese (30 g/1 oz)	12
Celery sticks with peanut butter (2 tbsp)	9
Cream soup (240 ml/8 fl oz milk)	8
Handful of peanuts (30 g/1 oz)	8

Stock up on snack foods that taste good and are nourishing. That way, when you don't feel like preparing a snack, you can grab a yogurt or drink a canned, high-calorie nutritional beverage, for example. When you do feel like preparing food, make extra servings to keep in the refrigerator or freezer for those times when you don't feel like cooking.

skimmed or semi-skimmed milk, yogurt and favourite fruits. For people with normal lipid levels, milk can be any type from whole to skimmed. People who are lactose intolerant can use lactose-free milk or a fortified soya milk. Chocolate syrup, malt powder and vanilla are also good flavourings. You can also add powdered skimmed milk or a protein powder; these can be low-priced, good protein sources.

High-calorie nutritional drinks also make convenient, easy-to-eat snacks between meals. To enhance your protein intake, you could consume a high-protein nutritional supplement drink.

Having a poor appetite when you have HIV/AIDS shouldn't be accepted as normal, Bell-Wilson says. 'If you've lost your appetite, consult your doctor or dietitian to try to figure out why. Is it the medications? Are you depressed? Are you having a lot of nausea and diarrhoea? Determining the root of the appetite loss can be very helpful.'

A Balancing Act

Despite being HIV-positive for 16 years, Maureen Cassidy of Boston is still struggling to eat enough nourishing foods every day, especially foods that include enough protein. 'Those of us who have HIV require more protein. We may have malabsorption problems that make it hard to get enough protein to maintain our muscle,' she notes.

'Our meds can make our cholesterol levels rise, so we're told to stay away from red meat and eggs and so on. Trying to eat right is like walking a tightrope. You have to balance what you can eat with the timing of your medications – some meds must be taken on an empty stomach three times a day. And you have to balance the job of getting enough protein and vitamins with finding foods that still taste good to you. It isn't easy. I've had a lot of mouth problems and, to me, many foods now have an unpleasant aftertaste,' Cassidy says. In addition, she notes that some HIV medications can make foods 'taste funny.'

The best solution she's found is to find foods she likes that are nourishing and stick with them. 'I tend to eat the same things over and over,' says Cassidy.

For example, tinned tuna is one of her protein standbys. She also finds that scrambled eggs made with one yolk and a double amount of egg white are another way of getting enough protein without raising her cholesterol.

When broccoli and cauliflower and other nutrient-rich cruciferous vegetables cause wind, Cassidy might eat them at night, when that could be less of a social problem. With this disease, trying to eat well 'is always a challenge, because nothing stays constant. Your system is always reacting to your meds or what you've eaten,' she notes.

MANAGING SIDE EFFECTS WITH DIET

HIV/AIDS and the drugs used to treat it can cause unpleasant side effects. Always talk to your doctor about new side effects and any old ones that have returned or are lasting for several days.

To ease common side effects, try the following hints gathered by nutritionist Phyll Ribakoff, RD, of Nutrition Works in Boston.

If you have nausea or a mildly upset stomach:

- Eat plain biscuits and other dry foods.
- Try cool, clear liquids such as water, ginger ale, ginger iced tea and flat colas.
- Avoid greasy foods, including many fast foods.
- Eat a little at a time, but eat often to avoid an empty stomach.
- Try an apple.

If your nausea is severe, talk to your doctor about taking B-complex vitamins, including folic acid, or a phenothiazine used to treat nausea and vomiting or vitamin B_6.

If you have diarrhoea:

- Eat starchy foods such as white rice, potatoes, noodles and bread.
- Try bananas, tinned fruit and clear soups, which are easy to digest.
- Avoid dairy products. Yogurt may be better tolerated than milk or ice cream because it contains less lactose.
- Avoid caffeine. Tea, decaffeinated coffee and guava juice are usually

Nutritional Supplements

When you're feeling fatigued or slightly nauseated, eating a big meal is probably the last thing you're in the mood to do. As a result, you may well find yourself eating less. Furthermore, drug therapy, medications and the infection itself can hamper your body's ability to absorb all the nutrients it needs.

This is where supplementary vitamins and minerals can compensate for any nutritional shortfalls in your food intake. Dietitians almost always well-tolerated.

• Salty foods such as Twiglets are fine, but stay away from sweets, particularly chocolate.

• Consider calcium tablets, which help some people. Follow the directions on the label.

• Don't forget your vitamins. Frequent diarrhoea prevents nutrients from being absorbed by your body. If the diarrhoea is severe, chewable vitamins might be better absorbed.

Ask your nutritionist or doctor about L-glutamine, folic acid, acidophilus, or other products for managing diarrhoea. The cost varies, so you'll want to find out which ones are least expensive and start with those.

If you are constipated:

• Eat at least two vegetables and two fruits daily.

• Drink 1.5 litres (2½ pints) of liquid daily, particularly apple and prune juices.

• Avoid white rice and bananas because they may aggravate the problem.

• Take long walks: exercise can get the digestive system working.

• Add ¼ to ½ teaspoon of psyllium or flaxseeds to hot cereals.

If your mouth hurts or you have difficulty chewing and swallowing:

• Avoid high-temperature foods and spicy foods.

• Liquidise foods through the blender with water or stock, and eat them with a spoon or drink them through a straw.

• Eat slowly. Pay attention to your eating to avoid choking.

recommend a balanced vitamin and mineral supplement for people with HIV/AIDS. More specific regimens should be based on personal needs, suggests Fields–Gardner.

Don't feel that you can skip a meal just because you're taking a vitamin and mineral supplement, however. Staying healthy also requires plenty of protein and carbohydrates every day. In addition, you need fruits and vegetables to provide trace amounts of minerals and vitamins and other important substances that may not be in your pills, and you

HERBS AND HIV DRUGS

Herbs are natural, but that doesn't mean that they're always free of negative side effects. Two herbal supplements often used by people with HIV/AIDS appear to limit the action of certain drugs. Inform your doctor of any herbs that you are currently taking.

St John's wort. Research at the National Institutes of Health Clinical Center has shown that St John's wort appears to reduce the effectiveness of indinavir, a protease inhibitor. When the drug and the herb are taken at the same time, the levels of indinavir drop sharply, according to Stephen C Piscitelli, PharmD, research scientist at the National Institute of Allergy and Infectious Diseases in Bethesda, Maryland. Low blood levels of protease inhibitors are a cause of drug resistance and treatment failure.

Garlic supplements. Dr Piscitelli also has reported that garlic supplements, commonly used to lower cholesterol in patients receiving antiviral drugs, appear to decrease the amount of the protease inhibitor saquinavir in the blood. Be cautious when combining garlic with saquinavir when the drug is the only protease inhibitor being taken, reports Dr Piscitelli.

also need food bulk to keep your digestive tract functioning well, advises Fields-Gardner.

Many nutritionists and dietitians prefer to choose a basic vitamin and mineral supplement to meet the needs of the individual in response to his or her reactions. Diet and dietary supplements will almost certainly have to be adjusted if, as is very likely, the client's health status or drug therapy changes.

Nutritionists and dietitians who work with HIV/AIDS patients generally agree that people with this infection should take:

• A multivitamin/mineral tablet that contains 100 per cent or more of the RDA for all vitamins and minerals, every day.

• Extra amounts of the antioxidant vitamins, including 500 mg of vitamin C and 250 mg of vitamin E. If the person is taking amprenavir (Agenerase), which includes vitamin E in its preparation, additional E should be avoided.

The Benefits of Exercise

Exercise is an important part of maintaining good health when you have HIV/AIDS. It helps you fight the loss of lean body mass, increases your energy and can improve your mood and appetite, says Bell-Wilson, who is pursuing a doctorate in exercise physiology.

'The hardest part of exercise is incorporating it into your lifestyle. You don't have to join a fitness club if that doesn't interest you. You can start at home. You just need to start,' Bell-Wilson says. 'Walking is the easiest and can provide excellent health benefits to your cardiovascular system, muscle development and bone health. If you haven't been exercising at all, start with a 10- to 15-minute walk every day, and increase when you are comfortable.'

Weight training, which is particularly good for maintaining lean muscle, can also be done at home. Start with two or three times per week, leaving a day of rest between each session. Visit your local library or book-shop for an illustrated guide that outlines exercises, for all muscle groups, that require a minimum of equipment. Many exercises can be done with light free weights, an exercise band, or a towel.

As with eating properly, exercising takes some commitment on your part. But a healthy, nutrient-rich diet and a regular exercise routine will boost your immune system, and many experts believe that a strong immune system can significantly affect how quickly your disease progresses. That's one benefit that's definitely worth the effort.

Chapter 17

INFECTIOUS DISEASES: WHAT MAKES US ILL?

On a mountain top in rural Pennsylvania, there is a cemetery with tombstones dating back to the 1700s. As visitors stroll on these peaceful grounds, they first pass through the area with the most recent graves. According to these tombstones, many of the people buried there lived to see their eighties and even nineties. As visitors keep walking, though, they come upon tombstones from the 1800s. The dates chiselled into these rough markers tell a very different tale: many of them span less than 50 years. In one particularly chilling area of the cemetery, there are row upon row of small, roughly hewn tombstones all dating within a 2-year span. The cemetery records tell the story: a particularly virulent strain of influenza led to the deaths of countless children, devastating families and no doubt leaving parents desperate to find a way to help their families evade this merciless killer.

Thankfully, medicine has come a long way since the 1800s. Antimicrobial medicines and vaccines have been developed that have proved successful in controlling disease outbreaks. Today, we can get 'flu jabs' that will help protect us from influenza infections, potentially saving thousands of lives each year. In fact, thanks to vaccines, once deadly diseases such as smallpox, diphtheria, typhoid and polio have virtually disappeared from our lives.

In addition, we have become more knowledgeable about how most diseases spread, and public health efforts based on that knowledge are effective. For example, water purification, good sewer systems, efforts to control the number of disease-carrying rodents and insects, quarantine of the infectious, better nutrition and improved personal and household cleanliness have helped to decrease the risks of infection.

Why We Still Fall Ill

Modern medicine has certainly waged a heroic battle against infectious diseases. Yet despite making great progress, it hasn't been able to conquer them completely.

There are a couple of reasons why we remain vulnerable to some infections. In certain instances, such as AIDS, we are dealing with a constantly changing virus. Other diseases are new, and, as yet, we have no immune defences or vaccines against them. Even diseases that were once effectively managed, such as tuberculosis, may now have become resistant to the antibiotics used to fight them. In addition, the tempo and stresses and bad habits of modern life may be compromising the effectiveness of our immune systems.

Finally, doctors warn that we may see even more infectious disease in the future if we continue to use antibacterial soaps and cleaners for everyday household use. These doctors caution that bacteria are developing resistance to these products, which is resulting in 'superbugs' that are even stronger than ever. 'We're very much against overusing antibiotics – it's really a very scary thing for us in paediatrics,' explains Susan B Ryan, MD, a paediatrician in the medically fragile children's programme at Palmetto Richland Memorial Hospital in Columbia, South Carolina. 'Adding antibiotics to soaps and disposable wipes, and even building it into plastic toys, has us concerned. I worry about the bacteria becoming resistant to the antibiotic.'

We cannot resist an invasion of pathogens unless our immune systems are in peak condition. If we do come down with an infectious disease, our

TUBERCULOSIS: STILL A THREAT

For most of us in the developed world, tuberculosis is a disease that has almost disappeared. *Almost* is the key word here. In the late 1990s there were about 6,000 reported cases of TB in the UK each year, and the number of cases worldwide is rising. This may seem like a small number, but it's important to realise that TB is a highly contagious disease easily spread through the air by a cough or sneeze.

It's equally vital to realise that today's TB often is resistant to virtually all the antibiotics that once were effective against it. Multidrug-resistant tuberculosis, as it's called, has become a major health concern throughout the world.

If you've been exposed to TB, in most cases your immune system will envelop and control the infection. All the bacteria aren't eliminated, however. If you're otherwise healthy, the germs will live in your body without making you ill. You won't even realise that you have a TB infection.

If, however, you've been exposed to TB and your immune system is already weakened by age, an immune deficiency disease, or a chronic illness of some kind, the number of TB bacteria that you carry may multiply and spread to another part of your body, such as your lungs, spine, or brain. In this case, the infection has become a fully-fledged, active disease – and now is very contagious.

Although many of us are exposed to TB bacteria, people who have alcoholism, who are chronically undernourished, or who are living in crowded conditions such as dormitories, homeless shelters and nursing homes are especially vulnerable to the active disease.

TB cannot be 'caught' from shaking hands, from unwashed glasses or cutlery, or from a toilet.

Symptoms develop slowly and at first may resemble the flu. A persistent cough is one of the most obvious signs. Poor appetite, fever, chest pains, night sweats, fatigue, weight loss and shortness of breath together may indicate active TB.

A carefully followed antibiotic programme that takes 6 to 9 months is necessary to beat this disease. Medication that is stopped too early encourages the development of drug-resistant TB microbes.

immune systems will be key to determining how severe the illness is and how long it takes for us to recover. It all depends on keeping our immune systems strong with good nutrition, enough rest, relief from stress, exercise and an optimum environment.

How Do You Avoid
Catching an Infectious Disease?

Diseases can be spread in myriad ways: through the air, by touch, during sex, through contact with infected blood. To prevent illness, we need to keep our immune systems healthy as well as foil the illness's methods of transmission. The strategies for preventing most illnesses are chiefly common sense, yet many of us neglect to take the simple precautions that could reduce the number of infectious diseases that we or our children contract every year. The following practical recommendations are from Dr Ryan.

Wash your hands. All of us carry germs from surfaces we touch to our faces or our children's faces, where they can find easy entry into our bodies. At work, wash your hands several times a day, particularly before you eat, even if you're just having a snack while at the computer. Wash them when you get home, after shopping and before you prepare a meal. Don't forget to wash them after changing the baby's nappy or wiping a toddler's runny nose.

Teach your children to wash their hands. For even the tiniest toddler, washing hands before a meal and after going to the toilet should be automatic. It should be a thorough wash, with scrubbing and lots of soapsuds spread all over the hands and wrists, not just a quick splash of water.

Always use tissues. Encourage everyone in your household to get into the habit of using tissues. Teach them to cover their mouths and noses when they cough and sneeze. Even small children can learn automatically to cover up with a tissue to prevent germs from flying through the air.

Use your dishwasher as your secret weapon. Anything that goes in a child's mouth – dummies, toys, teething rings, teats, bottles – should be washed often. Put plastic toys in the dishwasher and soft toys in the laundry, especially when colds and flu are making the rounds. If you don't have a dishwasher, use a bowl of hot, soapy water, and rinse with the hottest water that the plastic (and your hands) can stand.

Give your toothbrush some breathing room. Don't store your family's toothbrushes together in a glass. Put them in the sort of holder that doesn't let them touch each other. Shake them after using so that they dry quickly – germs don't thrive well on dry surfaces. Of course, don't share toothbrushes – it's a very direct way to share germs.

Change your toothbrush regularly. Because they tend to harbour infectious organisms, if you've had a cold or sore throat, throw out your toothbrush and use a new one. (For hygiene and tooth health, change to a new toothbrush every 3 months.)

Use plenty of hot water. After you or your family member has recovered from a bout of illness, wash the bedding and nightclothes in hot water. Wash down the cot or bed and all bedroom surfaces with hot water, and then open windows – even in the winter – to help fresh air circulate into the room.

Change the towels. Facecloths and towels should be changed every day. This is doubly important when someone in the house has a cold or the flu.

Observe kitchen etiquette. Change dish towels every day. Do not dry dishes with the same towel that you use for your hands. Even better, let your dishes air dry. Clean your sponges in the dishwasher and change them often.

TAKE THE **FIRST STEP**

The next time you go to the supermarket, make a point of buying soaps and cleaners that *aren't* labelled 'antibacterial'. Scientists fear that bacteria are becoming resistant to the antibiotics found in many products, which could result in 'superbugs' for which we have no cure.

Keep surfaces dry. Most infectious organisms don't thrive on dry surfaces. After you use soap and water on the sink and worktops in your kitchen, dry them with paper towels. This is a good practice for the bathroom, too.

Quarantine raw meat. To prevent food poisoning from salmonella and other organisms, keep your meat and salads apart. Use different areas of the kitchen if you can and different cutting boards and knives. Clear up spilled meat juices with soapy paper towels, not sponges. Store meat where its juices cannot leak on to other foods and never store raw meat and cooked meat together. Wash your hands after handling raw meat.

Think of the tips above as a gentle reminder of some basic household strategies for preventing infectious illnesses in general. In the remainder of this chapter, we'll discuss specific infectious diseases that take advantage of a weakened immune system, how they spread, and all the things you can do to avoid infection. You'll notice that in nearly every case, people who have strong immune systems are better able to fight off these illnesses, resulting in less severe symptoms and a faster recovery time. To boost your own immune system, read the Immune Boosters on page 106 and the MaxImmunity Plan starting on page 305.

Sore Throat

Most sore throats are caused by viral infections. Viral sore throats can be an early sign of a cold, flu, the measles or chickenpox. Most sore throats are mild and can be eased by using a vaporiser, gargling with salt water and using throat lozenges, and they disappear within a week.

A sore throat can also be caused by streptococcus bacteria. These bacteria require fairly intimate contact to be spread. You need to be sneezed or coughed on or touched by someone carrying it. Sharing a drinking cup, toys, or a toothbrush also transmits the infection.

If you have a severe sore throat that lasts longer than a week, or if it is difficult to swallow, breathe, or even open your mouth, call your doctor. You should also consult your doctor promptly if your sore throat is accompanied by a fever, joint pains, an earache, or a rash.

A sore throat needs to be treated right away, not only to avoid feeling rotten but also to prevent it from leading to rheumatic fever or kidney inflammation (nephritis). If the cause is bacteria, an antibiotic will be the most effective treatment.

To ease discomfort, gargle with warm salt water (½ teaspoon of salt to 120 ml/4 fl oz of water) every 4 hours, or with fenugreek and water (20 drops of extract to 240 ml/8 fl oz of water) three times a day. If your throat is so sore that you don't feel like eating, try an instant breakfast drink. Drink lots of liquids: chilled rather than very cold drinks cool the throat and make it easier to swallow.

Conjunctivitis (Pinkeye)

This extremely contagious infection inflames the conjunctiva of the eye, the clear membrane that lines your inner eyelid and covers the white part of your eye. The infection makes the eye look pinkish red and blood-shot and makes it feel irritated, gritty and itchy.

Bacterial conjunctivitis usually produces a thick, yellow discharge that can make your eyelids stick together; if a virus is the problem, however, the discharge will be watery.

Whether caused by a virus or bacteria, conjunctivitis is one of the most contagious infections around. It can be spread by sharing flannels, towels and cosmetics, or simply by being in the same room and breathing the same air as a person carrying the germ. One child can infect an entire classroom.

The virus that causes conjunctivitis also invades the upper respiratory tract, leading to swollen lymph nodes and a sore throat. It can travel down the trachea, or windpipe, into the lungs, resulting in viral pneumonia.

If you have the symptoms mentioned above, see your doctor to find out whether your conjunctivitis is bacterial or viral, and to take steps to avoid transmitting this disease to anyone else. Viral conjunctivitis can be eased by washing your eyes with warm water and by using warm compresses several times a day, advises Dr Ryan. Using soft paper towels or tissues on eyes, and then discarding them carefully, may help avoid spreading the contagion. Make the compresses as warm as you can bear them, which may discourage some infectious organisms.

To prevent conjunctivitis from spreading, change flannels and towels every day and do not share them. Also, do not share cosmetics. Use a clean pillowcase every night, and wash sheets and pillowcases in hot water. Finally, segregate your toothbrush and wash your hands often.

Bronchitis

The best way to prevent bronchitis is to take steps to avoid getting an upper respiratory infection, which often precedes bronchitis. Read Colds and Flu on page 168 for some practical strategies to avoid these illnesses.

The air you inhale enters your trachea, or windpipe, and then flows into your lungs via the bronchial tubes. Because of this, the bronchial tubes are susceptible to airborne irritants and infection.

Bronchitis is likely to be the diagnosis when the linings of the bronchi are inflamed and swollen and the bronchial glands overproduce mucus. You may have difficulty breathing and may wheeze and cough. You also may have a fever, fatigue, chest discomfort, a sore throat and sudden chills and shaking.

Bronchitis can be a miserable experience anytime, but it can be a serious illness in babies, the frail elderly and people with lung disease. It takes two forms: acute and chronic.

Acute Bronchitis

This form is caused by one of several infecting agents: viruses, bacteria and mycoplasmal or chlamydial organisms. It's also associated with asthma and allergies. Although it can be very uncomfortable, acute bronchitis usually doesn't last more than a week, which is why it's called acute. The cough may last longer, however.

Steam can help to relieve the discomfort of acute bronchitis. For quick relief, sit in the bathroom with a hot shower running. Another option is to run hot water into a sink, put a towel over your head, and breathe in the steam. (Be sure to stay about 30 cm/12 inches away from the water to avoid burning yourself.) Humidifying your entire living space – or the room you're in most of the time – can make breathing easier. You can use a humidifier or a less expensive vaporiser, which produces warm, moist air.

To ease the coughing, drink lots of fluids, especially water – 2–3 litres/4–6 pints a day. This will help thin the phlegm being coughed up and makes it easier to cough. Avoid very cold or dry air and dusty, polluted environments – anything that might challenge your ability to breathe.

Most acute cases clear up with no further trouble. You should call your doctor, however, if you also experience severe breathlessness or severe chills, if you don't improve after 3 days, if you cough up blood, or if you have a fever that isn't reduced by aspirin or paracetamol. You should also consult a doctor if you have a lung disease of any kind and come down with bronchitis.

'If bronchitis occurs as a reaction to an allergy, it's important to identify the allergen (the agent triggering the allergy) and reduce the frequency of allergic episodes,' advises Guy Pugh, MD, medical director of the Marino Center for Progressive Health in Cambridge, Massachusetts. Dr Pugh says that the same approach is needed if bronchitis follows asthma attacks.

Chronic Bronchitis

Chronic bronchitis is a perfect example of how your environment can affect your immune system. The condition results when the bronchial tubes are constantly irritated and inflamed by tobacco smoke or other inhaled pollutants. Allergies also can be a cause. Bronchitis is considered chronic if a person coughs up mucus almost every day for 3 months and this occurs during 2 consecutive years.

Perpetual irritation thickens the walls of the bronchial tubes, which makes the airways narrower. Mucus is constantly produced as the body tries to rid itself of the irritating pollutant. These changes make the exchange of oxygen and carbon dioxide between the lungs and the blood capillaries more difficult. The lungs and heart are forced to work harder, often leading to serious complications.

When chronic bronchitis first makes itself felt, the symptoms are a lot like those of acute bronchitis, except that they don't go away. If the symptoms are ignored, the lungs become permanently damaged. The condition steadily worsens, and eventually, the person's breathing is so compromised that he or she cannot move without using supplemental oxygen.

To relieve breathlessness, your doctor may prescribe the use of an inhaler that contains a drug that eases and expands your airways. Or you may need to have oxygen therapy.

Averting chronic bronchitis is more useful than trying to treat it. In most cases, you can avoid getting chronic bronchitis by not smoking and by staying away from polluted, dusty environments. If you have to be in an area where there are strong fumes or where there is a high degree of pollution, wear a mask called a chemical respirator that protects against such conditions.

Pneumonia

A major infection of the lungs, pneumonia can be caused by a number of different organisms, although viruses and bacteria are usually the cause. It may be preceded by a cold, flu, or the measles.

This infection causes the tiny air sacs in the lungs to inflame and fill with mucus and pus. It hinders the diffusion of oxygen from the air sacs into the blood capillaries, as well as the movement of carbon dioxide from the capillaries into the lungs.

Pneumonia can be particularly dangerous for children younger than 12 months, for those over the age of 60, and for people of any age whose immune systems are weakened. People with a chronic illness, such as diabetes, cardiovascular disease, HIV infection, sickle cell disease, or kidney failure, are at particular risk of contracting pneumonia.

Older people are five times more likely to die of pneumonia than younger adults because their lungs and immune systems are not as strong and they may not be well-nourished. Pneumonia is a particular risk to smokers, alcoholics, people who have had strokes and anyone with severe malnutrition. It also can occur if foreign material is sucked into the lungs.

WHO SHOULD BE VACCINATED?

You should consider getting a pneumonia vaccine and a flu vaccine if you have a medical history of frequent bouts of acute bronchitis, if you are over 60, or if you have a lung problem or a chronic disease such as diabetes or liver disease. If you don't fit this description but work or live with persons who do, you, too, should be immunised so that they can't catch these dangerous 'bugs' from you.

Today, more and more doctors believe that even healthy young adults should get a flu vaccine.

The type of microbe that causes the pneumonia can be a factor in its severity, but just how ill you become depends chiefly on your health at the time of the infection.

Bacterial pneumonia. This is the most dangerous form of pneumonia. It can appear without warning or as a complication of another illness. Medical help should be sought as soon as it is suspected.

Symptoms include:

- Shaking and chills

- High fever

- A cough that may be dry at first, then produce phlegm

- Phlegm that is yellow or greenish

- Sick, tired and achy feelings

- Chest pain and fatigue; sometimes, abdominal pain

- Rapid, hard breathing; shortness of breath (At any time, shortness of breath is a worrying symptom; it indicates that a large portion of the lung is affected. You should not be short of breath, no matter how ill – or well – you feel.)

Viral pneumonia. This form is considered less serious than bacterial, but if it isn't treated, it can worsen or lead to bacterial pneumonia. It can be caused by influenza and other viruses. The symptoms usually are the same as with bacterial pneumonia. Only your doctor can diagnose which form of pneumonia you have, so if you have these symptoms, seek medical attention within a day or two.

'Walking' pneumonia. Caused by a microorganism called mycoplasma, this type of pneumonia usually affects people under the age of 40. Although its symptoms generally are less severe and tend to be limited to a cough, chills and fever, it is highly contagious. It is called walking pneumonia because people often don't feel ill enough to retreat to bed.

If you have a mild case of pneumonia, you probably can be treated at home. Severe cases require hospitalisation.

The type of drug prescribed for this illness depends on the microbe causing it. Sputum (phlegm) and sometimes the blood are tested to reveal the cause. Aspirin or paracetamol can reduce fever. Some severe cases may call for oxygen therapy and the use of a ventilator.

Sexually Transmitted Diseases

The microbes that cause sexually transmitted diseases (STDs) are passed from person to person chiefly through anal, vaginal, or oral sex. The viruses that cause hepatitis B and C and AIDS circulate in the blood, which means that they're also spread when drug users share needles. Seafood contaminated with the hepatitis A virus also causes the disease.

If you are sexually active, you can get an STD – even if you have sex only once with an infected person. You may not notice any symptoms, and you easily can have one – or more – without knowing it. Furthermore, no one is immune to them: they can infect anyone of any social level, state of health, or age.

The infectious diseases that STD microbes cause may be limited to your genitals or may spread to your reproductive organs. HIV, which causes AIDS, spreads throughout the body. (See HIV and AIDS on page 261 for more information on how this virus spreads.)

STDs can impair a person's health and fertility and can be transmitted along to a baby before it's born. Some types, such as genital warts, can lead to cancer. Certain viral STDs, such as HIV, herpes simplex, hepatitis B and C and human papillomavirus (genital warts), are incurable and commonly

WOMEN MORE VULNERABLE THAN MEN TO STDS

When it comes to sexually transmitted diseases (STDs), things just aren't equal. Women are more likely than men to acquire a sexually transmitted disease, and women experience more severe and long-lasting repercussions, such as pelvic inflammatory disease, infertility, chronic pelvic pain and cancer of the cervix.

Pelvic inflammatory disease is caused by bacteria that pass from the man to the woman and can infect the fallopian tubes. If not treated, the microbes cause inflammation and the growth of scar tissue in the tubes, blocking them and leading to infertility, ectopic pregnancy, pelvic abscess or other complications.

become chronic diseases. Others can be treated successfully with antibiotics.

The state of your immune system may not have much effect on whether you get a sexually transmitted disease (though it can affect how the disease progresses). STDs are most common during the years when people are most sexually active, which usually is a time when they're very healthy.

The most common STDs seen by doctors today are chlamydia, gonorrhea, trichomoniasis, genital herpes (herpes simplex virus), genital warts (human papillomavirus), urethritis, HIV infection and pelvic inflammatory disease.

The following symptoms may indicate a sexually transmitted disease in men.

• Watery discharge from the penis, swollen testicles and pain when urinating may indicate chlamydia.

• Painless, cauliflower-like warts on the genitals are a sign of an infection with one of the many human papillomaviruses.

• Weeping sores and itching and burning in the genital area; a swollen, leaky penis; painful urination and swollen lymph nodes in the groin are signs of genital herpes.

• Inflammation of the head of the penis, clear urethral discharge, or uncomfortable urination may be signs of trichomoniasis.

Women should be aware of the following warning signs.

• Trichomoniasis usually exhibits few or no symptoms but sometimes produces painful inflammation and itching in the genital area, and an abundant, offensive, frothy vaginal discharge. Intercourse can be painful.

• Burning urination; painful intercourse; a white, thick vaginal discharge and itching can be signs of chlamydia, although this disease is another STD that often has no symptoms. (If not treated, chlamydia may lead to pelvic inflammatory disease and infertility.)

• Blisters anywhere in the genital area are signs of herpes, as are itching and burning. Discomfort while urinating and a watery discharge are also symptoms.

• As in men, painless genital warts can mean infection with one of the human papillomaviruses.

DON'T IGNORE GENITAL WARTS

Two of the human papillomaviruses (HPVs) that cause warts to develop around and in the genitals also are strongly associated with cellular changes that may develop into cervical cancer. Nine others in this large family of viruses carry a moderate risk of preceding a cancer. They are transmitted through oral, anal and vaginal sex and are highly contagious. Altogether, 30 strains of this virus can infect the cervix; most don't lead to cancer.

Currently, DNA testing can pinpoint which version of HPV is present. If it's one of the lower-risk HPVs, watchful waiting is usually the chosen approach. If it's a high-risk strain, the gynaecologist may use an illuminated magnifier to check the cervix (the neck of the uterus) for signs of cancer or precancerous tissue.

The following symptoms affect both men and women.

• Dark urine, jaundice, joint aches, weight loss, constant tiredness, fever and abdominal pain may be symptoms of hepatitis B or C. These viral infections often don't have symptoms even when the liver is inflamed.

• Headache, night sweats, unexplained weight loss, persistently swollen lymph nodes, a constant fever, recurrent vaginal yeast infections, chronic diarrhoea, recurrent lung infections, and a thick, white coating in the mouth and on the tongue (oral thrush) are signs of HIV infection.

Preventing STDs

Because sexually transmitted diseases are so insidious, the most reliable protection is abstinence, or having a mutually monogamous relationship.

Although mucous membranes and skin protect the body against microbe invasions, small cuts or scrapes permit germs to enter. The genitals and the anus are particularly susceptible to small, unnoticed abrasions.

All sexually active persons who are not in mutually monogamous relationships need to remember that the male and female condoms are the best protection against disease organisms. When used properly, condoms not only greatly reduce the possibility of pregnancy but also protect the vagina, cervix and genitals from microbes. Female condoms are an excellent alternative if a man refuses to use a male condom. Even if pregnancy isn't a concern, don't stop using condoms unless you've been mutually monogamous for 6 months and both of you have tested negative for HIV and other infections. This may sound unromantic, but it could save your life.

If you're allergic to latex condoms, you can use a male or female polyurethane condom instead. Be aware that 'skin' condoms made from treated lamb membranes don't protect against microbes. Don't think that oral sex is risk-free; be sure to use a male or female condom.

Of course, contraceptive pills, intrauterine devices (IUDs) and natural family planning do not protect against sexually transmitted diseases.

Treating STDs

The most important part of treating sexually transmitted diseases is identifying the infection. It's possible to have more than one STD at a time, and each one must be treated. Every sexual partner should be notified and treated as well.

The main thing to remember is that some STDs, particularly chlamydia, pelvic inflammatory disease and hepatitis B and C, do not produce symptoms. As a result, men and women who have these diseases may unwittingly pass them on to their sexual partners. Furthermore, if sexual infections aren't treated in their early stages, they can spread to other organs. Even if you're sexually active only occasionally, it's important to have regular medical check-ups, and to be frank with your doctor about the fact that you are sexually active.

Urinary Tract Infections

When bacteria invade the urethra, bladder, or kidneys, the resulting infection can be annoying and painful, and it can sometimes lead to complications. Women are especially susceptible to these infections if they are pregnant or using a diaphragm. A weakened immune system also leads to an increased vulnerability to urinary tract infections.

Bacteria from the digestive tract – usually *Escherichia coli* – linger around the rectum and sometimes get pushed toward the urethra opening. They then migrate up the urethra to the bladder or kidneys. Most urinary tract infections involve the urethra or bladder, often at the same time.

An untreated bladder infection may ascend the urinary tract and infect the kidneys. Women are more likely to experience bladder and kidney infections than men, because their shorter urethras provide a quick route to those organs.

Both men and women can get urethritis, an inflammation of the urethra. In men, the bacteria that cause it may migrate into the urethra from an infected prostate gland or be picked up from sexual intercourse.

Chlamydia organisms are commonly responsible for causing urethritis. The first symptom of this widespread disease is often a burning sensation when urinating. Similarly, a urinary tract infection can be a warning sign of an inflamed prostate, known as prostatitis.

Urethritis and other urinary tract infections also may result when an anatomical blockage, such as a tumour or a congenital condition, impedes the flow of urine.

Below is a list of common symptoms indicating a urinary tract infection.

- Pain in the lower back and around the hips can be a sign of a kidney infection. Swollen ankles and hands indicate the fluid accumulation that occurs when the kidneys aren't functioning properly. Smoky or red urine are symptoms of severe kidney disease. Chills, fever, bloating, nausea, vomiting and urinary urgency are also symptoms.

- The most notable sign of a bladder infection is the urgent and frequent desire to urinate, whether the bladder is full or empty.

- Urination is often painful. The urine may look cloudy, have some blood in it and have an unpleasant odour.

- Your lower abdomen may be painful, and you may feel unwell and have a low fever.

- The chief symptoms of urethritis are stinging and painful urination.

Preventing Urinary Tract Infections

There are a number of simple steps you can take to reduce your chances of getting a urinary tract infection. First, routinely drink a lot of water and other liquids to help move microbes out of your urinary system. Be sure to include cranberry juice in your diet, which will prevent bacteria from sticking to the urinary tract and multiplying. Also, eat plenty of fresh blueberries: scientists think that they may prove as helpful as cranberry juice in preventing urinary tract infections.

Make frequent visits to the toilet, too. In general, it's a good idea to try to urinate every 2 to 3 hours, since stagnant urine encourages the growth of germs. You should also try to urinate after intercourse to help flush out any microbes that may have been pushed into the urethra.

Be sure to practise careful personal hygiene. You might want to carry packaged wipes, which are effective and portable, along with you. In addition, shower or wash after intercourse.

Finally, wearing cotton underwear helps keep you dry and discourages the growth of the microbes that cause urinary tract infections. On the other hand, nylon pants and close-fitting jeans and trousers can aggravate urinary tract infections.

Treating Urinary Tract Infections

Most urinary tract infections are treated with antibiotics. It's important to take the drug for the entire length of time prescribed by your doctor.

In addition, try drinking up to 1 litre (2 pints) of cranberry juice each day. Natural diuretics in the form of birch or parsley tea can reduce some of the discomfort of a bladder infection, say herbalists. They may also relieve that false feeling of having to urinate every few minutes. Lots of filtered water – 240-ml (8-fl oz) glass every hour – will help keep your urinary tract flushed out.

To ease the irritation of a bladder infection and urethritis, soak in a warm sitz bath twice a day for 20 minutes. Some alternative practitioners suggest adding a cup of white vinegar to the bath once a day to discourage microbes.

Change your diet while you fight the infection. 'Avoid foods that stimulate your immune system unnecessarily,' suggests Glenn Rothfeld, MD, of WholeHealth New England in Arlington, Massachusetts. In so doing, he says, 'You lessen the load on your immune system and allow it to fight microbes better.' He suggests avoiding foods high in sugars, wheat, dairy products and yeast. It's also wise to eliminate alcohol, caffeine and carbonated beverages from your diet so that they can't irritate your bladder.

Dr Rothfeld finds that food sensitivities are often the culprit in frequent bladder infections because for some people, particular foods irritate the bladder. Discuss this possibility with your doctor if you suspect that you might have a food sensitivity.

To flush out germs, try to urinate fully every 2 to 3 hours during the hours when you're awake.

Finally, be aware that the active ingredient in the spermicides used with the diaphragm, cervical cap and condom is nonoxynol-9. Unfortunately, it also kills helpful bacteria that control the growth of *E. coli*. If you're experiencing frequent bladder infections, ask your doctor to test you for the bacteria that's causing them. If it's *E. coli*, consider a contraceptive method that doesn't require a spermicide.

Chapter 18

OTHER CONDITIONS THAT MAY HAVE AN IMMUNE CONNECTION

In the previous chapters, we discussed diseases that have a definite connection with the immune system, such as multiple sclerosis, lupus and AIDS. Unfortunately, when it comes to the complex cellular workings of the human body, establishing cause and effect is not always this easy.

In this chapter, we'll discuss conditions that some doctors and scientists believe may have an immune link. Some of these diseases may not be what come to your mind when you think of immunity – conditions such as heart disease, chronic fatigue syndrome, psoriasis and autism. More research needs to be done to determine whether the immune system does indeed play a direct role in conditions such as these, but in the meantime, understanding the avenues that scientists are exploring can help you gain a better sense of what might be affecting your health.

A Prime Suspect: The Immune System

Despite all the medical advances, in many ways, the human body still remains a mystery. Yet many scientists believe that the immune system may hold many of the answers to some currently unexplained diseases. They point to research indicating that weakened immunity can affect the body in ways not previously suspected. They also have evidence that the immune system is vulnerable to outside factors, such as stress, that were once ignored in research. For example, scientists have discovered that psychological stress can interfere with immune response by inhibiting the functioning of the T-cells, which normally help to fight infection and disease, and by interfering with antibody production.

'There is clear evidence that stress impacts immunity. Indeed, many studies have now shown pathways between the brain and the immune system, but, to date, nobody fully understands the clinical significance of relationships between these two systems,' says Anna L. Marsland, RN, PhD, a psychologist in the behavioural medicine programme at the Western Psychiatric Institute and Clinic at the University of Pittsburgh Medical Center.

However, this is about to change.

In a study, Dr Marsland and her colleagues evaluated the antibody levels in the blood samples of 84 young adults who received a standard course of three hepatitis B vaccinations.

First, the researchers measured antibody response based on personality traits revealed in psychological tests that the participants had taken earlier. Then, they measured antibody levels in reaction to a stressful situation: giving a 5-minute speech with little preparation time. The researchers found that those people who had negative outlooks and were highly stressed showed lower antibody responses.

'This is significant,' says Dr Marsland. 'These are only associations, but the findings suggest that individuals who are prone to stress may be at increased risk for some health problems and would benefit from learning ways of managing stress in their lives.'

Dr Marsland's study is relevant because it shows that there is a correlation between an outside factor – stress – and the functioning of the immune system. Yet stress is only one factor that scientists believe could be influencing immune function. There are many others, including genetics, diet and exposure to environmental toxins. More research needs to be done to determine how these factors (by themselves and in combination) might be influencing the immune system and, in turn, causing various diseases. In the remainder of this chapter, we shall take a look at some specific diseases and explore why scientists believe that they may have an immune connection.

Heart Disease

Scientists have long known that obesity can play a role in heart disease, but they have discovered that there may also be an immune link. In a joint study from Appalachian State University in Boone, North Carolina, and Loma Linda University in California, researchers concluded that people who are obese are more likely to have impaired immune systems than those who are not overweight.

The researchers found that the obese women in the study had elevated levels of specialised immune cells known as leucocytes and neutrophils. They believe that the higher levels of leucocytes might contribute to heart disease by encouraging plaque to build up on artery walls when those walls are affected by chronic infection, inflammation, or other damage. In addition, they say that high levels of neutrophils tend to clump, resulting in a release of free radicals and enzymes that could injure the walls of the arteries. This could lead to the development of plaque and, eventually, heart disease.

Myalgic Encephalomyelitis (ME) and Fibromyalgia

Not very long ago, when a person complained of weakness, fatigue and aching in her muscles and joints, doctors dismissed her complaints as imaginary. Myalgic Encephalomyelitis (ME) is now recognised as a real illness. It is characterised by severe fatigue lasting 6 months or longer and symptoms such as memory loss, sore throat, tender lymph nodes, muscle and joint pain and headaches.

Scientists aren't sure what causes ME, and some suspect that it may be the result of numerous factors. One of the factors being investigated is a dysfunctional immune system. Some studies have shown lower numbers of natural killer cells (cells that attack invading microorganisms) or decreased killer cell activity among people with ME. Other researchers believe that an outside factor such as stress or a viral infection might lead to an increase in the number of cytokines, soluble proteins released by cells of the immune system. Their secretion may drive specific responses in other susceptible cells. Some researchers theorise that this may lead to ME.

Many people who have ME also have fibromyalgia. This is often called the invisible illness because it's difficult to diagnose. The most common symptom is widespread muscle and skeletal pain. Other symptoms may include extreme fatigue, irritable bowel syndrome, headaches, heart palpitations, confusion, depression, joint swelling and total body pain. For many, the pain can become unbearable.

Although the exact cause of fibromyalgia is still unknown, some researchers suggest that stress may be a major culprit in compromising immune cells and allowing dormant viruses to flourish.

Psoriasis

An overactive immune system may be at the root of psoriasis, a skin disease affecting nearly 3 per cent of the population. We are constantly growing and shedding skin cells. As new skin cells develop, the cells above them move outward, eventually being shed in a cycle lasting 28 days. For people with psoriasis, however, this cycle happens in just 4 days. Because the cells are being produced so quickly, they begin to pile up on the skin's surface, causing thick, red patches of skin that are covered with silvery scales. These patches usually appear on the elbows, knees, scalp and face, lower back, palms and soles of the feet. The fingernails and toenails also thicken and grow very quickly. Ten to 30 per cent of people with psoriasis also develop arthritis symptoms.

Some researchers believe that psoriasis may be caused when the immune system produces too many T-cells. They speculate that an infection, certain drugs, smoking, a change in climate, or hormonal changes might trigger this overreaction.

Hormone and Pregnancy Problems

Scientists are studying autoimmunity as a women's issue because of a possible link to certain hormones that exist in higher concentrations in women than in men. Women are at greater risk for most autoimmune diseases, and part of the reason may be due to the hormonal differences between the sexes. At Mills College in Oakland, California, Elizabeth A Bachen, PhD, assistant psychology professor, is studying women with autoimmune diseases. 'We think there are hormonal factors involved with these diseases and that these hormones affect the immune system in a way that increases the risk for autoimmunity,' she says.

The immune system may also play a role in infertility or miscarriages early in a woman's pregnancy. Since the embryo is genetically foreign, scientists think that some miscarriages might be caused by an abnormal immune system response in the mother that rejects the developing embryo. Clinical trials are trying to assess whether immunisation with cells from the father may help enhance the mother's immune system. So far, there have been no significant findings.

Raynaud's Disease

Another disorder believed to have an autoimmune connection is Raynaud's disease, which is indicated by painfully cold fingers and toes and the colour of the skin changing to white, then blue, then red as they warm up again. The onset is triggered by a rapid change in temperature, particularly cold. Often, this trigger can be as minor as touching a package of frozen food.

During a Raynaud's attack, blood vessels in the fingers and toes go into spasm, cutting off bloodflow to the arteries or the small capillaries of the fingers. This is likely to be caused by an exaggeration of a normal mechanism that maintains the central body temperature by shunting blood away from our hands and feet when we're cold. Interestingly, Raynaud's may be a marker for diseases with a known link to the immune system, such as lupus, scleroderma and rheumatoid arthritis, but it may also occur without any connection to an autoimmune disorder.

Autism and Alzheimer's Disease

Scientists are investigating evidence that autism may have an autoimmune link. This developmental disorder is usually diagnosed before the age of 3 and is marked by numerous mental and physical problems, including impaired language, social interaction, imagination and behaviour. In studies, Vijendra Singh, PhD, research professor at the Biotechnology Center at Utah State University in Logan, has found autoantibodies in some children that react against a specific protein in the brain. He theorises that when this protein is attacked, structures in the brain don't develop properly, ultimately leading to autism.

In addition, there is some anecdotal evidence that autism may be linked to diet. One theory is that, in very rare cases, a child's immune system could be weakened by the measles-mumps-rubella vaccination (MMR), which is usually administered before a child turns 2. As a result of this weakening, according to the theory, the child's digestive system is unable to break down certain food proteins, leading to abnormal brain development. Proponents of this theory believe that putting the child on a diet that eliminates certain foods, such as wheat and dairy products, could in certain cases reverse the course of the disease. This theory remains speculative, however, and research needs to be done to determine its validity.

In fact, a 2001 report issued by an Institute of Medicine committee examining studies about the health effects of the MMR vaccine in young children suggests that there is no proven link between the vaccine and autism. The committee recommends that there be no change in immunisation practices that require children to be immunised during early childhood.

Another disorder affecting the brain, Alzheimer's disease, may also have an immune connection. Alzheimer's is a degenerative disease that slowly attacks nerve cells in the brain. It eventually results in the loss of all memory and mental functioning. Scientists are currently investigating the role that the immune system plays in producing an overabundance of the amino acid glutamic acid, a powerful nerve-cell killer. Another immune connection that researchers are investigating is the idea that Alzheimer's might be triggered, in part, by a virus. They suspect that people who are already genetically predisposed to Alzheimer's who also have a weakened immune system might become vulnerable to a virus such as herpes, leading to the onset of Alzheimer's. More studies need to be conducted to investigate these theories.

The Next Step

Much research remains to be done before scientists can hope to fully understand the immune system and its complex workings. Further, we are only beginning to understand the numerous other factors, such as genetics, environmental pollution and diet, that could influence the immune system and may play a role in diseases for which an immune connection has not yet been fully established. In addition, scientists acknowledge that conventional medicine has been more effective in discovering palliatives than in finding preventive measures or cures. Treatments that have been used successfully include steroids, such as cortisone and prednisone, to suppress the immune system. But since they can inhibit the entire system – not just the part that is malfunctioning – steroids can have significant drawbacks. Researchers are continuing to look for safer, more effective therapies.

Yet despite the research that remains to be done, there is also much hope. Researchers have made great strides over the last few decades in unravelling the mystery of the immune system, and they are currently pursuing exciting theories that may one day allow them to cure, or even prevent, some diseases.

In the meantime, remember that there is much you can do *today* to start taking control of your health. Whether or not you are at risk for any of the diseases discussed in this chapter, we strongly recommend trying the MaxImmunity Plan that begins on page 305. You'll strengthen your immune system by modifying your diet, improving your sleeping habits, managing stress better, getting exercise and becoming more in tune with your body. Scientists can't yet guarantee that these things will slow down the course of a disease or keep you from becoming ill, but it's fairly certain that the strong immune system you'll develop will have a profoundly positive effect on your general health.

PART
4

The

MaxImmunity
Plan

THE SIX-FACET
VITALITY DIAMOND

Your IMMUNE SYSTEM IS THE ULTIMATE DEFENDER OF YOUR BODY. It consists of trillions of cells with multitudes of talents to ward off invaders. As shown in earlier chapters, the miraculous gift of your immune system's cells is their ability to recognise toxins, bacteria, viruses, parasites, fungi and yeast. Your immune cells attack and kill or neutralise them, collaborating every step of the way with your nervous system, your endocrine glands, your liver and other organs. You, for the most part, are none the wiser for all the work accomplished. No matter what you're doing – even whether you're awake or asleep – your immune cells are always on patrol. Each cell accepts its responsibility. Born in your bone marrow, educated in your thymus and commissioned throughout your body, your immune cells work together like a magnificently tuned machine.

While earlier your immune system was compared to an army in the battlefield, another analogy is to describe your immune system as being a diamond. When the various facets of immune system function are honed with precision and care, it becomes a thing of beauty. You may feel as if your immune system is an unpolished piece of work, but with enough nurturing, it has the potential to become a precious and beautiful gem. With care and persistence, your immune system can become as strong, durable and brilliant as a perfectly chiselled diamond whose facets fit together flawlessly.

You need your immune system to have that sharp focus so that it can clearly distinguish the good from the bad. When it does identify a dangerous invader, you need your immune system to quickly and efficiently eliminate the threat. With such high performance expectations, your immune system welcomes everything you can do to enhance its power. In fact, when you do all that you can to work with – not against – it, you'll find that your immune system is your best friend.

The Six Shining Points

There are six elements (or facets) in the MaxImmunity Plan to help you transform that rough diamond into a long-lasting jewel of an immune system.

- Eating healthily
- Taking supplements where necessary to support nutrition
- Exercising
- Managing stress wisely and getting proper rest
- Approaching life with a sense of positive meaning
- Listening carefully to your body

You'll learn much more about each of these facets in the following chapters. We'll also provide you with specific ways that you can easily incorporate these facets into your lifestyle and create your own Vitality Diamond. (See page 379.)

The joy of this plan is its flexibility, unlike step-by-step programmes, which can become tedious and boring. At the end of part 4, there are lots of suggestions on how to construct your own Vitality Diamond. 'You may work on perfecting one facet at a time, or, if you prefer, incorporate all the facets into your lifestyle immediately,' says MaxImmunity Plan developer Keith Berndtson, MD, medical director at Integrative Care Centers in Chicago and Glenview, Illinois. You will discover that each time you polish a facet of your diamond – perhaps by walking for exercise or sprinkling antioxidant-rich sunflower seeds on your salad for your immune-enhancing diet – you are supporting your immune system's ability to guard your health.

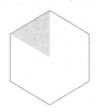

FACET 1:
THE MAXIMMUNITY
DIET

Somewhere along the road to good health, fat turned into a four-letter word. Yet research shows that certain fats – essential fatty acids and monounsaturated fats – are so good for you that you may be harming your immune system and general good health if you avoid them. Your body has more than 50 trillion cells, and every single one of them needs essential fatty acids, such as the omega-3s found in freshwater fish and walnuts, to keep its membranes strong and supple for the absorption and transport of nutrients. Monounsaturated fats, found in abundance in olive oil and nuts, can even help keep your heart healthier than a low-fat diet. Studies show that people who eat more omega-3 and monounsaturated fats get less cancer, heart disease, depression and even Alzheimer's disease. They are also better able to control their diabetes and high blood pressure problems.

The good fat, that is the monounsaturated fats found in nuts and seeds, should be an essential part of your diet. This may be a hard-to-swallow recommendation for good health, especially after you have read the nutrition label on something like a peanut butter jar: 16 g of fat for one 30 g (1 oz) serving.

In analysing the results of several studies on the benefits of consuming nuts, researchers at Loma Linda University in California reported that eating nuts frequently not only can protect your heart but also can increase longevity. The MaxImmunity Diet fully illustrates how this popular spread can be a delicious way to consume the best immune-boosting nutrients of nuts and seeds.

Nuts are Good for You

You cannot eat a whole jar of peanut butter at one sitting, of course. Nor do we advocate eating saturated fats found in meats and full-fat dairy products that can clog your arteries and damage your immune system. For optimal immune health, you need to limit your fat consumption to 25 per cent of total calories while consuming the right balance of foods, says Keith Berndtson, MD, medical director at Integrative Care Centers in Chicago and Glenview, Illinois. Balance is achieved with a variety of foods, and we all know that variety is the spice of life.

The MaxImmunity Diet, advocated by Dr Berndtson, is the *ultimate* diet that makes fruits and vegetables the foundation of your eating plan, with the added bonus of nuts and seeds to make sure that your immune system gets every ounce of power it craves to keep you healthy.

As members of the plant family, nuts and seeds are rich in flavonoids and phytochemicals, the nutrient-dense plant chemicals that act as antioxidants. One such phytochemical is tocotrienol, a form of vitamin E known to lower cholesterol and heart disease risk. But nuts are also special because they're high in phytosterols, which can inhibit cancer-causing hormones, and ellagic acid, which can neutralise the cancer-causing chemicals in tobacco smoke and processed foods. In addition, nuts contain the amino acid arginine, which can be used by the body to relax blood vessels. Together with generous amounts of copper and magnesium and a good supply of fibre, nuts are a powerhouse of health.

'All of these nutrients are working together,' says Paul Lachance, PhD, executive director of the Nutraceuticals Institute at Rutgers University in New Brunswick, New Jersey. It's no wonder, then, that studies show that people who eat nuts regularly have the best health records.

The only note of caution to heed when eating nuts is to pay attention to quantity. Nuts are packed with calories, so eating too many can lead to weight gain. Have a 30 g (1 oz) serving per day. That will be plenty to give your diet (and your health) a boost.

Suggestion: One simple way to incorporate nuts into your diet is to keep a jar of chopped nuts in your refrigerator, and sprinkle 30 g (1 oz) a day on cereal, yoghurt, or vegetable salads to give you the crunch and flavour that make eating enjoyable.

The MaxImmunity Diet

Unlike the traditional food pyramid, which is bottom-heavy with grains, the MaxImmunity Pie on page 312 (developed by the editors of *Prevention* magazine) gives you many more fruits and vegetables (and nuts and seeds) so that you'll be sure to consume the wide variety of plant chemicals your immune system needs to stay healthy.

In this plan, you get to eat nine servings of fruits and vegetables a day. If you're worried that you'll never be able to eat that much, bear in mind that the servings are only 50 g (2 oz) each – about the size of your fist. So, if you add 50 g (2 oz) each of blueberries and raspberries to your morning bowl of cereal, you've already eaten two servings before you leave for work.

Research continues to show that diets high in fruits and vegetables stave off diseases like cancer, heart disease and diabetes. To enhance your immune system, your diet should include whole grains, dark green and yellow and orange vegetables and fruits, and nuts, seeds and pulses. Your immune system is a big consumer of all the nutrients found in these foods, so if you rely on only one type of food, you can seriously compromise your immunity, says Dr Berndtson.

Day in and day out, your immune system's cells voraciously devour vitamins and minerals to ward off invading germs. Immune cells turn over rapidly, so after only a few days of poor eating, your immune system can go awry, Dr Berndtson adds.

That's why we can all learn from Mary's experience.

Mary, Mary, Quite Contrary

A successful management consultant, Mary joked that she couldn't work out when she had the time to get so fat and tired. 'I'm too busy,' she said. Besides, she thought that the multiple vitamins she took regularly would boost her flagging energy. What she didn't realise is that the vitamins alone couldn't save her immune system from her day-after-day junk food habit. She started each morning with doughnuts or pastries for breakfast, then ate hamburgers and chips or pizza for lunch and dinner. Snacks of chocolate, crisps and biscuits came from the vending machine. It seemed that the only vegetables she consumed were the few tomatoes scattered on her pizzas, or chips, which were cooked in saturated fat. At 45, Mary battled headaches, chronic sinusitis, constipation and high cholesterol.

'With my advice, she went to a clinical nutritionist on staff whose style is to educate and inspire changes in behaviour, rather than nag,' explains Dr Berndtson. 'Within 6 months, Mary's energy level was the best she experienced in years,' he says. 'Plus, she lost 15 pounds, her cholesterol level dropped 30 points and her headaches are rare now.'

Suggestion: Make a list of your favourite fruits and vegetables. Mary's list included kiwi fruit, mangoes and red grapes. She also learned that she could add olive oil, nuts, seeds and lean meats and fish to her diet.

A Cornucopia of Immune-Boosting Foods

Scientists are still uncovering the complex chemistry of the power of pigments – those that are responsible for the beautiful array of colours found in fruits, vegetables, nuts and seeds. They're discovering that the plant pigments might have some amazing health benefits, including helping to prevent cancer and heart disease and even slowing the ageing process. It takes more than just an apple a day to keep the doctor away; add blueberries, tomatoes, carrots, green peppers and oranges, too, to get

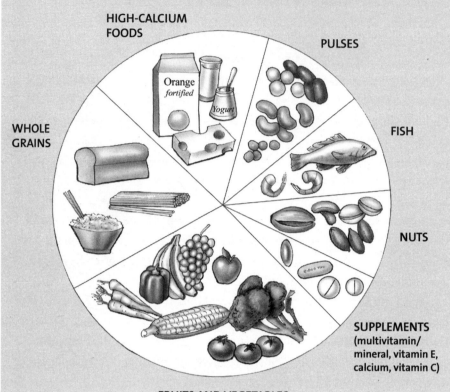

THE MAXIMMUNITY DIET

HIGH-CALCIUM FOODS

PULSES

WHOLE GRAINS

FISH

NUTS

SUPPLEMENTS
(multivitamin/
mineral, vitamin E,
calcium, vitamin C)

FRUITS AND VEGETABLES

DAILY SERVINGS

VEGETABLES AND FRUITS	WHOLE GRAINS	MEAT AND POULTRY
9 servings (5 vegetable/4 fruit)	3–6 servings	1 serving (optional)
	HIGH-CALCIUM FOODS 2–3 servings	2 LITRES (4 PINTS) WATER AND 1+ CUP TEA DAILY

your nine servings of fruits and vegetables daily.

In addition to a colourful array of fruits and vegetables, the MaxImmunity Diet includes three to six servings of whole grains, which are packed with bran and germ and provide protective fibre and nutrients. And

WEEKLY SERVINGS

PULSES
5+ servings

NUTS
5 servings

FISH
2 servings

SERVING SIZES

VEGETABLES AND FRUITS
1 serving = 60 g (2 oz) chopped fruit
60 g (2 oz) cooked or raw vegetable
115 g (4 oz) raw green leaves
80 ml (3 fl oz) vegetable or fruit juice
1 medium piece of fruit

WHOLE GRAINS
1 serving = 1 slice wholemeal bread
115 g (4 oz) brown rice or bulgur
60 g (2 oz) whole wheat pasta

HIGH-CALCIUM FOODS
1 serving = 240 ml (8 fl oz) skimmed or
semi-skimmed milk
240 ml (8 fl oz) fat-free or low-fat yoghurt
240 ml (8 fl oz) calcium-fortified orange juice
1 ounce reduced-fat cheese

PULSES
1 serving = 115 g (4 oz)
cooked dried pulses/lentils

NUTS
1 serving = 30 g (1 oz) ,
chopped

FISH
1 serving = 90 g (3 oz), cooked

MEAT AND POULTRY
1 serving = 90 g (3 oz), cooked

SUPPLEMENTS

MULTIVITAMIN/MINERAL
100 per cent RDA for most nutrients a day

CALCIUM
Under 50 years old: 500 mg a day
Over 50 years old: 1,000 mg a day

VITAMIN E
70–250 mg a day

VITAMIN C
100–500 mg a day

speaking of fibre, pulses are a top-notch source of fibre as well as folate. The MaxImmunity Diet recommends at least five servings of pulses a week.

To get the two to three servings of high-calcium foods a day recommended in this diet, turn to products such as skimmed and semi-skimmed milk, low-fat and fat-free yoghurt, and reduced-fat and fat-free cheese. Other good calcium sources include orange juice, grapefruit juice and soya milk that have been fortified with calcium.

Freshwater fish such as salmon, which are rich in omega-3 fats (healthy fats that keep your cell membranes strong for an empowered immune system) are next to the nuts on the pie. Add fish to your diet at least twice a week. You have the option of consuming one 90-g (3-oz) serving of lean meat or poultry a day (this is about the size of a deck of cards). In addition, eating up to seven eggs a week is permissible under most circumstances; if you have diabetes or high cholesterol or are overweight, however, you should limit yourself to no more than four eggs a week.

As you work on your immunity-boosting diet, don't forget to drink plenty of water. Not taking in enough water can allow waste to become concentrated, leading to painful kidney stones. You've probably heard that you should try to drink 2 litres (4 pints) of water a day, but you don't have to drink that entire amount straight from the tap. Eat juicy fruits such as watermelon, cantaloupe melon, oranges and grapefruit, which naturally contain a lot of water.

Suggestion: Poach fresh salmon one day, and serve it with spicy salsa. On another day, mix tuna with chopped celery, red peppers and almonds. Other fish high in the omega-3 category are mackerel, sardines, herring, anchovies and rainbow trout. Finally, always choose the caviar from the canapés tray.

Go Shopping

To start you on your immunity-boosting diet, here is a list of suggested fruits, vegetables, lean meats and fish, and seeds and nuts from which to build your meals. Mix and match these ingredients into your favourite combinations of tastes and textures, using the MaxImmunity Pie as a guide. With so much to choose from, we promise that it will be easy – and enjoyable – to eat a whole pie every day.

Keep a broad selection of fruits and vegetables on hand, so that you are more likely to reach for something healthy when hunger strikes. Fresh items are always tasty, but they're also perishable. So stock up with frozen and dried and tinned food as well. While there may be some nutrient changes in tinned fruits and vegetables, you'll still be better off than if you hadn't eaten any at all.

'I encourage my patients to think of how many machines have come into contact with the food before they put it in their mouths,' says Dr Berndtson. 'When a food has been heavily processed, it usually means that machines have stripped away some nutrients and added colourings and additives that have no business being in your body. Think "fresh".'

If food tends to spoil in your house before it's eaten, consider building meals around such vegetables as carrots, potatoes and cabbage, which last longer than most vegetables. You can also buy tomatoes, melons, and bananas before they're completely ripe, and eat them as they ripen.

Suggestion: To avoid food spoiling before you get a chance to eat it, go to your supermarket and stock up on just the amount of fruits and vegetables you need for a day or two. In addition, drink ½ litre (1 pint) of water about half an hour before breakfast to hydrate your body and flush out wastes.

Below is a list of immunity-boosting foods. Use this list to whet your appetite and before long you'll find yourself automatically reaching for the health-enhancing foods as you cruise through the supermarket.

Apples. The quercetin found in apples prevents blood platelets from sticking together and forming clots, which can trigger heart attacks. The fibre in apples helps lower cholesterol, relieves constipation and slows digestion, keeping blood sugar under control.

Apricots. These are high in beta-carotene, which helps protect your eyes from macular degeneration – a leading cause of vision loss in older adults. Three apricots have 12 per cent of the suggested daily intake of fibre.

Asparagus. This tasty vegetable contains folate, a B vitamin, as well as small amounts of vitamin E, which helps prevent heart disease.

Avocados. Just like nuts, these are rich in monounsaturated fats. They also contain potassium and folate. Avocado may be high in calories, but it's a healthy addition to a salad.

Bananas. One of nature's best sources of potassium (a nutrient found to lower the risk of high blood pressure, heart attack and stroke) this fruit also seems to help ease heartburn and indigestion.

Barley. This grain is one of the richest sources of tocotrienols, a form of vitamin E. It also contains selenium, which may help prevent cancer, and lignans, which may help prevent blood clots.

Beetroot. This vegetable gets its deep red from betacyanin, a powerful tumour-fighting agent. It's also a good source of iron and folate.

Berries. Choose your colour: blueberries, cranberries, raspberries, strawberries. They contain ellagic acid, a compound thought to prevent cancer, vitamin C, a powerful antioxidant and lots of fibre.

Broccoli. This bright green vegetable is packed with indole-3-carbinol and sulphoraphane, both cancer fighters, as well as beta-carotene, calcium, folate and fibre.

Brussels sprouts. Like broccoli, these green vegetables also contain indole-3-carbinol and sulphoraphane, as well as vitamin C, folate and fibre.

Cabbage. You can't go wrong with a vegetable that includes beta-carotene, vitamin C and folate: all cancer prevention and cancer-fighting ingredients.

Carrots. These bright orange vegetables get their colour from beta-carotene. They also have alpha-carotene, an antioxidant, and fibre.

Fish. The omega-3 fatty acids found in fish protect against a wide range of diseases, including heart disease and cancer. Choose fresh or tinned salmon, mackerel, rainbow trout, anchovies, herring or tuna.

Flaxseed. Packed with lignans, which may prevent or stop the growth of breast cancer tumours and help combat bacterial and fungal infections, this ground or cracked food helps protect against heart disease, high cholesterol, diabetes, constipation and kidney damage.

Garlic. This odoriferous vegetable contains allicin, S-allylcysteine, diallyltrisulphide and diallyldisulphide – all nutrients that lower cholesterol, thin blood and may help alleviate high blood pressure and fight infections.

Grapefruit. A good source of vitamin C, this tasty fruit also contains limonoids and naringin, which may stop breast cancer cells. It also contains lycopene, antioxidants and fibre.

Grape juice. Flavonoids are what give this beverage its rich purple hue, and they also strengthen your immune cells. Each glass contains significant amounts of potassium, too. Pick the darkest juice you can find for the most nutrients.

Greens. Eat plenty of them. Spinach, kale, Swiss chard, cabbage and cress are chock-full of heart-healthy minerals, including magnesium, potassium and calcium, as well as iron, folate and vitamin B_6.

Melon. Rich in vitamin C, this delicious fruit is also high in potassium. Pink-fleshed varieties contain beta-carotene.

Milk. Skimmed or semi-skimmed milk is the healthiest way to obtain calcium, vitamin D and potassium.

Mushrooms. A delicious addition to salads, white button mushrooms are a good source of niacin, a B vitamin that helps your body form enzymes needed to use fats, convert sugars into energy and keep tissues healthy. Also try shiitake mushrooms, which contain polysaccharides, complex sugars that boost your immune system; oyster mushrooms; and maitake mushrooms. Many other varieties are both delicious and nutritious, too.

Nuts. Choose from a wide variety, including pistachios, almonds and chestnuts. These are rich in vitamin E, ellagic acid, monounsaturated fats and arginine.

Oats. A source of three antioxidant compounds (tocotrienols, ferulic acid and caffeic acid), oats are rich in fibre, which helps lower cholesterol and keeps you feeling full. Oat bran has fewer calories than oatmeal.

Olive oil. This is a good way to replace saturated fats with monounsaturated fats. It is rich in vitamin E and polyphenols, which are antioxidants that help prevent cell damage by free radicals. Choose the extra-virgin olive oil; it's highest in disease-fighting polyphenols.

Onions. One of the dozens of compounds found in onions is quercetin, a cancer-fighting flavonoid. For different flavours and lots of flavonoids, try red onions and shallots. For a greater number of nutrients, eat several different kinds of onions.

Oranges. High in fibre, oranges also have lots of vitamin C. In addition, they contain hesperidin, which may help lower cholesterol, and limonene, which may fight cancer. Remember to eat the white, spongy layer below the skin. It's high in fibre and flavonoids.

Peppers. The redder the pepper, the more beta-carotene it has. They come in yellow and green, too, and are brimming with vitamin C.

Poultry. Whether you choose turkey, chicken or other fowl, this low-fat protein source is also rich in three essential B vitamins: niacin, B_6 and B_{12}. It also contains zinc and iron. Remove the skin, which is high in fat.

Pulses. All these high-fibre beans contain protein, folate, iron and potassium.

Sweet potatoes. Rich in beta-carotene and vitamins C and E, these deep orange vegetables also contain vitamin B_6 and folic acid.

Tea. The pulverised leaves in tea bags release lots of polyphenols, fluoride and tannin. Black tea has a slightly higher antioxidant level than green tea.

Tomatoes. These contain vitamin C, lycopene, which helps prevent damage to healthy cells, plus coumaric acid, chlorogenic acid, vitamin A and potassium. Add a touch of olive oil and the lycopene will be better absorbed.

Wholemeal bread. Like nuts, wholemeal bread is a good source of vitamin E and fibre, only with less fat.

Wine. Red wine contains quercetin and resveratrol, two powerful antioxidants. The same benefits can come from red alcohol-free wines. But moderation is the key: women should limit themselves to one small glass of red wine a day, and men should drink no more than two small glasses a day.

Yoghurt. Your immune system will appreciate the *Lactobacillus acidophilus,* beneficial bacteria that help keep yeast infections under control. Make sure that the label says 'live active cultures'.

Make Variety Your Motto

Just as a bright red or deep green scarf adds a touch of glamour to a black dress, bright red peppers and deep green spinach make an ordinary salad interesting. Take advantage of the wide variety of foods you are actually *encouraged* to eat as part of the MaxImmunity Diet. By doing so, you'll never feel bored with your meals. For example, every week, buy at least one fruit or vegetable you've never tried before to integrate into your meals. How about mango salsa with fish? Or red, yellow and orange peppers with coriander and some vinegar for a salad? Store the new foods you buy where you can see them in your refrigerator so that you can mix and match colours and flavours.

Suggestions: If you are always in a hurry, clean and slice fruits and vegetables before you need them. That way, you can grab a quick handful from the refrigerator. (But be aware that some nutrients will be lost or diminished in this process.)

When on the move, remember that grapes, bananas, dried fruit, cherry tomatoes and small cans of juice travel well.

Add extra crunch by sprinkling some chopped nuts on salads, pasta or soups.

Your Winning Plan

Here are the simple guidelines to begin eating for immunity. You might want to put a copy of them on your refrigerator door and tuck one into your handbag or pocket before you set out for the supermarket.

- Eat nine servings of vegetables and fruits every day.
- Each day, consume three to six whole-grain foods.
- Have two or three calcium-rich foods every day.
- Eat pulses five or more times a week.
- Serve fish twice a week.
- Don't forget the nuts, but be sure to get no more than 25 per cent of your calories from fat.

To help monitor your fat intake, look at the simple chart below. These are the suggested amounts of total fat, according to experts, when you are consuming 25 per cent of your calories from fat. Determine the number of calories you eat per day. Then, make sure that you get no more than the recommended number of grams of fat for that amount. (Of course, if you want to lose weight, you'll want to decrease the number of calories and fat you're consuming, along with increasing the amount of exercise you get. Consult a qualified health professional before beginning any weight reduction programme.)

MAXIMUM DAILY FAT ALLOWANCE

TOTAL DAILY CALORIES	GRAMS OF FAT
1,250	35
1,500	42
1,750	49
2,000	56
2,250	63

Polishing Facet 1 of Your Vitality Diamond

Just as the MaxImmunity Diet is all about consuming a wide variety of foods, so too is there a wide variety of people, each with unique cravings, health needs and tastes. Use the diet to create your own immunity-boosting masterpiece: a plan that is specially designed to meet your needs and those of your family. To get started, turn to page 383 for 50 delicious, immune-boosting recipes that are sure to please nearly everyone. If you're not in the mood to try a new recipe today, then try out one of the following simple tips instead.

• Top breakfast cereal or yoghurt with several kinds of fruit and a tablespoon of chopped walnuts or almonds.

• Fill an egg-white omelette with chopped vegetables and top it with salsa.

• Transform a simple turkey sandwich into something special by adding red roasted peppers, some avocado slices and shredded carrots.

• Add stir-fried vegetables and sunflower seeds to pasta, soups, stews and casseroles.

• Always think about the *pièce de résistance* when finishing off your meal preparation: chopped nuts, flavoured vinegar and sliced fruits add that extra flavour and crunchiness.

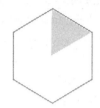

FACET 2:
THE MAXIMMUNITY
SUPPLEMENT PLAN

YOU AND YOUR FAMILY ALWAYS EAT A HEALTHY, BALANCED DIET. You eat oranges and strawberries, and make salads with lots of dark green vegetables mixed with olive oil and sprinkled with sunflower seeds. You drink skimmed milk and serve fish twice a week. Eating a vast array of fruits, vegetables and other healthy foods is your way of making sure that no nutrient is left off your plate.

If this is the case, why do you need to take vitamins?

Well, it's true that no pills can replace your MaxImmunity way of eating, but supplements give you an extra bit of nutritional insurance. Besides, if you relied on food alone for all your nutrients, you would be consuming far more calories than your body needs.

Then why not swallow multivitamin and mineral supplements and forget the healthy food part, instead eating whatever junk food you crave? The reason is that your immune system receives the lion's share of its nutrients from the variety of nutritional foods you eat. A diet high in saturated fats and calories, and low in nutrients, would harm your immune system. Supplements wouldn't even begin to be able to repair the damage.

As Ranjit Kumar Chandra, MD, PhD, director of the World Health Organisation's Center for Nutritional Immunology in St John's, Newfoundland, has shown in studies, your immune system improves greatly after only a few weeks of healthy eating and an appropriate supplement. Dr Chandra, also research professor at Memorial University of Newfoundland, advocates nutritional supplements, particularly as you age. Over time, your immune system slows down, and it makes fewer of the immune cells, such as T-cells and natural killer cells, that can fight off harmful invaders known as antigens. Taking supplements as you age may give your immune system the extra boost it needs. Even if you're still young, though, your immune system deserves a little extra insurance in the form of vitamin and mineral supplements to operate smoothly. Whatever your age, you are not immune to the harmful effects of stress, sleep deprivation and a less-than-adequate diet, so you should consider taking supplements to safeguard against nutritional deficiencies.

A Balancing Act

Think of taking supplements as another way to balance your life: to add a shiny facet to your Vitality Diamond, says MaxImmunity Plan developer Keith Berndtson, MD, medical director at Integrative Care Centers in Chicago and Glenview, Illinois. In this chapter, we'll recommend specific nutrients important both for overall good health and to boost immunity. It is the combination of these vitamins and minerals, from vitamin A to zinc, that enhances your immune system. Pay particular attention to getting the suggested amounts of vitamins and minerals, and to when you should take them. When you read the label on a bottle of supplements, look for the Recommended Daily Allowance (RDA).

Take your supplements at the same time every day, so that you will remember. When you're advised to split up the amounts (as with calcium and vitamin C), take one dose at breakfast and the other at dinner.

To make sure that you remember, invest in a pill container with the days of the week printed on it. Fill it once a week, and at the end of each day, you'll know that you have taken your vitamins.

Basic Supplements

A multivitamin/mineral supplement has close to 100 per cent of the RDA for most vitamins and minerals. Some experts, including Dr Berndtson, say that the only extra supplements most people need are calcium and vitamins C and E.

Look for a multivitamin that contains 100 per cent of the RDA for most essential vitamins and minerals. Take it at mealtimes with a small amount of fat so that you can absorb the fat-soluble vitamins A, D, E and K. For example, if you take it at breakfast, chop up a tablespoon of almonds for your cereal. The nuts will provide enough fat to help you absorb all the vitamins. It's also a good idea to drink some liquid to help the pill dissolve.

Your daily multivitamin/mineral supplement should include:

- Vitamin A (800 mcg)
- Vitamin B_6 (2 mg)
- Vitamin B_{12} (1 mg)
- Chromium (25 mcg)
- Copper (1.2 mg)
- Vitamin D (5 mcg)
- Folic acid (200 mg)
- Magnesium (100 mg; no multi contains 100 per cent of the RDA, 300 mg)
- Selenium (75 mcg)
- Zinc (15 mg)

Consult your doctor before beginning supplementation with any amount of magnesium if you have heart or kidney problems.

B Vitamins

Research shows that a lack of vitamin B_{12} raises levels of homocysteine, a substance linked to heart disease and memory loss.

In addition to B_{12}, vitamin B_6 and folic acid play a critical role in lowering the levels of homocysteine. Your body manufactures homocysteine, but if you're healthy, it's converted into amino acids, so there's no harm done. With a vitamin deficiency, however, the process may not be quick enough and the homocysteine levels can rise, leading to the build-up of cholesterol and damage to your arterial walls. In addition to levelling out the amounts of homocysteine in your body, these three B vitamins play important roles in various other immune functions. Because of this, you should make sure that they're included in your multivitamin.

Vitamin B_{12}

RDA: 1 mcg

This B vitamin, also known as cobalamin, helps create the protective lining of nerve cells, which is critical for a strong immune system.

A National Institute on Aging study found that disabled women over the age of 65 with a vitamin B_{12} deficiency were twice as likely to suffer from depression as those with a full store of the vitamin. A deficiency can lead to permanent neurological damage, disorientation and memory problems. The official group in the US that sets vitamin guidelines, the Food and Nutrition Board, recommends that everyone over 50 takes a vitamin B_{12} supplement. As you age, you absorb B_{12} much better from supplements than from food. In fact, 10 to 30 per cent of older adults lose their ability to absorb enough of this vitamin from food.

Vitamin B_6

RDA: 2 mg

Studies at Yale University found that people with diabetes who took 50 mg of vitamin B_6 three times a day for 6 weeks had fewer incidences of blood sugar sticking to proteins: a problem that can lead to kidney damage, nerve damage and cataracts. In addition, this vitamin, also known as pyridoxine, helps produce antibodies that fight infection.

Because most diets don't include enough vitamin B$_6$, it's a good idea to take it in a supplement. However, amounts exceeding the safe upper limit of 100 mg, such as were consumed in the Yale studies, can lead to nerve damage.

Folic Acid (Folate)

RDA: 200 mcg

Folate comes from natural sources; folic acid is the synthetic form used in supplements and fortified foods. Folic acid is about twice as potent as folate.

When folic acid is lacking, cells lose their ability to divide and multiply. This is one reason why folic acid is so critical for pregnant women; a deficiency can lead to serious birth defects. But whether you are pregnant or not, you need folic acid so that your cells can continue to multiply and divide healthily.

Experts recommend taking a multivitamin with 200 mcg of folic acid daily because this synthetic form is absorbed almost twice as well as the folate found in food.

Better Health with These Three

Among the vast number of vitamins and minerals, there are three that stand out. Doctors recommend that all adult men and women take supplements of vitamin E, vitamin C and calcium, even if they're already taking a multivitamin. Many experts feel that for optimal health, you may need more than the RDA. These recommendations are referred to in this book as the Suggested Daily Intake.

Vitamin E

Suggested Daily Intake: 70–250 mg

One of the marvels of the immune system is the ability of its cells to identify dangerous bacteria, viruses and other antigens and hunt them down. Those defensive weapons (the macrophages) need vitamin E to know when to go to battle. Vitamin E (RDA: 10 mg) becomes even more critical as you age because your immune system tends to become more sluggish and produces fewer cytokines, chemical messengers that arouse the immune defence.

In a study at Tufts University in Boston, researchers found that older adults who took 150 mg of synthetic vitamin E daily for 8 months reported fewer bouts of colds, flu and pneumonia. It's practically impossible to get that amount of vitamin E from food alone, no matter how healthy your diet. Fortunately, your body doesn't care whether the vitamin E you give it is synthetic or natural. You get the benefits either way.

Be sure to take vitamin E supplements with food, including some fat for better absorption.

Vitamin C

Suggested Daily Intake: 100–500 mg

This vitamin, whose RDA is 60 mg, is a powerful antioxidant that protects cells from free radicals, unstable molecules that may lead to cancer, heart disease and other health problems. It may help you cope with stress because it aids your adrenal glands in the production of adrenalin and noradrenalin – hormones that mobilise energy. Studies show that people who get the most vitamin C reduce their risk of cataracts. Finally, people who suffer from fatigue may be deficient in vitamin C, which allows the body to convert fatty acids into fuel.

The best way to maintain your levels of vitamin C all day is to take half the amount in the morning, and the other half at night.

Calcium

Suggested Daily Intake: 1,000 mg
(If over 50, the suggested daily intake is 1,200 mg)

Your bones will pay a price if you omit this mineral, which also plays a role in helping your blood to clot. So will your muscles and your heart. You need the healing power of calcium to help regulate your muscle function: the movement of calcium ions in the cells allows your muscles to relax and contract, and the calcium in your body interacts with potassium and sodium to help your heart beat, and to control its rhythm.

Take 500 mg of calcium at a time for maximum absorption. You may need to take calcium supplements several times a day to ensure that you get enough of this mineral. Take calcium carbonate with meals; calcium citrate can be swallowed on an empty stomach.

However, when you take supplements with calcium-rich meals, some calcium may be wasted. Consider breakfast, for instance. Foods such as cereal and orange juice are often fortified with calcium. In addition, there's calcium in the milk for your cereal and coffee, and there's some in your multivitamin. Add it up, and you could be near the maximum calcium your body can absorb at one time – 500 mg. Time your supplement for a meal with less calcium. This could be a good excuse to have a small snack before bedtime: if you take a calcium supplement before going to bed, you may help limit calcium loss from your bones while you sleep.

Note: If you are over 50, find a calcium formula with vitamin D, which is crucial to proper calcium absorption.

Essential Minerals

The following minerals are critical in helping you to boost your immunity and balance your whole system. Make sure that your multivitamin/mineral supplement contains these minerals, but also be aware that the amount you're consuming in foods (read the nutrition label to learn the specific amount that a food contains). These are powerful nutrients, and you don't want to overdo them.

Selenium

Suggested Daily Intake: 75 mcg

This mineral, found in varying quantities in meat, dairy products and grains, is a powerful cancer fighter. It protects your cells from harmful free radicals. Studies of people who took selenium supplements found that they had one-half the risk of cancer death, and one-third the risk of contracting any form of cancer, than those who took no selenium supplements.

The problem is that selenium levels in food aren't consistent, so a mineral supplement is a good idea – except that too much selenium can be toxic. The amount of selenium in most multivitamins is safe.

Zinc

RDA: 15 mg

This trace mineral is essential for the production of white blood cells, which produce the antibodies that protect your immune system. Zinc also promotes healing. In one study, people who sucked on zinc lozenges every 2 hours recovered from their cold symptoms almost twice as quickly as those who didn't take zinc. (For more information on zinc lozenges for colds, see 'The Right Zinc' on page 174.)

Copper

Suggested Daily Intake: 1.2–3 mg

Copper is a trace mineral that helps your white cells transform into fighting cells against germs. You may not need much to do the work, but the average woman gets only 0.96 mg a day, and the average man gets only 1.27 mg a day. Even a marginal deficiency can suppress the immune system.

Be aware that copper absorption can become impaired if your level of zinc is elevated. Make sure that your multivitamin supplement contains copper in the form of copper citrate or copper picolinate for the best absorption.

Iron

RDA: 14 mg

Your cells need this mineral for their oxygen supply and one indication that you're iron-deficient, or anaemic, is fatigue. Iron helps carry oxygen to all cells, including your immune cells. Without enough iron, your body produces fewer antibodies and your immune defences are slowed to the point that they don't go after invaders.

Caution: Take more than 14 mg a day *only* if you are diagnosed with an iron deficiency. Too much iron may be linked to heart disease. If you take iron supplements, or a multivitamin with iron, when you take a calcium supplement, the iron absorption will lessen.

Polishing Facet 2 of Your Vitality Diamond

Now that you know which are the most important vitamins and minerals for maintaining your immune system, take a careful look at your diet and try to identify where any nutritional gaps might exist. For example, if you're a vegetarian, you might not be getting adequate amounts of vitamin B_{12}, zinc or calcium. In addition, consider what your body may be trying to tell you. If you've been feeling tired lately and you can't identify an obvious reason why, you could be anaemic. Work with your doctor to see whether you should take iron supplements. If you are a post-menopausal woman who lives in a region where there is often too little sunshine, consider adding some vitamin D to your supplement schedule. If you have no specific health concerns, try taking a multivitamin/mineral supplement as extra nutritional insurance. Be sure to select one that contains the nutrients we've identified in this chapter as being vital to your health. If you're already taking a multivitamin, try adding vitamin E, vitamin C and calcium and see how you feel.

When you fill in your own Vitality Diamond at the end of part 4, write down your supplement choice for Facet 2. Remember, you can replace what is written in this facet with something else whenever you like. As long as you choose supplements from the list in this chapter and pay attention to our dosage guidelines, you will be enhancing your immune system.

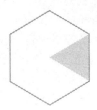

FACET 3:
THE MAXIMMUNITY
EXERCISE PLAN

THE SECRET TO A LONG, HEALTHY LIFE HAS BEEN AFFIRMED — AND it is exercise.

Exercise is one of only a few activities known to improve your quality of life and help you live longer, declares S. Jay Olshansky, PhD, professor in the School of Public Health at the University of Illinois at Chicago and author of *The Quest for Immortality: Science at the Frontiers of Aging*. Exercise can be as simple as putting one foot in front of the other and going for a walk in your neighbourhood or your local park, and it can be as relaxing as it is invigorating. This is the facet of your Vitality Diamond that can be polished at any age for strength, balance and agility.

From planting flowers in your garden to running a marathon, every type of exercise enhances your immune system. When you work out, your immune cells respond with a kind of enthusiasm: the natural killer cells flourish, building up your resistance to viruses and germs and other invaders.

'There is almost nothing better than exercise,' says Bruce S Rabin, MD, PhD, director of the Brain, Behavior, and Immunity Center at the University of Pittsburgh School of Medicine, and author of *Stress, Immune Function, and Health: The Connection*. After only 10 minutes of walking, you can boost your energy and reduce your stress level for up to an hour later.

Researchers at Duke University Medical Center in Durham, North Carolina, report that aerobic exercise is just as effective as medication in treating major depression in middle-aged and elderly people. With the increased activity, the heart pumps blood more effectively, improving the flow of oxygen-rich blood to specific areas of the brain. Aerobic exercise also enhances the immune system. White blood cells circulate throughout the body more quickly, which means they have more opportunities to combat viruses and bacteria.

Another study conducted by researchers at the Appalachian State University in Boone, North Carolina, found that over a 12- to 15-week period, people who walked briskly almost daily reduced their number of sick days by half compared with the sick days taken by those who were inactive.

Researchers at Temple University in Philadelphia asked a group of 22 healthy obese women to participate in a weight-reduction and exercise programme to evaluate the reduction of natural killer cell activity associated with weight loss from low-calorie diets. After 8 weeks, the study revealed that a combined programme of diet and light- to moderate-intensity aerobic exercise stabilised powerful natural killer cells responsible for combating illness. This study confirms the importance of incorporating exercise as part of any weight-loss programme.

To take advantage of the immune-boosting effects of exercise, follow the advice below.

Stand Tall

The first step to incorporating movement into your life is to pay attention to your posture. Good posture will make you feel better about yourself, says Lisa Dorfman, MS, RD, a sports nutritionist and certified

Olympic-level triathlon/track and field coach in Miami. Most people with backaches, headaches, stiff necks, restricted breathing and sore thighs, legs and ankles can attribute these maladies to slumping. When you slump, your muscles and ligaments become strained and your lungs and other organs have no 'breathing room' of their own. You hurt and may become stressed by the aches and pains, which sets off a gush of stress hormones that can hamper your immunity.

We have been supporting ourselves against the force of gravity since we learned to stand on two feet. It sounds like a lot of work, but by standing and sitting tall, you can breathe more easily and move more easily – without pain and stress, says Dorfman. Your spine will lengthen, your neck will relax and your joints and muscles will operate with less tension.

To take advantage of the health benefits of good posture, try the following tips, recommends Dorfman.

• Stand or sit with your shoulders back. Hold this position, taking slow, deep breaths. You can do this any time during the day.

• Practise tightening your abdominal muscles. Hold for a count of three (keep breathing), and then relax. Do this two or three times every 2 to 3 hours. Try it while standing in a queue at the supermarket or bank, when you're stopped at a red light in your car and even while you're watching television.

• Think about how you're standing, especially when you're forced to stand for a long time. Balance yourself on both feet. If you become tired, shift your weight from one foot to the other.

• If you sit at a desk for long periods of time, choose a straight-backed chair. Sit back in it so that your shoulders are against the chair. Keep your chest lifted and your upper back straight. Keep your weight evenly divided on your right and left buttocks. Keep your feet flat on the floor. If your chair is too high and cannot be adjusted, place your feet on a book or footstool.

• Regardless of the length of your trip, fix the driver's seat in your car so that you can easily reach the steering wheel, accelerator and brake. Occasionally switch the seat position, tilting it forward or back and change your posture from time to time to alleviate postural fatigue.

Think of an imaginary wire attached to the top of your head that's keeping your head up. This will help you to maintain a healthy posture. If you're on a long trip, stop every 2 hours to stretch.

In addition to the tips above, try the following routine created by Suki Munsell, PhD, president of the Dynamic Health and Fitness Institute in Corte Madera, California. When you do this routine, called the short shirt-pull, you imagine that you're taking a shirt off.

Cross your arms at your wrists in front of you, as if to pull a shirt off over your head. Gradually raise your crossed wrists upward until they're high above your head, fully stretching your arms overhead. Remember to lift your face into a smile as you inhale, while raising your arms. Lengthen your torso as you reach toward the sky. Exhale, and return your arms to your sides while continuing to grow taller through your spine. While keeping your head level, imagine that you're lifting your head into a sparkling crown. Repeat.

As you lower your arms, drop your shoulders like a shirt resting on a

Short Shirt-Pull

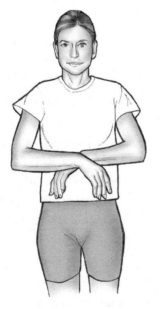 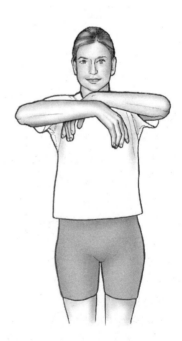

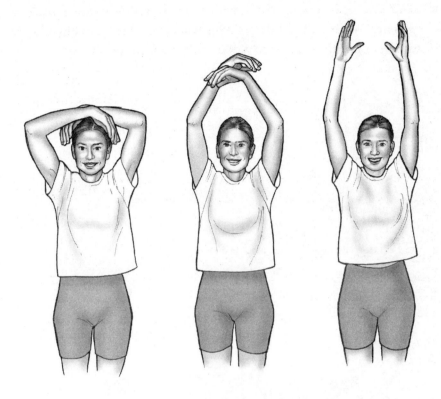

hanger. Repeat several more times, imagining that you're pulling off your old body, revealing a lighter, brighter you. Resist the urge to arch your back. Keep your head level, as if you were scanning the road ahead – the way you would while driving a car.

You can do this standing still or while walking. In a 15-minute walk, do this 6 to 10 times.

Use Your Breath to Relax

'The breath functions like a flywheel that drives all other involuntary functions, setting the tone for good health,' says yoga expert Rolf Sovik, PhD, PsyD, senior instructor at the Himalayan International Institute of Yoga Science and Philosophy in Honesdale, Pennsylvania. 'The first goal in systematic breath training is to create a relaxed breath that is both deep and smooth. With only a little practice, you can feel the breath naturally cleanse and nourish you as it moves through your body.'

Try the following two yoga poses provided by Dr Sovik. They'll help you to relax, which will boost your immunity.

For the Corpse posture, also known as *savasana*, lie on your back on a firm, flat surface. Rest your arms 15–20 cm (6–8 in) from your sides, with your palms up. Spread your feet 23–30 cm (10–12 in) apart, allowing them to drop open on the sides. Support your head and neck with a thin cushion if you want to. Bring your shoulder blades slightly together and draw them down, away from your ears, opening your chest, then relax. Close your eyes. Let the feeling of stillness in your body grow. Relax your abdomen and feel the rise and fall of your stomach with each breath. Let the muscles of your chest wall soften, and gradually deepen each breath. Lie resting for 6 to 10 minutes, relaxing your body, breath and mind.

Corpse Posture

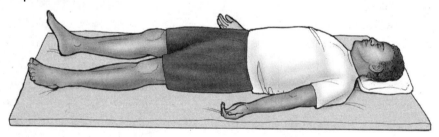

For the Crocodile posture, lie face down with your arms folded under your head. Your chest is slightly off the floor and your forehead rests on your crossed forearms. Your torso is slightly raised and supported by your elbows. Your legs should be 45–60 cm (18–24 in) apart, with your toes turned out. This posture will help you better use your diaphragm, which is below your lungs and is the principal muscle of breathing. You will feel the sides of your ribs expand and contract as you breathe. Once you've settled into this pose, stay there for 5 to 7 minutes. Let your breath soothe you.

Crocodile Posture

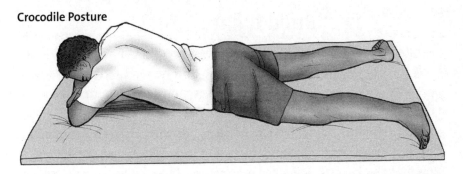

Now that you are relaxed you are ready to move on to the other elements in your exercise routine.

Exercise Basics

When you think of exercise, you undoubtedly think of physical activity such as walking, running, swimming and cycling. With these kinds of activities, you're increasing your heart rate to strengthen your heart and lungs.

How long do you need to exercise each day to get these benefits? The standard recommendation is 30 minutes a day, but many doctors believe that you can divide this amount into three 10-minute sessions. 'I find that my patients aren't as intimidated when we say it's just 10 minutes, three times a day,' says Keith Berndtson, MD, medical director at Integrative Care Centers in Chicago and Glenview, Illinois, and adviser to this book. 'This shows them that it's not so hard to be active.'

To get the full benefit from physical activity, you also need to work on your balance, improve your flexibility and agility and strength train, says Dr Berndtson. We'll explain the benefits of each of these in detail in the rest of the chapter and give you some practical tips for incorporating these elements into your exercise routine and for making time for exercise in general.

Finally, set realistic goals, and find activities that you enjoy, Dr Berndtson recommends. 'You don't have to do everything all at once. Start one foot at a time.'

Build Balance First

Now that you're relaxed and have good posture you need to work on your balance. Falls are the leading cause of injury-related deaths among people over the age of 65. One out of every three adults in that age group falls each year, breaking hips and other bones.

It's no wonder, then, that fear of falling increases with age, and this fear can be a major deterrent to participating in activities, says Dr Rabin. To improve your balance, you need to exercise. 'The equation is a simple one: exercise equals better strength and balance, which equals fewer fractures,' say John W Rowe, MD, and Robert L Kahn, PhD, in their book *Successful Aging*.

To improve your balance, start with the 'clock leg reach' exercise.

Pretend that there is a clock face drawn on the ground. Stand in its

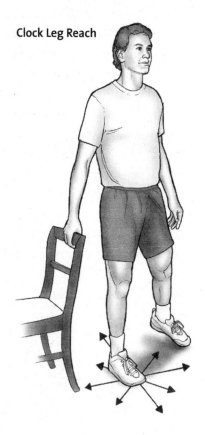

Clock Leg Reach

centre while holding on to a table or the back of a chair for support with your right hand. Keep your left arm relaxed at your side. While looking ahead with your shoulders slightly back, lift your left foot off the ground and, without changing the direction you're facing, touch the floor with your toes as you point to all of the hours on the clock. Alternate directions as you get better, pointing first, for example, at the 10:00, then the 5:00, then the 2:00, and finally the 12:00. Then, turn around and support yourself with the opposite hand, and repeat. Do this once for each leg. Having a partner call numbers randomly to catch you off guard will increase the difficulty.

Here are some additional tips for easy exercises recommended by

Dorfman to help you improve your balance.

• Stand in front of a wall, keeping your feet about hip-width apart. Without bending your knees, roll your weight on to the balls of your feet as far as you can. If necessary, touch the wall to steady yourself, but try not to tip or let your heels leave the floor. Then, roll your weight backwards on to your heels, without lifting your toes. Do this on a daily basis.

• Stand with the side of your body next to a wall. While bending your knee, lift one foot. If necessary, touch the wall to steady yourself. How long does it take before you start to teeter? This will help you practise building balance until you can stand on one foot at a time for 1 minute. Remember to change sides.

Stretch for Flexibility and Agility

As your balance improves, you should also work on stretching your muscles. Stretching keeps your muscles flexible, helping you to increase your range of motion so that you don't injure them. It's important, therefore, to stretch for about 5 to 10 minutes before and after workouts. Stretching also relaxes you, which banishes stress and damaging hormones. Here are some stretching exercises some experts say that you can do almost any time. Remember not to bounce but to move slowly and evenly into your stretch, so that you feel resistance. Hold each stretch for 10 to 20 seconds, always breathing. Do each stretch two to four times.

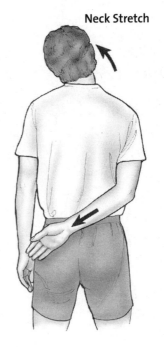

Neck Stretch

Neck stretch. Lean your head sideways towards your left shoulder as you reach your right arm down and across, behind your back. Keep your left arm relaxed at your side. Hold an easy stretch for 10 seconds. Then repeat on the right side. You can do this stretch standing, sitting on the floor, or on a chair.

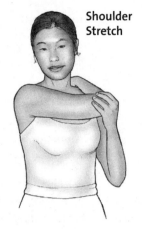

Shoulder Stretch

Shoulder stretch. Hold your right arm across your chest at shoulder level, with your palm facing back behind you. Grasp your right elbow with your left hand, then press the crook of your elbow towards your chest. Repeat with your left arm.

Hamstring stretch. Lie on your back, keeping your lower back pressed to the floor. Bend both knees and keep your feet flat on the floor. Bring your hands to the back of your left thigh and slowly straighten and raise your left leg. Gently pull your left leg in towards your torso until you feel a stretch in the back of your leg. Hold for 10 seconds, then repeat with your right leg. Repeat one or two times with each leg.

Hamstring Stretch

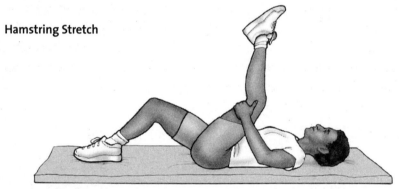

Calf Stretch

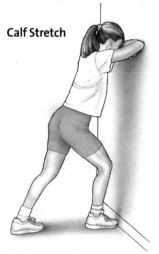

Calf stretch. Stand a few feet from a wall. Rest your forearms against the wall, and bring your right leg out in front of you with the knee bent. Your knee should not extend past your toes. Keep your left leg straight and your foot flat on the floor. Slowly lean forwards on your right leg until you feel a stretch in the back of your left calf. Then slightly bend your left knee to extend the stretch. Hold for 10 to 15 seconds. Switch legs and repeat. Remember to do this exercise very slowly.

Become Strong

To build stronger muscles and burn more calories even when you're not working out, exercise experts say that you need to incorporate strength-building exercises into your exercise routine. Here are a few to get you started.

Biceps curl. Stand with your feet shoulder-width apart. Grasp a dumbbell in each hand and hold them at your sides with your palms facing forwards. While keeping your arms at your sides and your elbows tucked in against the sides of your body, raise the weights by bringing your lower arms up until you're holding the weights at shoulder height. Your elbows should be pointing down. Lower slowly. Repeat this exercise 8 to 10 times using 1.5–2.5 kg (3–5 lb) weights. Do 3 sets. Begin with the lighter weight and gradually build up to more weight and repetitions.

Biceps Curl

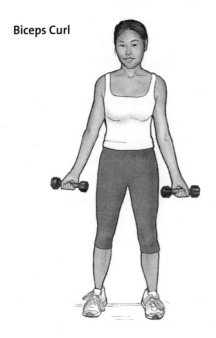 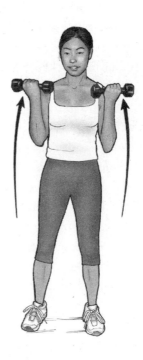

Lateral Shoulder Raise

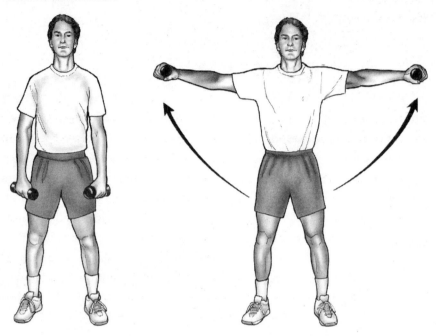

Lateral shoulder raise. Stand with your feet shoulder-width apart. Grasp a dumbbell in each hand and hold them at your sides with your palms turned inwards, facing your thighs. Keeping your elbows bent slightly but not locked, your arms straight, raise the weights out to the sides until your elbows are just slightly higher than your shoulders. Lower slowly. Do 3 to 5 repetitions and 2 sets using 0.5–1.5 kg (1–3 lb) dumbbells. Begin with the lighter weight and gradually build up to more weight and repetitions.

Inner-thigh lift. Lie on your left side with your head resting on your folded left arm. Place your right hand on the floor in front of you, palm down, for balance. Bend your right leg and rest your right knee on a rolled-up towel in front of you at hip level. Raise your left leg about 15–20 cm (6–8 in) off the floor and hold for 3 to 5 seconds, then lower. Do 3 sets of 8 repetitions each, then switch sides.

Curl-up. Lie on your back with your pelvis tilted to flatten your back against the floor, arms at your sides, knees bent at about a 90-degree angle,

Inner-Thigh Lift

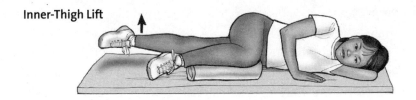

and feet flat on the floor. Using your upper abdominal muscles, raise your head and shoulders from the floor. Your arms should be extended out in front. Hold for 2 seconds, then lower your shoulders to the floor in a slow, controlled motion, touching your shoulders lightly to the floor. Do 8 to 12 repetitions per set, progressing to 3 sets as you advance.

Curl-Up

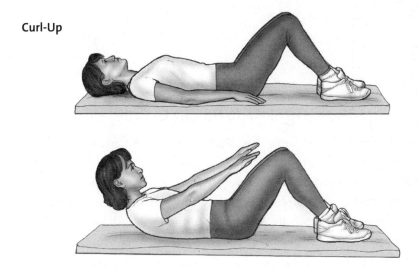

Make Aerobics Simple

All it takes to get fit is putting one foot in front of the other – and what better way to do that than walking? Walking is one activity that you can incorporate into everything you do, says Dr Berndtson. Yet one study found that the first thing to go when women are too busy and stressed is aerobic exercise.

If you can just manage to continue walking, though, you'll do yourself a world of good – *particularly* when you're stressed. Studies show that walking reduces the production of stress hormones, making you feel calmer and happier. It also helps keep your bones strong, helps reduce your levels of bad cholesterol and strengthens your heart muscles. Here are some tips for increasing your steps.

• If you can't find the time to walk until after dark, walk around your living room instead of going outside. Get up during every commercial break for a couple of laps. Or, if you can, invest in a treadmill and walk while you watch TV.

• Walk early in the morning before the rest of your household is up. This will give you time to yourself to think about your day.

• Take it easy. You aren't out to win the fastest-time medal. Keep your walks leisurely to avoid the stress of competition – even against yourself.

Making Time for Exercise

If you're worried that you're too busy to fit exercise into each day, remember that you can break up the recommended 30 minutes a day into three 10-minute segments. If even carving just 10 minutes at a time out of your schedule seems impossible, simply incorporating movement into your everyday routine can still make a big difference, says Dr Berndtson. The problem with many of our lifestyles is that movement is no longer a natural part of our day. For example, we work at desks where we have everything we need – computers, telephones, fax machines – so we never have to get out of our chairs. And with e-mail, many of us don't even have to walk to our colleagues' offices any more when we have a question. Furthermore, we find it easy to hop in our cars, even when our destination is only a few streets away.

When Tracey Perles started her own public relations firm at home in Upper St Clair, Pennsylvania, she didn't know when she would ever be able to fit in her two favourite activities: running and walking. Finally, it dawned on her that she could run and/or walk to the post office, the office supplies shop, even the supermarket. 'There isn't a day I don't have to run out to do something,' she says. 'I put on my backpack and, depending on my mood, I walk or run. If I don't have to meet with anyone that day, I can stay in my workout clothes until I feel like changing after I get home!'

Virginia Linn, a health editor in Pittsburgh, has a different kind of work schedule. With three children under the age of 10, she is up early to get them ready for school and watch them board the school bus. She meets them at the bus in the afternoon and then has to rush them to piano lessons, gymnastics and other activities. Then, dinner. She had no time to indulge in her favourite exercise, running. 'I was wondering when I'd ever be able to fit exercise into my schedule again,' she says. She did – at home with a skipping rope.

The moderate impact of a skipping rope can help build strong bones. Since blood cells are primarily made in the bone marrow, there may be a link between healthy, strong bones and a strong immune system. You can split the workout into 2- to 3-minute sessions, three times a day, for a good workout while watching the children. (They will probably want to join in.) Gradually build up to three 10-minute sessions.

Use Tracey and Virginia as your inspiration to find ways to incorporate more movement into your schedule. Here are some ideas to get you started.

• Park far from your office, and walk.

• If you must park close to your office, then walk up the stairs to your office. If you're on the 20th floor, walk to the fifth floor and take the lift the rest of the way. In a few weeks, you'll be able to tackle several more flights.

• Take the bus. You can walk to and from the bus stops, and leave the rush-hour driving to someone else.

• Drink lots of water, but only use water fountains on different floors.

• As often as possible, instead of sending e-mails from your desk to a colleague in another office, go in person.

• If you can't get away from your desk for lunch, walk around the office for 10 minutes, at least.

At home, think of domestic chores – scrubbing floors, vacuuming, mowing the lawn, raking leaves – as opportunities. By the end of the day, you will have added a few minutes here and a few minutes there into your exercise routine.

Of course, exercise is not all about work. Try gardening, playing tennis, fast dancing, swimming and volleyball.

Polishing Facet 3 of Your Vitality Diamond

Adding exercise into your lifestyle doesn't require a huge time commitment. As little as 30 minutes a day is enough to boost your immune system and improve your overall health.

Start by paying attention to your posture. Good posture will help ease muscle aches caused by slumping, and it will improve your general outlook. Also, pay attention to your breathing. Try our suggested yoga poses, which will help you to focus on your breath and to notice when you're breathing shallowly. Then, move on to improving your balance. Simply standing on one foot and, over a number of days, trying to increase the amount of time you can do this without teetering will help you to focus on your balance and give you more confidence as you begin to exercise.

Before and after working out, make sure you stretch your muscles for about 5 to 10 minutes. This will improve your range of motion and help prevent injury. It can also help you to relax. Finally, make sure you include both weight training and aerobic exercise in your workouts. Weight training will tone and strengthen your muscles, increase your bone density and improve your metabolism, while aerobic exercise will help you to burn calories and improve your cardiovascular health. Furthermore the fact that you are moving, releasing stress and becoming more in tune with your body will boost your immune system immeasurably.

Start your exercise programme today by filling in Facet 3 of the Vitality Diamond provided on page 379 with your first steps.

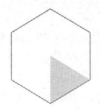

FACET 4:
THE MAXIMMUNITY
STRESS RELIEF
AND SLEEP PLAN

TAKE A MOMENT NOW, IF YOU WILL, TO LIST SOME OF THE THINGS you've done lately to make you feel better about yourself: actions as simple as lending a sympathetic ear, calling a friend just to say hello, holding a door open for someone carrying packages, or taking a bubble bath.

1.

2.

3.

4.

If you can't think of anything, perhaps you were too tired to do anything, or too stressed, or maybe you've simply forgotten what you did.

When Stress Makes You Forget

When you're stressed, your body releases the hormone cortisol, which, in high levels over prolonged periods, is toxic to the nervous system. Over time, cortisol kills neurons by keeping them from using oxygen and glucose. The result: memory loss. In fact, the hippocampus (the part of the brain directly related to short-term memory) has been found to be smaller in highly stressed people than in those who aren't extremely stressed.

If you're among the millions of people today who feel extremely stressed, this news about memory loss may seem discouraging and frightening. But don't give up hope. In this chapter, we'll introduce you to some practical steps you can take to improve your ability to both relax and sleep better and, in so doing, enhance your immune system and stave off the memory-harming effects of stress.

Even though we'll be working in small steps, the joy of following these stress and sleep cure tips is that every time you master one, you will feel better, says Keith Berndtson, MD, medical director at Integrative Care Centers in Chicago and Glenview, Illinois. You already know that when you are stressed and tired, immune-busting agents create a cascading effect, attacking your immune system and making you more vulnerable to illness and disease. 'Fortunately, you get a positive hormonal cascading effect when you do something nice for your body – like watching a funny movie with a good friend, or getting a good night's sleep,' says Dr Berndtson.

Take Control of Your Time

Too often, we lose precious time – and lose sight of our priorities – just trying to gain a sense of control over our daily lives. When we're constantly working in emergency mode, our bodies and our health pay the price. Here are some practical strategies for regaining control over your time. As you make them part of your life, you'll begin to feel less stressed and anxious, and your immune system will become stronger and stronger.

Budget your time. At some point, you've probably made a list of your family's expenses so that you could create a budget that would help you save money. You can use this same technique to help manage your time. Think of your time as money, and prepare a 'time budget'. First, write down *everything* you do: consider it your inventory. There's commuting time, errands, housework, watching television, cooking, talking on the telephone and helping your daughter with her science project – even sleeping. Now that you have your inventory, you can take the next step.

Schedule yourself. When you schedule activities – even enjoyable ones – into your day, you will find that you have more control over your time. On the other hand, when you skip your favourite walk in the park or forget to eat lunch, you become tense and tired. Remember that one of the best things you can do for your immune system is to enjoy yourself. With a schedule, you'll be able to go out for that walk.

Put white space in your calendar. You've made a schedule; now make it flexible. This will encourage you to think of priorities so that you don't blindly add one more thing to your day. Are you spending too much time at work? 'No one is ever going to be eulogised for working himself to death,' points out Bruce S Rabin, MD, PhD, director of the Brain, Behavior, and Immunity Center at the University of Pittsburgh School of Medicine and author of *Stress, Immune Function, and Health: The Connection*. 'They'll think he's a jerk because he didn't know how to relax. It was an opportunity lost.'

Make a to-do list and stick to it. Make a list of the really important things you need (and want) to do, giving each a priority level. Then ask your family for help in getting them done. If necessary, hire a professional organiser to get you on the right track.

Remember: be realistic. So you're not going to write a work of literary genius by the time you're 50. Instead, write letters to your friends and family. You'll have the satisfaction of knowing that they will be cherished. Even e-mail is a helpful way to promote connectedness with others. Though these things are not a substitute for real, human contact, they can combat the immune-dampening effects of social isolation.

Changing your day-to-day lifestyle does not occur overnight, but it also doesn't happen if you keep putting things off. Start with this: every hour, take 5 minutes for yourself. Close your eyes and visualise something pleasant, like a visit to the zoo with your children, a sailing adventure, or a walk in the park. By taking 5 minutes, you can begin to understand that stress relief is not a time robber: it is an immunity enhancer.

More Tips on Stress Relief

Once you've used the tips above to gain a little more control over your daily schedule, you can begin to think about how you can work some stress relievers into your calendar. Here are some suggestions from Dr Berndtson to get you started.

Become friends with your diary. Buy a diary and write in it every day, listing the things that made you feel stressed and out of control. How long did you feel that way? What were your reactions? How often did you snap at your son? What did he say or do to make you react angrily? What did you say? Over time, this will help you look at the triggers that cause you to be upset, and allow you to brainstorm better ways of handling them.

Try progressive muscle relaxation (PMR). This technique uses no special equipment and can be practised practically anywhere. When no one is home or the children are asleep, try this: lie down on a comfortable surface. Take a few deep breaths. Slowly tighten, then relax, different muscles in your body, starting at your head and going all the way to your toes. As you tighten the muscles, inhale deeply, then hold the tension for several seconds. Relax and exhale slowly. This exercise can help you enhance your own awareness of where muscle tension builds up in your body. Then, when you're in a stressful situation and you feel your body becoming tense, you can use what you've learned to help yourself relax.

'If you think PMR sounds right for you but want some expert advice on the technique, consult with a psychologist who specialises in stress management,' says Dr Berndtson.

Explore other relaxation techniques. Try yoga, meditation, or guided imagery – or even daydreaming – to take your mind off the daily problems that lead to stress. Some studies show that relaxation techniques such as these heighten the natural killer cell activity in your immune system.

These techniques don't have to be complicated. For example, you might sit comfortably with your eyes closed and imagine a warm beach, a waterfall, or the rolling waves of the ocean. Let the hot sand warm up your hands, a sign that bloodflow is being redirected to your skin and that you are releasing tension. Or sit comfortably, with your eyes focused on a single object, such as a flower. Breathe deeply as you look at this flower. Think about nothing else except the flower.

Another option is to lie down, close your eyes and breathe deeply and slowly, letting your stomach expand outwards with each inhalation. Focus on your breathing. As you inhale, concentrate on one word. Say the word slowly. Try saying the word *calm* as you inhale. Repeat the word *calm* as you exhale. Continue this until you feel relaxed. Practise this technique for about 5 minutes, or 60 calm breathing cycles.

Avoid negativity. There are only so many hours in a day, so make an effort to surround yourself with positive people. Negative people have a way of sapping your energy. If you must be around them, acknowledge their negativity to yourself so that you can mentally deflect it. Remember that you can limit the time you spend with people who sap your energy. When a negative person approaches you, stand up while talking to her. That way, you can cut the conversation short, walking away for another commitment (you don't need to explain what it is) after a short period. If it is someone you must spend time with, take short but frequent breaks from him or her.

Become attuned to the power of prayer. In studies at Duke University Medical Center in Durham, North Carolina, researchers have shown that prayer enhances the immune system. When you pray, you're actually engaging in a form of visualisation, so it's no surprise that prayer can leave you feeling renewed and calm.

Learn about essential oils. You can relieve stress by stopping to smell the rosemary. Certain essential oils (distilled from roots, leaves, flowers and other plant material) have energising effects on the nervous system. Place one drop of essential oil on a compress or a handkerchief and take a whiff. Try rosemary, basil, pine, hemlock, spruce, eucalyptus, or grapefruit.

Colour your surroundings. A new coat of paint on the walls can do a lot to improve your mood, according to colour behaviourists. Shades of green evoke serenity and are thought to help lower the heart rate. Blue encourages daydreaming and fantasising. Pink, violet and other shades of purple also have calming effects.

Try to find the funny side. It might sound trite, but trying to find the humour in a stressful situation really can help you get through it. Humour has been shown to improve blood circulation, suppress stress hormones and boost the immune system. In addition, it may release the body's feel-good chemicals, the endorphins. To take advantage of humour's health-boosting effects, try turning a stressful situation into a comedy routine in your mind. It's hard to take those gossipy colleagues in your department seriously, for example, when you picture them as a comedy double-act.

Change the scenery. If you can't take a 'real' holiday, at least try to get yourself away from your usual stressful environment for a day – or even a few hours. A trip to the zoo or a museum may help you take your mind off stressful problems. Or take a class for fun, such as dancing lessons: the exercise will help relieve your stress, and you'll meet other people who enjoy dancing, too.

Fill a worry box. A shoebox will do to start with. As the year progresses, fill it with items that represent the stresses in your life: office memos, newspaper clippings, meeting agendas. When you put them in the box, you're stashing away worries that soon won't matter. When the box fills up, you can throw them away and start anew, collecting worries that magically disappear for no other reason than the passing of time.

Sleep Like a Baby

Once you've taken steps to reduce – or at least cope with – the stresses in your life, you may find that sleeping better comes naturally. If not, Dr Berndtson offers these tips to help ensure that your time between the sheets leaves you feeling refreshed and renewed.

Make breakfast your biggest meal of the day. Digesting food takes energy, so if you eat a heavy meal late in the day, your body will have to work hard to digest it while you're trying to go to sleep. Many people sleep better if they have protein at breakfast and lunch, and a light dinner with some carbohydrates.

Cut back on the sleep robbers. Cut out caffeine after 2.00 p.m., and refrain from drinking alcohol within 3 hours of bedtime. You may become drowsy after a couple of glasses of wine, but too much alcohol will make you wake up frequently during the night. In addition, although coffee is the most obvious source of caffeine, don't forget that there's also caffeine in colas, chocolate, tea and some medications.

Seek out the light. Get outside when it's sunny, or at least turn on the lights at home in the morning. This will help you reset your awake-sleep cycle.

Drink like a fish. Even mild dehydration – losing as little as 120 ml (4 fl oz) of body water – could turn into low-grade chronic fatigue. Drink eight to ten 240 ml (8 fl oz) glasses of water a day, and add four to six more glasses when you exercise. To prevent unnecessary trips to the bathroom at night, empty your bladder before going to sleep, and don't drink more than 120 ml (4 fl oz) within an hour of going to bed.

Exercise earlier in the day. Regular exercise first energises, then relaxes you. If you start doing calisthenics or aerobics just before bed, nerve-stimulating hormones will be released and will raise your body's core temperature, preventing you from falling asleep. Do your exercise earlier in the day.

Walk into sleep. You don't have to walk far to get sleep-enhancing benefits. People who walked for about 10 minutes a day at a normal pace were one-third less likely to have trouble sleeping, according to one study of more than 700 men and women. Those who walked at a fast pace had even better sleeping habits. You get the same benefits with walking that you'd get with sleep medication but without the medication's side effects, such as grogginess, increased snoring, risk of sleep apnoea and possible addiction.

Take a nap. A brief sleep is fine, especially if you didn't sleep well last night. Research has found that people who nap for 15 minutes feel more alert and less sleepy, even after a bad night's sleep.

Go to bed only when you're sleepy. If you can't fall asleep within 15 to 20 minutes, get up and leave your bedroom. Go into the living room and read until you're tired again. Or sit in a chair and think pleasant thoughts: a dream holiday, standing by a waterfall. This should help calm you so that you can return to bed and sleep.

Move the television out of your bedroom. Your bed and bed-room are for sleep and sex, nothing else. No reading, no talking on the telephone, no worrying.

Create a sleep schedule and stick to it. You put together a de-stressing schedule. Now, set a sleep schedule. You may not be able to go to bed at the same time every night, but you can establish a regular wake-up time. Get up at the same time every morning, even on weekends.

Watch your night-time posture. For a restful night, try these strate-gies.

• Relieve lower-back pressure by putting a pillow under your knees. The pillow comfortably flexes your lower spine.

• Try a pillow made with down instead of a foam pillow. You want a pillow that is low enough to support your head without flexing your neck, to avoid neck and shoulder aches. Orthopaedic pillows with a scooped-out hollow for your head help support the neck and can also be helpful, especially if you have chronic neck problems.

• Put enough covers on your bed to stay warm. You may otherwise unconsciously curl up to keep warm, which can leave you with a sore back.

• Allow yourself enough room to be able to move your arms and legs and roll over during the night. This is a natural way to prevent your joints from getting stiff.

Take special measures when you're on the night shift. You weren't designed to work the night shift, or rotating shifts, but you may have no choice. So, here are some tips for when you have to work while everyone else is asleep.

• Use bright lights to mimic daylight, to keep you awake.

• Try to stay on the same shift, but if you must rotate, do it by the clock: from days to afternoons to nights.

• If you can't sleep when you get home in the morning, don't force yourself. Wait till early afternoon when you have an energy dip.

Try a herbal soother. Instead of sleeping pills, you might want to try valerian, a herb that can improve your quality of sleep without leaving you feeling groggy the next morning. You need to allow about 2 weeks for valerian to build up in your system. Try taking between 150–300 mg at bedtime as needed, but take a break now and then to allow your sleep patterns to develop without help. You don't have to buy the more expensive valerian supplements that have other ingredients or herbs.

Polishing Facet 4 of Your Vitality Diamond

Reducing stress and getting a good night's sleep sound like good ideas, but if you're thinking that this is easier said than done, don't be discouraged. This facet may require the smallest time commitment of them all: just 5 minutes spent writing in your diary or visualising a peaceful place can make a huge difference in your stress levels.

Nearly everyone has made a budget at some point in their lives to help manage their finances. Apply this same philosophy to your most valuable resource: your time. Take a few minutes tonight to plan your day tomorrow. Look specifically at what you can eliminate: could you shorten that meeting with your colleague to half an hour instead of a full hour? Could your daughter get a lift to her football match with the neighbour down the street whose daughter is also on the team? Could you make a double batch of vegetable stir-fry so that you don't have to cook two nights in a row? Then, schedule some stress-relieving time just for you with those 'extra' minutes you've just uncovered. Try a few yoga poses. Say a silent prayer. Do whatever helps you to relax and unwind.

While you're planning your day, also take a look at what you can do during your waking hours to ensure that you have a peaceful night's sleep. Get out in the sunlight for a few minutes. Plan some exercise for the morning hours. Make your bedroom an oasis of calm by removing the television set or desk where you write out your bills. With simple changes like these, you're sure to have a less stressful day and a more peaceful night.

Resolve to make a change, however small, in the way you spend your time, and write it into your Vitality Diamond on page 379. You'll see why people say, 'Little things mean a lot.'

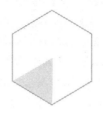

FACET 5:
THE MAXIMMUNITY EMOTIONAL QUOTIENT PLAN

Laugh and the world laughs with you,
Weep, and you weep alone;
For this brave old earth must borrow its mirth,
But has trouble enough of its own.

FROM THE POEM 'SOLITUDE', BY ELLA WHEELER WILCOX

BETH WESTBROOK REMEMBERS HOW DISTRAUGHT SHE WAS THE day her daughter's doctor explained to them that having an amputation was the only way to save Katie's life from the growing malignant tumour in her leg. Beth put her arm around Katie, who was only 12, as the doctor solemnly described the treatment. Suddenly, Katie stood up and shouted, 'Stop!'

No one spoke.

'The least you can do is tell a joke,' she said.

Silence. Then her parents started laughing. Her doctor joined in. Katie finally laughed, too. The tension was broken with the laughter. Everyone felt better – at least for the moment.

Good things happen when you laugh. Your pulse and respiratory rates rise, and then, when you stop, there is a brief period of relaxation, says Keith Berndtson, MD, medical director at Integrative Care Centers in Chicago and Glenview, Illinois. You feel good because the muscles you used while laughing had a light workout. If you laughed heartily, you involved a large mass of muscle tissue, so that your total body response provided some conditioning exercise. The relaxation that follows eases muscle tension. Your blood pressure drops. In short, laughter enhances your immune system.

'From that point, we took our cue from Katie. Every day, we look for the humour in a situation,' says Beth. 'I really believe that Katie's positive emotions have helped her. I know they've helped me cope.'

How It All Started

It is only in the past 30 years that the medical community has taken seriously the connection between the brain and the immune system. Robert Ader, PhD, remembers all too well the disdain from scientists when he reported a connection between the mind and conditioned immune changes in the body.

'They decided we had to have done something wrong,' says Dr Ader, director of behavioural and psychosocial medicine at the University of Rochester, New York, and co-author of *Psychoneuroimmunology*. 'Everyone knew there were no connections between the brain and the immune system.'

Undeterred, Dr Ader first coined the term *psychoneuroimmunology* in a paper in 1980. The term refers to the relationships among behaviour, nervous and endocrine functions and the immune system. In 1980, as president of the American Psychosomatic Society, he talked about his new work in psychoneuroimmunology. 'It was important,' he recalls. 'The data were good. It was consistent with my background in psychosomatic medicine – that you can't separate the mind from the body, and you can't separate one system from another. It's all one integrated system.'

Your Emotional Map

Dr Ader's self-described stubbornness paid off for all of us. Since he first spoke out on his theories, the scientific community has made remarkable progress in exploring the complex system of physiological, cognitive and emotional connections to the immune system.

Researchers have identified specific cells – such as the T-cells, B-cells, neutrophils and macrophages – that have specific duties in warding off the bacteria and viruses that are constantly attacking the body. The ability of these cells to do their job is influenced by your emotions. When you are anxious or agitated, stress hormones are secreted that interfere with your immune cells' ability to ward off infections.

When it comes to your immune system, your emotional outlook is as important to overall health as what you eat and how much you exercise.

Check Your Emotional Quotient

The place to start boosting your emotional outlook is at the beginning: with a self-assessment, says Dr Berndtson.

Take a moment to review the 15 questions below, suggests Dr Berndtson. They require only yes or no answers.

1. I am a happy person.
2. I have frequent crying spells.
3. I feel good about myself.
4. I can't stop feeling depressed.
5. I enjoy my friendships.
6. I feel alone in a crowd.
7. I work well with my colleagues.
8. I am tense all the time.
9. I have outside hobbies and interests.
10. I cannot concentrate.
11. I am hopeful about the future.

12. I cannot bear to read or listen to the news.
13. I control my time; it doesn't control me.
14. I feel out of control.
15. I believe that the glass is half-full.

If you answered yes to the positive statements (the odd numbers) and no to the negative statements (the even numbers), you have a healthy view of yourself and the world, and your immune system is enhanced because of that. More likely, your responses are mixed, meaning that you could do with some help in working out ways to have a more positive outlook.

Studies show that people who have negative outlooks – those who are depressed, hostile, cynical, hopeless, unempowered, or lonely – have suppressed immune systems and become ill more often than those who have a more positive view of their lives. One 30-year study at the Mayo Clinic in Rochester, Minnesota, found that pessimists were at a higher risk of dying early than optimists.

The same kind of immune response occurs when you are continually depressed. 'When someone is depressed or suppressing justified anger, the message sent from the mind to the body is: 'I guess we're not worth fighting for,' says Dr Berndtson.

Some researchers contend that there may be a connection between optimism and good health because people who have a rosier view of the world tend to take better care of themselves than those who are distressed. In her research, Anna L Marsland, RN, PhD, a psychologist at the Western Psychiatric Institute and Clinic at the University of Pittsburgh Medical Center, has found that there can also be other direct or indirect mitigating factors. Poor nutrition, smoking, drug and alcohol intake, lack of exercise and poor sleep are surefire ways to impair your immune system, she notes.

If you suspect that your mental outlook is negatively affecting your health, you need to take the time to closely examine your life – including the frustrations and joys – and reconnect with what makes you happy. 'Fortunately, the prescription for things you can do to empower your immune system includes a long list of emotional health strategies,' says Dr Berndtson. With these strategies, you'll not only gain a new perspective, you'll also be able to boost your immune system and make improvements to your overall health and well-being.

Faith Heals

Researchers believe that we can boost our mental outlooks – and improve our health – by nurturing our spiritual sides.

At Duke University in Durham, North Carolina, Harold G Koenig, MD, director of the Center for the Study of Religion/Spirituality and Health, says that his research demonstrates that prayer may neutralise negative emotions. Gaining the health benefits of spirituality takes more than attending services at your place of worship every week, however.

'Anyone can become religious and potentially reap the benefits,' says Dr Koenig, author of *The Healing Power of Faith*. 'But they can't become religious just to improve their health. They're going to have to become religious for some other reason. A side effect of becoming devoutly religious may be that your health improves.'

On a personal level, Dr Koenig, also author of *The Healing Connection*, says that he has been able to use his faith to help patients understand that there is always hope.

'Faith combines different modalities,' explains Dr Koenig. 'All social organisations are based upon a kind of a barter system. You do for other people, they do for you. But it's different in religious communities. There, people provide support to each other even when the other person can't return the favour. The social element is so important – the element of getting your eyes off of yourself and on to others.'

Indeed, some of the healing benefits of religion may have to do with the sense of connectedness we feel when we're part of a religious community. This sense has been sorely lacking in many people's high-tech lifestyles. 'In an age like this, where we have departed from human connection, where we're focused on using computer technology and e-mail and voice mail, we're distancing ourselves, and we're harming our immune systems,' says neurologist Barry Bittman, MD, chief executive officer and medical director of the Mind–Body Wellness Center in Meadville, Pennsylvania. By becoming part of a religious community, we can sometimes overcome this high-tech remoteness and put less distance between ourselves and others.

Control Your Anger

You've seen it in the films: the outraged man punches a hole in the wall. If it's a comedy, it might be funny to watch him writhe in pain. Except that there's nothing funny about venting your anger with aggression. It could be dangerous. Further, when people believe that they have 'permission' to react aggressively, they are more likely to do so. A study at Iowa State University in Ames found that when participants read material claiming that aggressive behaviour is a good way to relax and reduce anger, they became more aggressive than those who read messages saying just the opposite.

Acting out your frustrations only exacerbates the situation and can be counterproductive, says George Solomon, MD, a pioneer in psychoneuroimmunology and emeritus professor of psychiatry at UCLA. When your anger is uncontrolled, your immune system releases cytokines that bind to cells, leading to any one of a number of problems that can slow down or frustrate your immune system, including kidney, liver, lung and heart damage.

Diverting your energy into suppressing your anger is not a healthy thing to do either, however. Dr Solomon has documented immune-boosting advantages in HIV-positive patients who are assertive. Long-term survivors with AIDS are better able to express anger and say no when pressed than a control group of persons with AIDS. Immunologically, they also show high activity of their natural killer cells when compared to the control group.

A healthy immune system loves to triumph over adversity. You can help it do this by consciously making an effort to react in a balanced way to anger and frustration, neither lashing out nor meekly resigning yourself to unfair situations.

Music to Your Ears

Whether you have the voice of an angel or are completely tone-deaf, sing. Music is one of the most soothing ways to enhance your immune system. In fact, your brain may actually be wired for music. Researchers believe that the steady beat and rhythm of music can elicit a positive hormonal response. According to Dr Bittman, certain music stimulates the mind so that it can lower anxiety, lower your blood pressure, ease depression and help you focus.

The research on the practical uses of music in the health field has produced some intriguing results. For example, studies show that patients who listen to music during and after surgery need fewer sedatives for pain relief. Furthermore, a study at Colorado State University in Fort Collins showed that people with Parkinson's disease walked more steadily and with better balance and speed if they practised walking while listening to music.

Here are a few ways to put music into your life.

Keep your favourite CDs in your car. Listen to music while you're stuck in a traffic jam. Sing along and encourage your passengers to join in.

Keep a portable CD player in your handbag. The next time you're waiting in a long queue at the supermarket, pull out the headphones and listen to music while you wait.

Add music to household tasks. One woman puts on her favourite Christmas carols while she's cleaning her house. 'Even if it's July, I clean to Christmas carols. They keep me inspired,' she notes.

Dance. It doesn't matter if you do it alone or with a friend. You'll still get health-boosting benefits.

Child's Play

Children often amaze grown-ups with their carefree, spontaneous ways. Of course, they don't have mortgages, difficult bosses and home repairs to worry about. Still, we can learn some excellent outlook-improving strategies from them.

Buy some coloured chalk. With it, you can turn into a pavement artist. Since the next rainstorm will wash away your work, you can let your creativity loose. You can also use the chalk for your next game of hopscotch.

Memorise nursery rhymes. Then recite them to a friend. For an even bigger boost, skip while you chant the nursery rhymes.

Tell some jokes. There are dozens of humour websites on the Internet, and nearly every public library has books on humour. Entertain children with the silly jokes you find. They'll love you for it.

Read aloud. If you don't have a child, read aloud to yourself. Or visit a nearby nursing home and read to the residents.

Display your youth. Instead of packing away toys from childhood, show them off throughout your house. A stuffed animal here or comic book there will serve as reminders that you are still a child at heart.

Don't Be an Island

Take every opportunity to be sociable. Here again, when you feel connected to other people, your immune system responds favourably. It doesn't matter whether your social interaction makes you feel particularly happy or whether you simply don't feel lonely: you'll still be boosting your immune system, says Bruce S Rabin, MD, PhD, professor of pathology and psychiatry and director of the Brain, Behavior, and Immunity Center at the University of Pittsburgh School of Medicine, and author of *Stress, Immune Function, and Health: The Connection*. Your immune cells will be enhanced, which means that they'll be better able to protect you. Also, when you feel better about yourself, you will probably eat more healthily, sleep better, exercise and cut back on alcohol and cigarettes.

Not everyone can easily become the centre of the social whirl. Here are a few simple strategies from Dr Rabin to get you started.

Start small. You don't need to immediately begin throwing dinner parties for 20 to increase your level of social interaction. Try taking small steps to get more human contact into your everyday routine. For example, talk to people in shops or to the person on the checkout at the supermarket.

Make your commute 'people time'. Instead of driving alone, start up a car pool. Even better: take the bus. Take a sketch pad and draw those around you. It's almost guaranteed that someone will strike up a conversation with you.

Show an interest in other people's lives. Send an amusing card to a friend, then follow up with a telephone call. Or make friends with a nursing home resident and visit regularly.

Adopt a dog from the local animal shelter. Take him for long walks, and you'll find yourself stopping to talk to other dog owners in the neighbourhood. If you can't keep a dog, volunteer to take other people's dogs for a walk instead.

Use the dining room. Eat dinner with your family at the dining room or kitchen table – not in the living room in front of the television. 'How you eat is as important as what you eat,' says Leslie Bonci, RD, MPH, spokeswoman in Pittsburgh for the American Dietetic Association and the director of the sports medicine nutrition programme at the Center for Sports Medicine at the University of Pittsburgh Medical Center Health System. 'Taking the time to enjoy your food and your family and friends is part of eating healthily.'

Learn to play bridge. In one study, researchers at the University of California, Berkeley, had 12 women from Orinda, California, play bridge for 1½ hours. When the researchers took blood samples from the women before and after the bridge sets, they found an increase in their protective white blood cells in the post-game readings. Bridge involves skills stimulating the dorsolateral cortex, a part of the frontal lobe of the brain that may play a role in the immune system.

Have sex. In a recent study at Wilkes University in Wilkes-Barre, Pennsylvania, researchers found that regular sex can boost your immune system and keep colds and flu away. In addition, if you've been feeling like you've been drifting away from your partner, scheduling regular time to be intimate – even if you end up simply talking about how you've been feeling lately – will help you reconnect.

Random Acts of Kindness

You've heard of them: the person who spontaneously puts money in an expired parking meter for the car owner she will never meet; the friend who babysits so that the new mother can run errands; the neighbour who plants flowers in an elderly person's garden.

People who take the time for the little things seem to instinctively know what makes them – and others – feel good. They certainly don't fit the profile of the type A personality, the one who is so driven, so much the perfectionist, that he is more prone to disease. As studies show, negative emotions – hostility, resentfulness and anger – damage your immune system.

'We know that when people feel better, the biological effects are beneficial,' says Elizabeth A Bachen, PhD, assistant psychology professor at Mills College in Oakland, California.

Look for ways that you can randomly incorporate some kindness into your life. These don't need to be huge, time-consuming tasks. Try simple things like holding open a door for the person behind you, allowing someone with a few items to go ahead of you in the supermarket checkout queue when you have a full trolley, or offering to do some shopping for a housebound elderly neighbour or friend.

A Wake-Up Call

The way you start your day can be a deciding factor in how it goes. Dr Rabin suggests that you try the following mood-boosting strategies to make the day go well.

Start with a scent. Before you go to bed tonight, place some citrus, vanilla, or rosemary potpourri in a covered jar and put it on your bedside table. In the morning, before you get out of bed, open it and smell. Think of fresh fields of flowers.

'Your immune system produces a hormonal milieu that protects you, warding off disease,' says Dr Rabin. That fresh smell communicates with the area of your brain that helps to regulate memory, emotion, body temperature, appetite and sexual responsiveness.

Make your shower luxurious. A quick morning shower can still be a pleasant one. Surround yourself with aromatic bath gels and soaps. Use thick, soft sponges and loofahs to scrub. Spoil yourself with enormous, fluffy towels. Turn on the music. Sing, if you want.

Change your morning routine. Do you, without thinking, eat the same brand of breakfast cereal every day? For a delicious change of pace, toast wholemeal bread and serve it with blackcurrant jam and peanut butter. The monounsaturated fat from the peanut butter will give you an energy boost.

Write It Down

Katie wrote and illustrated a book that described how sad she felt when she learned that she had bone cancer. She also kept a diary, as did her mother.

In research at the University of Texas at Austin, scientists found that students who expressed their feelings had higher levels of infection-fighting lymphocytes. The researchers monitored two groups of medical students. One group wrote diaries for 20 minutes a day, 3 to 5 days a week, focusing on an emotional issue meaningful to them. The other group wrote, too, but about events of the day. In each group, some were asked not to think about what they wrote, while others were asked to mull over what they had penned.

Those who tried to suppress their thoughts showed impaired immune systems, while those who did not were rewarded with a rise in infection-fighting cells, researchers said.

Stay connected to your thoughts and emotions by writing them down. Don't forget to thoroughly record – and congratulate yourself – when you notice your outlook changing for the better.

There is one more thing you can do to help your immune system – and very likely someone else's too:

Hug someone.

'I hug Katie every chance I get,' says Beth. 'We both feel better every time.' *

Polishing Facet 5 of Your Vitality Diamond

Of all the facets, the benefits of polishing this one are the least quantifiable. That's not to say, however, that they aren't important. The connection between your brain and your health – and, specifically, your immune system – is only now starting to be understood.

If, after doing the self-assessment in this chapter, you believe you could benefit from a more positive attitude, take some time to brainstorm practical things you could do to change your outlook. Jot them down on a piece of paper as you think of them. Then, read over the list and try to focus on on three or four of the ideas that really speak to you.

Perhaps you might choose to volunteer for a worthy cause, such as a literacy campaign, an animal shelter, or a hospice organisation. Perhaps you'll decide that you want to learn more about or renew a religious faith. Perhaps you'll find that you've been so busy worrying about bills that you haven't actually *laughed* in ages. If so, you might want to read a few jokes each day from a humour website or rediscover childhood activities you used to enjoy, whether that means getting the family together for a game of football or buying a CD of your favourite music from when you were a teenager. Whether they're big or small, do those things that bring you joy and make you feel connected to others. Those positive feelings may benefit not only your general outlook but your overall health as well.

Start today by noting the steps you have taken on your Vitality Diamond on page 379.

* *Katie died peacefully at home on 3 June, 2001.*

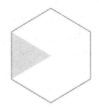

FACET 6:
LISTEN TO YOUR BODY

This chapter, which discusses the sixth – and final – facet of your Vitality Diamond and summarises the entire plan, was written by Keith Berndtson, MD, medical director at Integrative Care Centers in Chicago and Glenview, Illinois.

Iꜰ ᴏɴʟʏ ᴡᴇ ᴄᴏᴜʟᴅ ᴄʟᴏɴᴇ Dᴀᴋᴏᴛᴀ.

Dakota is a lovable golden retriever so sensitive to his owner's body that he has saved the Alabama man's life more times than Mike Lingenfelter can count.

Dakota is a service dog trained to help keep Mike from falling again into the deep depression that overtook him after a series of heart attacks several years ago. The two bonded so well that Dakota instinctively knew before his owner did that Mike was about to have an angina attack, and that he needed to take his prescribed medicine to stave it off. The first time, Mike didn't pay attention as Dakota pawed him, licked him and then jumped on him. Within a few minutes, Mike collapsed from the chest pains and had to be rushed to the hospital for treatment.

'Dakota knows me better than I know myself,' says Mike, 64, a transportation consultant.

When your body is stressed, chemicals are released into your bloodstream, and traces of them show up in your sweat. So it's no surprise that dogs can smell or taste chemicals on your skin. Still, Mike understandably calls Dakota his angel. The dog performs a particular task in an extraordinary way. But unless you have a special need for a service dog, there really is no reason for you to acquire a Dakota to alert you to what your body is trying to tell you.

You can listen to your body yourself.

You can become attuned to what your body is saying: you have the ability to listen for cues and then take steps to enhance your immune system to stay healthy for life. Your immune system is the sum of its parts: your whole body.

That may be a difficult concept to grasp in this age of specialisation. We learned by speciality in medical school. At no time during my training did anyone bother to piece it together: to put the whole body into perspective. That's starting to change, but not at all too soon.

Check the Oil

When you hear a noise under the bonnet of your car, you have a couple of choices. You can turn up the radio to drown out the clunks, or you can check under the bonnet.

When you don't pay attention to what your body is trying to tell you, you're doing the medical equivalent of turning up the radio. Perhaps you're afraid to get a troublesome symptom investigated by your doctor because you fear that he'll tell you that you have a serious health condition. Or perhaps you're overwhelmed by the vast amount of medical information out there, and you feel paralysed. Or perhaps you consider that since you can't change your gene pool, what's the point? But the truth is that by listening to your body and acting on the information it's giving you, you can empower your immune system for optimum health.

Let's say there's breast cancer in your family. You might begin eating a diet high in phytonutrients and antioxidants (found in fruits, vegetables and nuts), which have been found to help protect against cancer. You may also choose to take vitamin and mineral supplements, like vitamin E and selenium. Because selenium levels in food aren't consistent, a mineral supplement is a good idea – except that too much selenium can be toxic. The amount of selenium in most multivitamins is safe.

Of course, it is incumbent upon us – your health professionals – to help you filter the information. It's not just listening to your body that is important, but understanding what it is telling you and making the changes that it needs: transforming your life from a diamond in the rough into a Vitality Diamond.

They Did It, and So Can You

As you work on establishing your own Vitality Diamond, you will no doubt notice some immediate changes in how you feel, your attitude and perhaps even how you look. But visualising the complete, polished Vitality Diamond can sometimes be difficult when you're just getting started. To help strengthen your resolve, read on to find out how some of my patients have established their own Vitality Diamond plans. You will no doubt notice that they faced similar obstacles to what you are now facing. Just like them, though, you will succeed.

Ben's Vitality Diamond:
College Student Beats Nagging Health Problems

Ben was a 22-year-old college student who for the most part ate a healthy diet. Breakfast was usually oatmeal, fruit and wholemeal bread. Lunch was either a tuna sandwich, pasta or a salad, and dinner usually meant lean meats, potatoes and vegetables. He took yoga classes twice a week, and slept well. He had strong relationships with his family and friends.

The problem? Ben had recurring flu-like symptoms, fatigue, headaches and muscle aches. He was constantly worrying about his academic performance, and the continual stress taxed his immune system.

Despite a healthy diet, supportive relationships, good sleep and regular yoga, the stress of Ben's academic workload – combined with his tendency to worry more than he should – and a roommate whose pack-a-day smoking habit filled his room with secondhand smoke caused him to use up certain nutrients faster than usual. We placed him on a high-potency multivitamin without iron, taken both morning and evening. We also added an antioxidant combination that included moderate doses of vitamins C, E and selenium (for general antioxidant support) as well as vitamin A and quercetin. Vitamin A provides targeted antioxidant support to mucous membranes, and quercetin, a bioflavonoid with potent antioxidant properties, concentrates in the thin layer of fluid that lines the respiratory tissues.

Ben became more assertive, asking his roommate not to smoke around him. He also bought a HEPA (high-efficiency particle arrestor) filter, which recirculated the air in his room several times an hour, trapping most of the smoke-related particulates and irritants. Finally, Ben gathered information about breathing awareness and mindfulness practice and applied some relaxation techniques to help him worry less and go with the flow more easily.

Within 6 months of making these changes, Ben's recurrent respiratory infections and feelings of fatigue were gone. He was one of the top students, and he was learning not to worry about the unimportant things in life.

Harriet's Vitality Diamond: A New Lease of Life

Harriet, 50, the mother of three grown-up children, suffered from recurring urinary tract infections and depression. She seldom ate breakfast, and drank at least five cans of carbonated drinks every day. She played tennis once a month. She complained of overall lack of energy, and of loneliness and cynicism about life in general.

Harriet had entered the menopause within a year of her youngest child leaving home for college. In addition, marital discord was threatening to lead to divorce. She had virtually no sex drive. It was no surprise when screening revealed that she was moderately depressed.

Fortunately, Harriet agreed to seek counselling, which got her to focus on herself and what she could do to get her life back on a positive track. She was able to vent her anger with her husband. She reconnected with her religious faith and put more energy into cultivating her relationships with her husband and her children.

A bone density exam revealed osteopenia, or early bone thinning. Harriet's oestrogen and progesterone levels were clearly in the post-menopausal range. Because she had a family history of breast cancer and was fearful of hormone replacement, she was willing to make dietary changes and to begin an exercise programme that would gradually build strength, endurance and agility.

Harriet switched from carbonated drinks to purified water. She started eating a light breakfast every day in the form of a smoothie made with skimmed milk, yoghurt, ground flaxseeds, soya protein and fruit. She also added a multivitamin and a bone-building formula, which gave her additional calcium, magnesium, vitamin K and trace minerals.

She took a brisk 30-minute walk at least five times a week, and she began playing tennis on a weekly schedule. She also started doing special exercises known as Kegels to strengthen her pelvic and bladder muscles.

Within 3 months, Harriet's efforts were rewarded with considerable feelings of enhanced well-being. Her energy levels and mood were improved, and her attitude toward life grew positive again. Her husband, not wanting to be left behind, agreed to marriage guidance.

After returning to an intimate relationship with him, she experienced some mild vaginal discomfort. In addition, her urinary symptoms were only partially improved. When she began using a vaginal oestriol pessary nightly, these symptoms resolved as well. (Because a pessary is a local application of oestriol, there's little systemic effect to fuel concerns about cancer risk.)

Within a year, a repeat bone density measurement showed that Harriet was back in the normal range. Her bones were looking younger, and, according to her family and friends, so was she.

Jane's Vitality Diamond:
She Realised Her Risk before It Was Too Late

Jane, a 38-year-old married mother of two with a law practice, complained of incessant fatigue and irritability as well as a sore throat, cough and postnasal drip. She couldn't remember how many glasses of wine she had every night to calm down. Her father was an alcoholic. She said that she was too busy to exercise.

Jane did it all: she ran the software licencing division of an up-and-coming law firm serving the high-tech industry. She packed the lunches for her two secondary-school-age daughters and attended their music recitals and sports days. By all accounts, she was a wonderful mother and a great lawyer. But these accolades came at a price. Her body was threatening to collect a big toll.

Jane's drinking insidiously increased from a glass of wine to an entire bottle on most nights. Her sleep, as a result, became less refreshing. It was increasingly hard for her to get going in the morning. She relied on a coffee jolt every morning, and another every afternoon. Jane was dehydrated but looked puffy, particularly around her eyes. She put on 9 kg (20 lb) in 2 years.

Jane knew that her health was sinking fast. She agreed to share some of her supervisory responsibilities with a colleague at work. This led to a 5 per cent pay cut, but it freed up 5 desperately needed hours a week. She also negotiated a schedule with her family to divide up domestic chores. This gave her another 4 hours a week.

With those added hours at her disposal, Jane allocated 4½ hours a week to go to her local gym, where she worked with a personal trainer on strength, flexibility and endurance. She now had more time to spend with her children before they went to bed, to engage in night-time conversations with her husband, and to enjoy an occasional dip in the hot tub or quiet reading time for herself. She and her husband scheduled time together, too: a monthly date.

Jane also acknowledged her own risks for alcoholism. She stopped drinking.

She started taking a multivitamin with iron, with an additional 350 mg of magnesium gluconate and 2 g of flaxseed oil every day. (Check with your doctor before beginning supplementation with any amount of magnesium if you have heart or kidney problems. Doses exceeding 350 mg a day may cause diarrhoea in some people.) She steered her diet away from simple sugars and increased her intake of fresh vegetables, fish and poultry.

Within 3 months, Jane lost 4.5 kg (10 lb) and was sleeping like a baby. She was happy about the quality time she had with her husband and children, and she enjoyed her job more. Her postnasal drip had gone, and her optimism and confidence were back.

Randall's Vitality Diamond: Former Couch Potato Transforms His Life

Randall, 35 and single, is an accountant who had gained 18 kg (nearly 3 stone) in 2 years. He slept poorly and complained of constant fatigue. He also had frequent wind and bloating. Randall's nasal allergies were getting worse, and he had developed eczema on his chest and arms. His diet consisted of various junk foods, especially his favourites: cake, ice cream, crisps and fizzy drinks. He was bored at work. Rather than socialising after work, he would go home, eat and watch television until after midnight. The thought of exercise led him to the biscuit tin and the couch.

Randall found it increasingly difficult to drag himself out of bed each morning. He felt isolated and disconnected.

While Randall wasn't showing signs of depression, he was socially withdrawn and had a hard time motivating himself. Fortunately, he wanted to feel better, physically and emotionally. He realised that he had a responsibility to change his diet, become more active and develop social connections.

We began with nutritional counselling to teach him how to take the guesswork out of shopping, ordering from a restaurant menu and preparing meals. He took high-strength multivitamins without iron. In addition, I prescribed 2 g of fish oil and 2 g of borage oil every day for his eczema.

Randall sought psychological counselling to help him deal with his social anxieties and to begin removing obstacles to getting out and doing things with other people. He agreed to restrict television viewing to his favourite programmes, occasional specials and sporting events.

Randall joined a local gym and began a weight-lifting programme. He took a class on low-fat cooking at the community centre, and he began dating.

Within 6 months, his energy, sleep and digestion had all improved, and his eczema had cleared. All of these were signs that his immune system was functioning better. He lost 10 kg (1½ stone) and was proud of his ability to bench-press 90 kg (200 lb). He was dating a woman steadily and had started a second class on gourmet cooking.

Not too long ago, I asked Randall, 'So, how's life these days?'

Randall replied, 'Life is good, doc. And I'm not afraid to die, either. I just don't want to be there when it happens.'

We both laughed.

Polishing Facet 6 of Your Vitality Diamond

The people I described above listened to their bodies and initiated changes in their lives that gave them the opportunity to strengthen their immune systems. You can, too.

Pay attention to what your body is trying to tell you. If you're already keeping a diary, you might want to record in it how you're feeling – both mentally and physically – each day. That way, you can identify stresses and brainstorm ways to eliminate or reduce them. If you're experiencing physical symptoms, you may be able to identify a pattern in when they occur and what may be triggering them.

Finally, make an appointment with your doctor for your annual physical check-up *now*. You'll want to write down any changes you've noticed in your body or symptoms you've been having so that you won't forget to ask about them on the day of your appointment. Make sure that your doctor knows about your family's medical history. That way, he or she will be better able to assess your risk and advise you on screenings.

Putting It All Together: Your Vitality Diamond

You now have all you need to complete your Vitality Diamond. How you go about doing that is, of course, up to you. You might choose to concentrate on one facet a week, perhaps beginning by selecting a week's worth of healthy meals built on the MaxImmunity Diet principles. If so, you could spend next weekend shopping for the freshest fruits and vegetables and tasty nuts and seeds so that you're ready to begin cooking. Or perhaps you prefer to work on a few facets at a time, or maybe all six simultaneously. Remember: there is no wrong way to construct your Vitality Diamond. It is truly *your* plan, so customise it to fit your needs.

On page 378, we have given you an example of Jane's filled-in Vitality Diamond. Read it: it will give you ideas for filling in your own diamond. Then, when you're ready, copy the blank diamond on page 379. Use it to construct your very first Vitality Diamond.

If you want a starting point, here are some ideas for each facet to get you going.

Facet 1: Diet. In fond memory of the peanut butter sandwiches of your childhood – but with some added sparkle – make yourself a peanut butter sandwich (2 tablespoons of peanut butter, 2 slices of wholemeal bread) topped with half a banana. Or slice up an apple and spread the 2 tablespoons of peanut butter on each slice. Or find as many different kinds of green salad leaves as you can, and toss them together with 2 teaspoons of olive oil and flavoured balsamic vinegar. Add 1 tablespoon of sunflower seeds for a tasty crunch. Remember that you want to make sure that your diet includes nuts, seeds, vegetables and fruit for maximum phytochemical power.

Facet 2: Supplements. Leave yourself notes – in your bedroom, in the bathroom, on the coffee table in your living room – so that you will remember to take your multivitamin. You can write reminders to add vitamin E, vitamin C and calcium to your daily multivitamin.

Facet 3: Exercise. Start with the simple moves. This week, for instance, get up from your computer every hour and walk around your office building for 5 minutes. Or get up and stretch. If you need to go to the toilets, walk to the cloakroom on the floor above you. Park at the far end of the company car park. Every minute counts; soon you'll find that you're incorporating 30 minutes of extra moves into your day.

Facet 4: Stress Relief and Sleep. Pick a time to go to bed, and go at the same time every night this week. Wake up at the same time. But before you head for bed, take 20 minutes or so to wind down. Listen to soothing music, or start reading a book you've been meaning to read for some time. With these steps, you will start on the road to eliminating stress from your life and sleeping more soundly.

Facet 5: Emotional Immunity. Pull out the Monopoly game, or Cluedo – or any entertaining board game that you played growing up. Enlist your family or friends to sit with you at the dining room table, and start rolling the dice. You're guaranteed to have more fun – and feel better about yourself – even if you don't buy Mayfair or guess who dunnit.

Facet 6: Listen to Your Body. Pay particular attention to how you're feeling today. Are you carrying tension in your body? Do your muscles feel tight? If so, spend some time doing light stretches followed by a few minutes relaxing in a comfortable chair, simply focusing on your breathing.

One of the most satisfying aspects of being a doctor is working with my patients as they discover the different facets of their health – their Vitality Diamonds. As they come to understand what it is to have and maintain a strong immune system, they know what it is to create the Immune Advantage. I wish the same for you.

Jane's Vitality Diamond

Below is an example of how Jane filled out her Vitality Diamond for one day. As you will recall, Jane is a 38-year-old lawyer with two daughters. Her stressful career and jam-packed schedule were leading to her deteriorating health, including fatigue and a chronic sore throat, cough and postnasal drip. But by identifying her risk factors and taking positive steps to reduce stress, Jane was able to improve her health and rediscover the joys in her life.

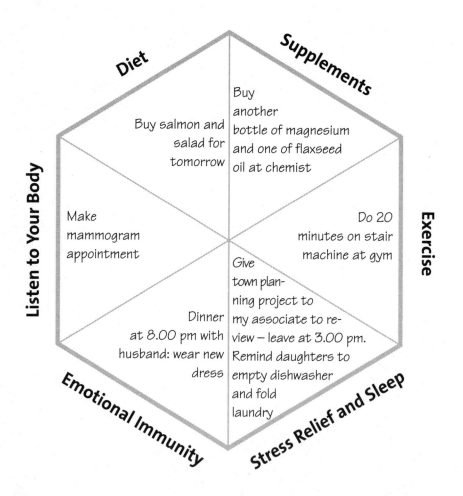

Your Vitality Diamond

Use this page to create your own Vitality Diamond. You may want to make copies of it so that you can constantly customise your plan to fit your needs.

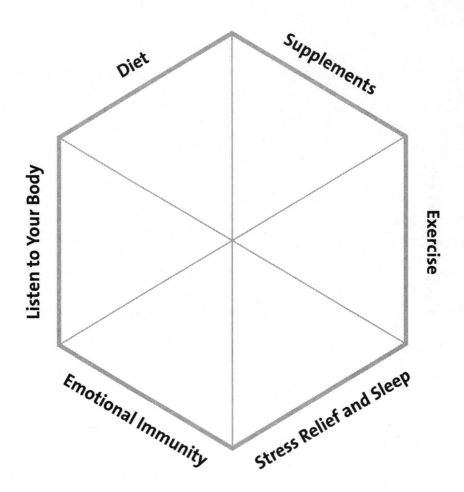

PART
5

Immune
Resources

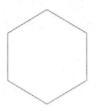

50 DELICIOUS IMMUNE-BOOSTING RECIPES

Forget all your preconceptions: eating for good health and a strong immune system means consuming a wide variety of delicious, colourful foods. It means eating the freshest, most tender vegetables, the juiciest fruit, even decadent nuts. As you'll see from the 50 recipes that follow, you can give your immune system the nutrients it needs to keep your body running at a high level while still eating soul-satisfying meals.

You're sure to find a recipe for any occasion among this collection of immune-boosting recipes. When you and your family are enjoying a leisurely Saturday morning, whip up a batch of Multigrain Blueberry Scotch pancakes (page 384). For a quick dinner on a busy weeknight, try Asian-Style Chicken and Broccoli Stir-Fry (page 406). It's as fast as a take-away, but much healthier. On a cold winter evening, try Roasted Garlic and Vegetable Soup with Pasta (page 389). And when you're in the mood to celebrate, treat yourself to Peanut Butter–Chocolate Mousse (page 428). Eating for good health never tasted so good!

MUFFINS, SCOTCH PANCAKES AND OTHER BREAKFAST FOODS

Multigrain Blueberry Scotch Pancakes

Blueberries are a superior source of antioxidants, and there are few more delicious ways to enjoy them than in these decadent Scotch pancakes.

115 g (4 oz)	plain flour
60 g (2 oz)	wholemeal flour
50 g (1¾ oz)	rolled oats
½	teaspoon baking powder
½	teaspoon bicarbonate of soda
½	teaspoon salt
450 ml (¾ pt)	skimmed milk
2	egg whites
3	tablespoons soft light brown sugar
1	tablespoon vegetable oil
200 g (7 oz)	blueberries
170 g (6 oz)	maple syrup

Preheat the oven to 110°C/225°F/gas ¼. Coat a baking sheet with cooking spray.

In a large bowl, combine the plain flour, wholemeal flour, oats, baking powder, bicarbonate of soda and salt.

In a medium bowl, combine the milk, egg whites, brown sugar and oil. Add to the flour mixture. Whisk until a smooth batter forms. Fold in the blueberries.

Coat a griddle or frying pan with cooking spray. Preheat.

Pour 120 ml (4 fl oz) of the batter onto the centre of the griddle or frying pan. Cook until the batter has set, then flip the pancakes and cook for about 1 minute on the other side. Transfer the pancakes to the prepared baking sheet. Place in the oven to keep warm. Repeat with the remaining batter to make a total of 8 pancakes. Serve drizzled with maple syrup.

MAKES 8

Per pancake: 230 calories/961 kJ, 6 g protein, 47 g carbohydrate (of which sugars 29 g), 3 g fat, 3 g dietary fibre, 301 mg sodium

Breakfast Wrap

Rather than stopping at the local café for a greasy egg and bacon breakfast sandwich with all the (fried) trimmings, try this delicious alternative instead. Though it still contains egg, the amount of cholesterol has been reduced by limiting the number of yolks used. Plus, these wraps are the best way to get immune-enhancing vegetables such as tomatoes and mushrooms into your first meal of the day.

2	**eggs**
6	**egg whites**
¼	**teaspoon salt**
115 g (4 oz)	**mushrooms, sliced**
4	**plum tomatoes, chopped**
1	**small courgette, chopped**
1	**small onion, chopped**
	A few leaves of basil, torn
4	**wholemeal tortillas (20 cm/8 in diameter)**
60 g (2 oz)	**grated low-fat mozzarella cheese**

In a medium bowl, whisk together the eggs, egg whites, salt and 2 tablespoons water.

Coat a large nonstick frying pan with cooking spray. Set over medium-high heat. Add the mushrooms, tomatoes, courgette, onion and basil. Cook, stirring occasionally, for 4 to 5 minutes, or until the vegetables are soft.

Add the egg mixture. Cook, stirring often, for 3 minutes, or until the eggs are cooked. Remove from the heat.

Meanwhile, wrap the tortillas in a paper towel and place in the microwave oven. Cook on high power for 30 seconds to heat. Place the tortillas on a cutting board. Spoon some of the egg mixture down the centre of each tortilla. Sprinkle with the mozzarella. Roll into cylinders and cut in half diagonally.

MAKES 4 SERVINGS

Per serving: *215 calories/899 kJ, 15 g protein, 14 g carbohydrate (of which sugars 6 g), 11 g fat (of which saturates 5 g), 3 g dietary fibre, 468 mg sodium*

Orange Bran Flax Muffins

Flaxseed is hard to beat. It's nature's richest source of lignans, which may help prevent cancer. Plus, it's full of heart-healthy omega-3 fats and soluble fibre. These orange-flavoured muffins just may be the most delicious way to incorporate flaxseed, which you should be able to buy at your local health food shop, into your diet.

150 g (5½ oz)	oat bran
115 g (4 oz)	plain flour
170 g (6 oz)	flaxseed, ground
100 g (3½ oz)	wheat bran
1	tablespoon baking powder
½	teaspoon salt
2	oranges, quartered and seeded
200 g (7 oz)	brown sugar
240 ml (8 fl oz)	buttermilk
125 ml (4 fl oz)	rapeseed oil
2	eggs
1	teaspoon bicarbonate of soda
230 g (8 oz)	sultanas

Preheat the oven to 190°C/375°F/gas 5. Line two 12-cup muffin tins with paper cases or coat the tins with cooking spray. In a large bowl, combine the oat bran, flour, flaxseed, wheat bran, baking powder and salt. Set aside.

In a blender or food processor, combine the oranges, brown sugar, buttermilk, oil, eggs and bicarbonate of soda. Blend well.

Pour the orange mixture into the dry ingredients. Mix until well-blended. Stir in the sultanas.

Divide the batter evenly among the muffin tins. Bake for 18 to 20 minutes or until a skewer inserted in the centre comes out clean. Cool in the tins for 5 minutes before removing to a rack.

MAKES 24

Per muffin: 210 calories/878 kJ, 5 g protein, 25 g carbohydrate (of which sugars 17 g), 10 g fat (of which saturates 2 g), 4 g dietary fibre, 139 mg sodium

Recipe courtesy of Flax Council of Canada and Saskatchewan Flax Development Commission

Papaya Smoothie

When you need a quick breakfast, this fruit smoothie is the way to go. It's packed with vitamins A and C and folate, all of which boost the immune system. For variety, replace the papaya with a mango, peeled, stoned and cut into strips.

1	papaya, peeled, seeded and cut up
240 ml (8 fl oz)	natural yoghurt
½	banana
100 g (3½ oz)	fresh pineapple chunks
½	teaspoon dried mint or 12 fresh leaves
4	ice cubes, slightly crushed

Combine the papaya, yoghurt, banana, pineapple, mint and ice in a blender and process until smooth.

Makes 4

Per smoothie: 74 calories/309 kJ, 4 g protein, 14 g carbohydrate (of which sugars 14 g), 0.5 g fat (of which saturates 0 g), 2 g dietary fibre, 52 mg sodium

SOUPS

Scallop and Sweetcorn Chowder

Scallops are a good source of immune-strengthening zinc, and they're also rich in magnesium, potassium, vitamin B_{12} and vitamin E. This mouthwatering chowder manages to taste creamy while still being low-fat.

1	tablespoon olive oil
30 g (1 oz)	onion, chopped
1	small green pepper, chopped
250 g (9 oz)	shucked scallops
2	large potatoes, peeled and chopped
¼	teaspoon dried thyme or 2 teaspoons fresh, chopped
¼	teaspoon salt
500 g (1 lb 2 oz)	fresh, frozen or tinned sweetcorn kernels
750 ml (1¼ pt)	skimmed milk
60 g (2 oz)	dried skimmed milk powder
30 g (1 oz)	superfine flour
	Ground black pepper (to taste)
	Cayenne pepper (to taste)

Warm the oil in a large pan over medium heat. Add the onion and pepper and cook, stirring frequently, for 3 minutes or until tender.

Drain the scallops, reserving the liquid. Set them aside. Add enough water to the liquid to make 240 ml (8 fl oz); add to the pan. Add the potatoes, thyme, and salt. Bring to the boil. Reduce the heat, cover, and simmer for 7 minutes. Lightly mash the potatoes with a wooden spoon or potato masher. Add the sweetcorn and simmer for 5 minutes.

Whisk together the milk, milk powder and flour. Pour into the pan. Stirring constantly, bring the soup to the boil. Reduce the heat to low and simmer for 1 minute. Add the scallops and simmer for 3 minutes or until the edges curl. Season with the black and cayenne pepper.

MAKES 6 SERVINGS

Per serving: 300 calories/1254 kJ, 19 g protein, 49 g carbohydrate (of which sugars 20 g), 4 g fat (of which saturates 1 g), 4 g dietary fibre, 570 mg sodium

Roasted Garlic and Vegetable Soup with Pasta

Studies have shown that garlic has a protective effect against numerous types of cancer. When it's added to the vitamin-A-rich vegetables in this soup, it becomes part of a sumptuous, immune-boosting meal. This soup is also a very good source of vitamin B_{12}, zinc, selenium, vitamin C and potassium.

1	bulb garlic, separated into cloves
1	tablespoon olive oil
1	onion, chopped
1	red pepper, chopped
1 l (1¾ pt)	defatted chicken stock, or stock made with bouillon powder or cube
500 ml (18 fl oz)	water
2	carrots, thinly sliced
1	tablespoon tomato purée
	A few leaves of basil, chopped (optional)
¼	teaspoon black pepper
115 g (4 oz)	shredded crisp lettuce, such as Cos
170 g (6 oz)	tiny broccoli florets
115 g (4 oz)	macaroni
	Salt (optional)
	Grated Parmesan cheese (optional)

Preheat the oven to 200°C/400°F/gas 6. Wrap the garlic in foil and place in a small baking dish. Bake for 45 to 50 minutes or until soft when squeezed.

Warm the oil in a large pan over medium heat. Add the onion and red pepper and cook, stirring frequently, for 5 minutes, or until tender. Add the stock, water, carrots, tomato paste, basil, if using, and black pepper. Bring to the boil. Reduce the heat, cover, and simmer for 10 minutes.

Remove 250 ml (9 fl oz) of the liquid. Mash the garlic into the liquid. Stir into the pot. Add the lettuce and simmer for 7 minutes. Add the broccoli, cover, and turn off the heat.

Cook the macaroni separately according to the package directions. Drain, and stir into the soup. If desired, season with the salt and Parmesan.

Makes 6 servings

Per serving: 28 calories/535 kJ, 6 g protein, 21 g carbohydrate (of which sugars 6 g), 3 g fat (of which saturates 0.5 g), 3 g dietary fibre, 263 mg sodium

Carrot, Tomato and Walnut Soup

Nuts in soup? Yes, when they're in a tasty version such as this. Not only do they provide extra flavour, but they also add vitamin E. You'll also be getting a healthy dose of beta-carotene from the carrots and vitamin C from the tomatoes.

1	tablespoon olive oil
1	large onion, chopped
2 x 400 g	tins chopped tomatoes (with juice)
6	carrots, thinly sliced
2	large potatoes, peeled and chopped
1	teaspoon ground coriander
1	teaspoon ground cumin
¼	teaspoon ground black pepper
⅛	teaspoon ground cinnamon

500–750 ml (18 fl oz–1¼ pt) defatted chicken stock, or stock made with
bouillon powder or cube
Salt (optional)
40 g (1¼ oz) chopped toasted walnuts (see note)

Warm the oil in a large pan over medium heat. Add the onion and cook, stirring frequently, for 3 minutes or until soft. Add the tomatoes, carrots, potatoes, coriander, cumin, pepper and cinnamon, and 500 ml (18 fl oz) of the stock. Bring to the boil. Reduce the heat, cover, and simmer for 15 minutes or until the vegetables are tender.

If the soup is too thick, add the remaining stock and heat. If desired, season with the salt. Serve garnished with the walnuts.

Makes 6 servings

Per serving: *181 calories/756 kJ, 5 g protein, 26 g carbohydrate (of which sugars 13 g), 7 g fat (of which saturates 1 g), 5 g dietary fibre, 220 mg sodium*

Note: To toast walnuts, bake at 180°C/350°F/gas 4, for 5 to 10 minutes.

Black Bean Soup

At 6 grams per serving, this soup is good for providing fibre. If desired, you can add 4 tablespoons of sherry along with the beans and garnish each bowl with chopped onion, fresh coriander, or a dollop of low-fat sour cream or crème fraîche before serving.

1	tablespoon olive oil
1	large onion, chopped
3	carrots, chopped
2	sticks celery, chopped
3	cloves garlic, finely chopped
2	rashers back bacon, cut into bite-size pieces
1	jalapeño chilli pepper, seeded and chopped (wear plastic gloves when handling)
1	tablespoon ground cumin
1.5 l (2½ pt)	defatted chicken stock, or stock made with bouillon powder or cube
250 ml (9 fl oz)	water
2 x 400 g	tins black beans, rinsed and drained
½	teaspoon salt

Warm the oil in a large pan set over medium heat. Add the onion, carrots, celery and garlic. Cook, stirring occasionally, for 4 minutes, or until the onion starts to soften. Add the bacon, chilli pepper and cumin. Cook for 3 minutes, or until the bacon is lightly browned. Remove the bacon and set it aside.

Add the stock and water to the pot. Increase the heat to high. Bring to the boil. Reduce the heat to medium-low. Cook for 15 minutes, or until the vegetables are tender. Add the beans. Cook for 5 minutes, or until heated through.

Ladle 750 ml (1¼ pt) of the soup into a food processor or blender. Purée until smooth. Return to the pot. Add the reserved bacon and salt. Cook for 5 minutes, or until heated through.

MAKES 8 SERVINGS

Per ungarnished serving: 145 calories/606 kJ, 10 g protein, 22 g carbohydrate (of which sugars 5 g), 3 g fat (of which saturates 0.5 g), 6 g dietary fibre, 348 mg sodium

Creamy Gingered Carrot Soup

For a change from the ordinary, try this tasty soup. Carrots are packed with beta-carotene, which is converted into vitamin A in the body. And vitamin A plays an important part in enhancing white blood cell function and increasing resistance to carcinogens.

1	tablespoon groundnut oil
455 g (1 lb)	baby carrots
2	sticks celery, chopped
1	large onion, sliced
1.2 l (2 pt)	water
500 ml (18 fl oz)	skimmed milk
2	large baking potatoes, peeled and sliced
75 g (2½ oz)	smooth peanut butter (with salt)
2	tablespoons finely chopped fresh ginger (or 2 teaspoons ground ginger)
1½	teaspoons salt
1½	teaspoons white pepper

Place a large pan over low heat. Add the oil, carrots, celery and onion, then cover. Stir occasionally for 8 minutes, or until the onions are translucent.

Add the water, milk, potatoes, peanut butter, ginger, salt and pepper. Cover and bring to the boil. Reduce the heat. Simmer, uncovered, until the vegetables are tender, about 25 minutes.

In a blender, purée the soup in batches. Return the puréed soup to the clean pan. Adjust the seasonings. Heat through over low heat.

MAKES 6 SERVINGS

Per serving: 208 calories/869 kJ, 8 g protein, 25 g carbohydrate (of which sugars 12 g), 9 g fat (of which saturates 2 g), 5 g dietary fibre, 702 mg sodium

Blue-Ribbon Blueberry Soup

It's a toss-up whether this soup most deserves a blue ribbon for its delicious taste or for its cancer-fighting ability. After all, blueberries are Mother Nature's number one source of antioxidants. Either way, this cold soup is sure to be a treat on a hot summer day.

570 g (1¼ lb)	**fresh or frozen blueberries**
250 ml (9 fl oz)	**unsweetened apple juice**
2	**tablespoons sugar**
2	**wedges lemon**
1	**cinnamon stick**
½	**teaspoon vanilla extract**
125 ml (4 fl oz)	**low-fat vanilla yoghurt**

Place the blueberries, apple juice, sugar, lemon, cinnamon and vanilla in a heavy saucepan. Bring to the boil over high heat, stirring to dissolve the sugar. Reduce the heat to low and simmer for 20 minutes. Remove the lemon wedges and the cinnamon stick and discard.

Allow the soup to cool to room temperature (about 45 minutes). Purée the soup in batches in a blender or food processor until smooth.

Chill the soup. Serve it cold, topping each serving with 2 tablespoons of yoghurt.

MAKES 4 SERVINGS

Per serving: *116 calories/484 kJ, 3 g protein, 26 g carbohydrate (of which sugars 26 g), 1 g fat (of which saturates 0.5 g), 7 g dietary fibre, 30 mg sodium*

SALADS

Spinach-Orange Salad with Sesame

Spinach, navel oranges and kiwi fruit are all top sources of cancer-fighting antioxidant power. Furthermore, spinach is loaded with lutein, which helps protect the eyes against the effects of ageing. This sunny salad is quck to make – you need just 15 minutes.

1	teaspoon sugar
½	teaspoon cornflour
80 ml (3fl oz)	orange juice
1½	tablespoons rice wine vinegar
1	teaspoon grated fresh ginger or ¼ teaspoon ground ginger
1	clove garlic, chopped
1½	teaspoons toasted sesame oil
285 g (10 oz)	baby spinach leaves
2	navel oranges, peeled and separated into segments
1	small red onion, thinly sliced
1	kiwi fruit, sliced

Place the sugar and cornflour in a small saucepan. Gradually add the orange juice and vinegar, whisking to dissolve the dry ingredients. Add the ginger and garlic. Cook, stirring, over medium-high heat for 2 to 3 minutes, until the mixture boils. Remove and whisk in the oil. Allow to cool.

In a large bowl, combine the spinach, orange segments, onion and kiwi fruit. Add the dressing. Toss to coat evenly.

MAKES 4 SERVINGS

Per serving: *91calories/381 kJ, 4 g protein, 15 g carbohydrate (of which sugars 13 g), 2 g fat (of which saturates 0.5 g), 5 g dietary fibre, 109 mg sodium*

Roasted Vegetable Salad

With its green beans, red peppers and onion, this salad is packed with vitamins. In addition, it contains cancer-fighting garlic and heart-healthy olive oil. Serve it warm or chilled.

685 g (1½ lb)	small red potatoes, quartered
340 g (12 oz)	green beans, cut into 2.5 cm (1 in) pieces
2	red peppers, thinly sliced
1	red onion, thinly sliced crosswise and separated into rings
125 ml (4 fl oz)	defatted chicken stock, or stock made with bouillon powder or cube
2	cloves garlic
2	tablespoons red wine vinegar
1½	tablespoons olive oil
1	teaspoon crushed dried rosemary or 1 tablespoon fresh, chopped
¼	teaspoon ground black pepper
8	Kalamata olives, pitted and sliced
1–2	tablespoons lemon juice

Preheat the oven to 220°C/425°F/gas 7.

Coat a 23 x 33 cm (9 x 13 in) baking dish with cooking spray. Add the potatoes, beans, peppers, onion stock and garlic. Mix well. Roast, stirring every 10 minutes, for 20 to 30 minutes, or until the vegetables are tender. Set aside.

Transfer the garlic to a small bowl and mash. Whisk in the vinegar, oil, rosemary and black pepper.

Place the vegetables in a large bowl. Add the dressing and olives. Toss to mix well. Sprinkle with the lemon juice just before serving.

MAKES 4 SERVINGS

Per serving: *228calories/953 kJ, 7 g protein, 39 g carbohydrate (of which sugars 11 g), 6 g fat (of which saturates 1 g), 7 g dietary fibre, 317 mg sodium*

Sweetcorn, Tomato and Mozzarella Salad

This side salad is simple to prepare, and the flavours are pure summer. Not only do you get calcium from the mozzarella, but this salad also provides folate and vitamins C and B_{12}.

4	cobs of sweetcorn (see note)
455 g (1 lb)	cherry tomatoes, halved
¼	teaspoon salt
⅛	teaspoon ground black pepper
115 g (4 oz)	low-fat mozzarella cheese, cut into 1 cm (½ in) cubes
2	tablespoons prepared pesto sauce

Husk the sweetcorn and blanch in a large pot of boiling water for 1 minute. Drain. Let cool slightly, then cut the kernels from the cobs.

In a large bowl, mix the corn, tomatoes, salt and pepper. Stir in the cheese and pesto. Serve at once, or cover and refrigerate for up to 24 hours.

Makes 4 servings

Per serving: 278 calories/1162 kJ, 9 g protein, 37 g carbohydrate (of which sugars 16 g), 11 g fat (of which saturates 5 g), 7 g dietary fibre, 800 mg sodium

Note: If fresh sweetcorn is not available, you can use 640 g (1 lb 6 oz) frozen corn, thawed.

Mediterranean Chickpea Salad

Chickpeas contain both vitamin B_6 and vitamin B_{12}. They're delicious in this salad, which also contains cancer-fighting tomatoes and garlic. Allow the salad to stand at room temperature for 10 minutes for the flavours to blend.

1 x 400 g	tin chickpeas, rinsed and drained
½	small red onion, quartered and thinly sliced
½	cucumber, peeled, seeded and chopped
1	roasted red pepper, chopped
3	plum tomatoes, chopped
2	tablespoons chopped parsley
2	cloves garlic, chopped
3	tablespoons lemon juice
2	teaspoons extra-virgin olive oil
¼	teaspoon salt

In a large bowl, combine the chickpeas, onion, cucumber, pepper, tomatoes, parsley, garlic, lemon juice, olive oil and salt. Toss to mix.

Makes 8 servings

Per serving: 74 calories/1309 kJ, 4 g protein, 10 g carbohydrate (of which sugars 3 g), 3 g fat, 2 g dietary fibre, 191 mg sodium

Chinese Chicken Salad with Peanut Butter Dressing

Once you try this Asian-inspired salad, it will become a mainstay of your meal repertoire. The leafy greens are a good source of cancer-fighting carotenoids, and the peanut butter provides a healthy dose of heart-healthy monounsaturated fat.

Peanut Butter Dressing

2	teaspoons groundnut oil
2	teaspoons toasted sesame oil
60 g (2 oz)	smooth peanut butter (with salt)
4	tablespoons rice vinegar
	Juice of 1 lime
1½	tablespoons soy sauce
1	tablespoon clear honey
1	clove garlic
2.5 cm (1 in)	piece fresh ginger, peeled (or 1 teaspoon ground ginger)
1	teaspoon chilli powder

Chinese Chicken Salad

4	small (approximately 400 g/14 oz total) grilled or baked boneless, skinless chicken breasts, sliced into long, bite-size pieces
250 g (9 oz)	mixed salad leaves
2	tablespoons chopped fresh coriander

To make the dressing: In a blender, purée all the dressing ingredients.

To make the salad: Combine the chicken, leaves and coriander.

Just before serving, toss the salad with the dressing. Garnish as desired.

Makes 4 servings

Per serving: 265 calories/1107 kJ, 26 g protein, 8 g carbohydrate (of which sugars 6 g), 15 g fat (of which saturates 3 g), 2 g dietary fibre, 449 mg sodium

Couscous-and-Vegetable Salad

When you're in the mood for something different, try this unusual salad. It boasts an amazing 12 grams of dietary fibre, and it's an excellent way to work a few nutritious – and delicious – nuts into your meal. With the vibrant colours of the carrot, tomato and pepper, it's also pleasing to the eye and the palate.

375 ml (13 fl oz)	water
¼	teaspoon salt
1	teaspoon + 1 tablespoon olive oil
75 g (2½ oz)	couscous
90 g (3 oz)	tinned chickpeas, drained and rinsed (reserve the liquid)
75 g (2½ oz)	frozen peas, thawed
1	medium carrot, coarsely shredded
1	small tomato, chopped
1	small red or yellow pepper, chopped
2½	tablespoons currants
2½	tablespoons finely chopped fresh chives
1½	tablespoons pistachio or pine nuts
1½	tablespoons lemon juice
¼	teaspoon dried thyme, or 1 tablespoon fresh, chopped
¼	teaspoon dried marjoram, or 1 tablespoon fresh, chopped
	Dash of Angostura bitters (optional)

In a medium saucepan over high heat, bring the water, salt, and 1 teaspoon of the oil to the boil. Stir in the couscous. Remove from the heat, cover, and let stand for 5 minutes, or until the liquid is absorbed. Fluff with a fork.

Transfer the couscous to a large bowl. Add the chickpeas, peas, carrot, tomato, pepper, currants, chives and nuts. Toss gently until mixed.

In a small bowl, whisk together the lemon juice, thyme, marjoram, bitters (if using) and the remaining 1 tablespoon oil. Add 3 tablespoons of the reserved chickpea liquid. Mix and pour over the salad. Toss to mix well.

Cover and let stand at room temperature for 30 minutes.

MAKES **4** SERVINGS

Per serving: 258 calories/1078 kJ, 7 g protein, 37 g carbohydrate (of which sugars 18 g),10 g fat (of which saturates 1 g), 5 g dietary fibre, 274 mg sodium

Pan-Seared Salmon Salad

Salmon contains omega-3 fatty acids, which fight both heart disease and cancer. But when you start eating this unique, savoury salad, all you'll be thinking about is the taste!

3	tablespoons chopped dry-packed sun-dried tomatoes
3	tablespoons balsamic vinegar
2	teaspoons extra-virgin olive oil
1½	teaspoons dried basil or 2 tablespoons fresh, chopped
1	teaspoon Dijon mustard
⅛	teaspoon salt
1	roasted red pepper, cut into small strips
455 g (1 lb)	mixed salad leaves
115 g (4 oz)	button or shiitake mushrooms, sliced
1	small onion, finely chopped
4	salmon fillets 90 g (3 oz) each, skin removed
1	teaspoon mixed dried herbs

Place the sun-dried tomatoes in a small bowl. Cover with boiling water. Allow to soak for 10 minutes, or until soft. Drain and discard the liquid.

In a large bowl, whisk the vinegar, oil, basil, mustard and salt until smooth. Place the pepper, salad leaves and sun-dried tomatoes in the bowl but do not toss. Set aside.

Lightly coat a medium nonstick frying pan with cooking spray. Add the mushrooms and onion. Coat lightly with cooking spray. Cook over medium-high heat for 5 to 7 minutes, or until soft. Remove to a plate to cool.

Wipe the pan with kitchen paper. Coat with cooking spray. Set over high heat. Lightly coat the salmon with cooking spray. Sprinkle with the dried herbs. Add the salmon to the pan. Cook for 3 minutes on each side, or until the fish flakes easily. Check by cutting into 1 fillet.

Add the mushrooms and onion to the reserved bowl. Toss to mix. Spoon the salad onto 4 plates. Top each with a salmon fillet.

Makes 4 servings

Per serving: 238 calories/995 kJ, 20 g protein, 10 g carbohydrate (of which sugars 9 g), 9 g fat, 5 g dietary fibre, 241 mg sodium

SIDE DISHES

Sautéed Spinach and Mushrooms

Spinach is a top source of beta-carotene, and when beta-carotene is converted in the body, it plays a major role in the development and maintenance of the immune system. This side dish is so tasty that even your children may come to love spinach.

1	teaspoon olive oil
1	teaspoon toasted sesame oil
90 g (3 oz)	sliced mushrooms
1	sweet onion, thinly sliced
2	cloves garlic, sliced
285 g (10 oz)	frozen chopped spinach, thawed and squeezed dry
½	teaspoon finely chopped ginger
2	teaspoons soy sauce

In a medium saucepan over low heat, warm the olive oil and sesame oil. Add the mushrooms, onion and garlic. Cook, stirring frequently, for 15 to 20 minutes, or until the onion and mushrooms are soft.

Add the spinach, ginger and soy sauce. Cover and cook for 10 minutes, or until the spinach is hot.

MAKES 4 SERVINGS

Per serving: *53 calories/221 kJ, 3 g protein, 5 g carbohydrate (of which sugars 3 g), 3 g fat, 3 g dietary fibre, 250 mg sodium*

Roasted Glazed Beetroot

An immune-boosting diet is a colourful diet, and this dish is one of the tastiest ways to add some new hues to your meals. Beetroot is an excellent source of folate.

685 g (1½ lb)	beetroot, peeled and sliced 5 mm (¼ in) thick
100 g (3½ oz)	raspberry jam
2	tablespoons red wine vinegar
125 ml (4 fl oz)	cranberry-raspberry juice
1	tablespoon chopped fresh thyme or 1 teaspoon dried

Preheat the oven to 200°C/400°F/gas 6. Coat a medium baking dish with cooking spray. In the baking dish, combine the beetroot, jam, vinegar, juice and thyme. Stir to blend well. Cover with foil. Bake for 45 minutes. Remove the foil and bake for 10 to 15 minutes longer, or until the beetroot is soft and tender and the juice is syrupy.

Makes 6 servings

Per serving: 94 calories/393 kJ, 2 g protein, 23 g carbohydrate (of which sugars 22 g), 0 g fat, 3 g dietary fibre, 80 mg sodium

Almond Carrots

Carrots are brimming with beta-carotene, and this almond version gives them a unique twist that you and your family are sure to love.

455 g (1 lb)	carrots, sliced into 5 mm (¼ in) rounds
15 g (½ oz)	butter or polyunsaturated margarine
1	small onion, chopped
1	teaspoon grated fresh ginger
4	tablespoons orange juice
3	tablespoons almond liqueur or ½ teaspoon almond extract
⅛	teaspoon salt
1	tablespoon toasted slivered almonds, chopped

Set a steamer rack in a medium saucepan filled with 2.5 cm (1 in) of boiling water. Place the carrots on the rack. Cover and cook over high heat for 10 minutes, or until tender.

Meanwhile, in a medium frying pan set over medium-high heat, melt the butter or margarine. Add the onion and ginger. Cook until soft. Add the orange juice, almond liqueur or almond extract, and salt. Cook until reduced by half. Add the carrots and toss to coat. Sprinkle with the almonds.

Makes 4 servings

Per serving: 149 calories/622 kJ, 2 g protein, 16 g carbohydrate (of which sugars 15 g), 7 g fat (of which saturates 2 g), 4 g dietary fibre, 157 mg sodium

Maple-Stuffed Sweet Potatoes

Sweet potatoes are a top-notch source of beta-carotene, and they also boost your intake of fibre and vitamin C. In this dressed-up version, the flavours of orange and maple serve as the perfect accent to the comforting flavour of the sweet potatoes.

4	large sweet potatoes
4	tablespoons natural yoghurt
3	tablespoons maple syrup
3	tablespoons orange juice
½	teaspoon ground nutmeg

Preheat the oven to 190°C/375°F/gas 5.

Place the sweet potatoes on a nonstick baking sheet. Bake for 1¼ hours, or until easily pierced with a fork (see note). Slice them in half lengthwise. Scoop out the pulp, leaving a 5 mm (¼ in) shell. Set aside the shells and transfer the pulp to a large bowl.

Using a potato masher or fork, mash the pulp. Stir in the yoghurt, maple syrup, orange juice and nutmeg. Mix well. Spoon the filling into the reserved shells.

Return to the oven and bake for 5 minutes, or until heated through.

Makes 4 servings

Per serving: *158 calories/660 kJ, 3 g protein, 37 g carbohydrate (of which sugars 21 g), 0.5 g fat (of which saturates 0 g), 2 g dietary fibre, 801 mg sodium*

Note: To cut the baking time, microwave the sweet potatoes, pricked, on high power for a total of 8 to 10 minutes, or until tender; turn them over halfway through the cooking time.

Brussels Sprouts with Dill

Think of brussels sprouts as little balls of phytonutrients that fight cancer and boost immunity. Specifically, this dish is a very good source of vitamin C, folate, potassium, vitamin B_6 and vitamin A. Don't be discouraged if you don't usually like brussels sprouts: In this delicious version, they have a fresh, even sweet flavour.

455 g (1 lb)	small brussels sprouts, trimmed
15 g (½ oz)	butter
2	tablespoons finely chopped fresh dill or 1 teaspoon dried
2	tablespoons snipped fresh chives

Remove any discoloured or wilted leaves from the brussels sprouts, and neatly trim the bottoms. Steam the brussels sprouts for 5 minutes or just until tender when pierced with a sharp knife. Do not overcook.

Melt the butter in a large nonstick frying pan over medium heat, and stir for 2 minutes or until it starts to brown lightly. Add the brussels sprouts, dill and chives. Toss and stir for 2 minutes.

MAKES **4** SERVINGS

Per serving: 75 calories/313 kJ, 4 g protein, 5 g carbohydrate (of which sugars 3 g), 3 g fat, 4 g dietary fibre, 35 mg sodium

Soya Beans with Sesame Oil and Spring Onions

Soya beans are true immune-boosting stars. They lower bad cholesterol levels, protect your heart and may help in the fight against cancer. This dish is also a very good source of vitamin C and fibre.

400 g	tin soya beans, drained
1	tablespoon reduced-sodium soy sauce
125 ml (4 fl oz)	water
1½	teaspoons sesame oil
	Dash of hot-pepper sauce (optional)
2	tablespoons finely chopped spring onions
⅛	teaspoon salt
⅛	teaspoon ground black pepper

Bring the soya beans, soy sauce and water to the boil in a medium saucepan over high heat, stirring once or twice. Lower the heat and simmer until the soya beans are tender, about 12 minutes. If any liquid remains, cook over medium-high heat, stirring occasionally, until the liquid has evaporated.

Remove from the heat. Stir in the oil, pepper sauce (if using), spring onions, salt and black pepper.

MAKES **4** SERVINGS

Per serving: 94 calories/393 kJ, 6 g protein, 14 g carbohydrate (of which sugars 3 g), 7 g fat, 7 g dietary fibre, 400 mg sodium

POULTRY

Citrus Chicken Breast with Mint and Toasted Almonds

With its orange-juice-flavoured sauce, this tasty dish is a good source of vitamin C. In addition, it uses chicken breast, which has less than half the fat of most cuts of meat. Finally, the almonds are a delicious source of monounsaturated fat.

750 ml (1¼ pt)	calcium-fortified orange juice
4	boneless, skinless chicken breast halves
1	medium onion, quartered
3	cloves garlic, halved
½	teaspoon salt
2	teaspoons rice wine or cider vinegar
15 g (½ oz)	butter or polyunsaturated margarine
2	tablespoons chopped fresh mint or 1 teaspoon dried
30 g (1 oz)	sliced almonds, toasted

Place the orange juice, chicken, onion, garlic, salt, vinegar and butter or margarine in a large saucepan. Bring to the boil. Reduce the heat to low. Simmer for 15 minutes, or until a thermometer inserted in the thickest portion registers 72°C (160°F) or the juices run clear. While the chicken is simmering, chop the mint and toast the almonds. (Sliced almonds can be toasted in a small pan over medium-high heat, stirring occasionally, for 5 minutes or until lightly browned.) Remove the chicken from the pan and set aside, keeping it warm.

Allow the juice mixture to cool slightly, then purée in a blender. Return to the saucepan over high heat. (If using dried mint, mix it into the orange sauce while its reducing.) Boil the mixture for 20 minutes, or until it is reduced by at least half, stirring as needed to make up to 500 ml (18 fl oz) of sauce. (Reduce the heat to medium-high if the mixture begins to boil over.)

Divide the chicken among 4 plates. Top each piece with 4 tablespoons of the orange sauce. Garnish with the mint (if using fresh) and almonds. Serve any remaining sauce on the side for topping side dishes, such as brown rice pilaf and green beans or asparagus.

MAKES 4 SERVINGS

Per serving: 270 calories/1128 kJ, 25 g protein, 20 g carbohydrate (of which sugars 18 g), 10 g fat (of which saturates 3 g), 1 g dietary fibre, 414 mg sodium

Baked Chicken Thighs with Peppers and Olives

It's true that chicken thighs contain more fat than chicken breasts, but because this dish is served with rice, a little chicken goes a long way. In addition, this dish uses garlic and onions, which contain phytochemicals that boost the immune system, and peppers, which contain vitamin C.

1	teaspoon olive oil
170 g (6 oz)	sliced onions
1	tablespoon finely chopped garlic
1	green pepper, thinly sliced
1	red or yellow pepper, thinly sliced
5	pitted black olives, sliced
$\frac{1}{4}$	teaspoon dried thyme, or 1 tablespoon chopped fresh
$\frac{1}{4}$	teaspoon dried rosemary or 1 tablespoon chopped fresh
	Pinch of chilli pepper flakes
570 g ($1\frac{1}{4}$ lb)	boneless, skinless chicken thighs, trimmed of all visible fat
2	teaspoons lemon juice
$\frac{1}{8}$	teaspoon ground black pepper
1	tablespoon grated Parmesan cheese
340 g (12 oz)	hot cooked rice

Preheat the oven to 220°C/425°F/gas 7. Coat a nonstick frying pan with cooking spray. Add the oil and warm over medium heat. Add the onions and garlic and cook, stirring frequently, for 4 to 5 minutes, or until the onions are nearly tender.

Add the green pepper and red or yellow pepper and cook, stirring frequently, for 5 to 6 minutes, or until tender. Add the olives, thyme, rosemary and chilli pepper flakes and cook, stirring frequently, for 1 minute.

Coat a shallow, 3.5 l (6 pt), nonstick baking dish with cooking spray. Arrange the chicken in a single layer in the baking dish. Drizzle with the lemon juice and sprinkle with the black pepper. Spoon the vegetables over the chicken and sprinkle with the Parmesan.

Bake for 25 to 30 minutes, or until the chicken is cooked through. Serve with the rice.

Makes **4** servings

Per serving: 311 calories/1300 kJ, 27 g protein, 34 g carbohydrate (of which sugars 6 g), 19 g fat (of which saturates 3 g), 3 g dietary fibre, 174 mg sodium

Asian-Style Chicken and Broccoli Stir-Fry

Instead of ordering a takeaway, whip up this fast-cooking stir-fry. Not only is it delicious, but the broccoli is also packed with immunity-enhancing vitamins and minerals such as beta-carotene, calcium and folate.

455 g (1 lb)	boneless, skinless chicken breasts, cut lengthwise into thin strips
1	tablespoon cornflour
2	teaspoons brown sugar
3	tablespoons soy sauce
1	tablespoon dry sherry (optional)
2	teaspoons toasted sesame oil
1	tablespoon corn oil or vegetable oil
1	teaspoon chopped fresh ginger
400 g (14 oz)	broccoli florets
4	tablespoons water or defatted chicken stock

Place the chicken strips on a plate and dredge with the cornflour and brown sugar. Sprinkle with the soy sauce, sherry (if using) and sesame oil. Toss well with 2 forks to coat strips evenly.

Place a wok or nonstick frying pan on a burner over high heat. When the pan is hot, add 1 teaspoon of the corn or vegetable oil. Turn the heat to medium-high, add the chicken, and cook until no longer pink and the juices run clear. Remove the chicken and set aside.

Lower the heat to medium. Add the remaining corn or vegetable oil and ginger, and stir for 30 seconds. Add the broccoli and cook, stirring constantly, for 2 minutes.

Add the chicken and water or stock. Stir for 1 minute or until the sauce is thickened. Remove from the heat. Serve with steaming hot brown rice.

MAKES 4 SERVINGS

Per serving: 222 calories/928 kJ, 30 g protein, 11 g carbohydrate (of which sugars 4 g), 6 g fat (of which saturates 2 g), 4 g dietary fibre, 737 mg sodium

Oven-Fried Chicken Fingers
with Tropical Peanut Butter Dipping Sauce

These garlicky finger lickers contain groundnut oil to perk up the 'good' monounsaturated fat. The sauce is packed with phytochemicals and fruity flavour.

Chicken Fingers

2¹⁄₂	tablespoons groundnut oil
90 g (3 oz)	plain flour
1¹⁄₂	teaspoons garlic salt
¹⁄₂	teaspoon cayenne pepper
¹⁄₂	teaspoon ground black pepper
1	large egg + 2 large egg whites
2	tablespoons cold water
115 g (4 oz)	unseasoned dried breadcrumbs
455 g (1 lb)	boneless, skinless chicken breasts, sliced into 16 strips

Dipping Sauce

60 g (2 oz)	smooth peanut butter (with salt)
75 g (2¹⁄₂ oz)	apricot jam
4	tablespoons tropical fruit juice
¹⁄₄	teaspoon grated orange zest

To make the chicken fingers: Preheat the oven to 200°C/400°F/gas 6. Pour the oil into a 23 x 33 cm (9 x 13 in) baking dish. In a shallow bowl, combine the flour, ¹⁄₂ teaspoon of the garlic salt, and the cayenne and black peppers. In a second shallow bowl, whisk the egg and egg whites with the cold water. In a third shallow bowl, mix the breadcrumbs with ¹⁄₂ teaspoon of the garlic salt. Season the chicken with the remaining ¹⁄₂ teaspoon garlic salt. Dip the chicken into the flour mixture, then into the egg mixture, then roll it in the breadcrumb mixture. Place the chicken in the baking dish and turn to coat with the oil. Bake for 22 to 25 minutes, rotating after 15 minutes.

To make the dipping sauce: Mix sauce ingredients in a saucepan and stir over medium heat until the mixture starts to bubble. Remove from the heat.

Serve the chicken warm or at room temperature with the warm sauce.

MAKES 4 SERVINGS

Per serving: *524 calories/2190 kJ, 37 g protein, 50 g carbohydrate (of which sugars 16 g), 21 g fat (of which saturates 5 g), 3 g dietary fibre, 1267 mg sodium*

Note: For an extra-crispy, lower-fat option, instead of using groundnut oil, just coat the chicken with cooking spray prior to baking.

Spinach-Turkey Burgers with Corn Salsa

When you're in the mood for a burger, throw a few of these family-friendly turkey burgers on the grill. They're moist and full of flavour, so even kids will love them, and they're a very good source of folate, vitamins A and B₆, niacin and vitamin C.

Burgers

455 g (1 lb)	minced turkey
285 g (10 oz)	frozen chopped spinach, thawed and well-drained
1	medium onion, grated
50 g (1¾ oz)	instant porridge oats
1	egg white
½	teaspoon dried sage or oregano or 1 tablespoon chopped fresh
½	teaspoon salt
	Pinch of pepper

Salsa

455 g (1 lb)	seeded and chopped tomatoes
250 g (9 oz)	fresh, cooked corn kernels
1	spring onion, finely chopped
1	tablespoon finely chopped coriander
	Pinch of salt and pepper

To make the burgers: Heat the grill. In a medium bowl, mix the turkey, spinach, onion, instant oats, egg white, sage or oregano, salt and pepper. Shape into 4 patties.

Cook for 6 to 8 minutes on each side or until the meat is cooked through and no longer pink.

To make the salsa: In a medium bowl, mix the tomatoes, corn, spring onion, coriander and salt and pepper. Serve with the burgers.

MAKES 4 SERVINGS

Per serving: 291 calories/1216 kJ, 34 g protein, 32 g carbohydrate (of which sugars 12 g), 4 g fat (of which saturates 1 g), 8 g dietary fibre, 742 mg sodium

MEATLESS MEALS

Stir-Fry with Tofu and Vegetables

Made from soya, tofu may help to reduce your cancer risk. Your family will never miss the meat when they tuck into this appetising dish with the taste of the Orient.

455 g (1 lb)	firm tofu, drained and cut into 1 cm (½ in) cubes
2	tablespoons soy sauce
1½	teaspoons groundnut oil
2	tablespoons finely chopped fresh ginger
1	tablespoon finely chopped garlic
½	teaspoon chilli pepper flakes
170 g (6 oz)	mushrooms, sliced
1	large red pepper, seeded and cut into thin strips
6	spring onions, cut into 4 cm (1½ in) diagonal slices
455 g (1 lb)	pak choi, coarsely chopped
400 g tin	baby corn, drained
1½	teaspoons toasted sesame oil
500 g (1 lb 2 oz)	hot cooked white or brown rice

In an airtight container, marinate the tofu in the soy sauce for 10 minutes. Shake gently every few minutes to baste the tofu.

Warm a wok or large nonstick frying pan over medium-high heat. Add the oil and tilt the pan in all directions to coat it. Add the ginger and garlic. Stir-fry for 10 seconds. Add the chilli pepper flakes, mushrooms and red pepper. Stir-fry for 2 to 3 minutes, or until the mushrooms release their liquid and the liquid has evaporated.

Stir in the spring onions, pak choi, tofu and tofu marinade. Cover and cook for 1 to 2 minutes, or until the pak choi is crisp-tender.

Stir in the baby corn, sesame oil and additional soy sauce to taste. Serve over the rice.

MAKES 4 SERVINGS

Per serving: 456 calories/1906 kJ, 19 g protein, 71 g carbohydrate (of which sugars 16 g), 12 g fat (of which saturates 2 g), 8 g dietary fibre, 682 mg sodium

Vegetable Cobbler

You'll never miss the meat in this appetising cobbler. It's pretty enough to serve to company, and since it's filled with a cornucopia of different vegetables, you're sure to be getting a wide array of vitamins and minerals.

Vegetable Filling

115 g (4 oz)	chopped onions
½	deseeded and sliced red pepper
2	cloves garlic, finely chopped
500ml (18 fl oz)	vegetable stock, or vegetable stock made with bouillon powder or cube
1	medium baking potato, scrubbed and cut into medium-sized cubes
2	small courgettes, sliced 1 cm (½ in) thick
1	large carrot, sliced
1	medium parsnip, sliced
75 g (2½ oz)	fresh or frozen peas
75 g (2½ oz)	fresh or frozen corn
½	teaspoon dried rosemary or 1 tablespoon chopped fresh rosemary
½	teaspoon dried tarragon or 1 tablespoon chopped fresh tarragon
¼	teaspoon dried thyme or 2 teaspoons chopped fresh thyme
3	tablespoons plain flour
80 ml (3fl oz)	cold water
2	tablespoons dry white wine (optional)
	Salt and ground black pepper

Crust

115 g (4 oz)	plain flour
¼	teaspoon baking powder
¼	teaspoon salt
3	tablespoons vegetable oil or cold polyunsaturated margarine, cut into pieces
4–4½	tablespoons iced water
1½	teaspoons skimmed milk
2	teaspoons grated Parmesan cheese

To make the vegetable filling: Coat a large saucepan with cooking spray. Warm over medium heat until hot. Add the onions, sweet peppers and garlic. Sauté for 5 minutes, or until the vegetables are tender.

Add the stock, potato, courgette, carrot, parsnip, peas, corn, rosemary, tarragon and thyme. Bring to the boil over high heat. Reduce the heat to low, cover, and simmer for 10 minutes or until the vegetables are tender.

Return to the boil over medium-high heat. In a small bowl, whisk together the flour and water. Stir into the vegetable mixture and cook, stirring constantly, until thickened. Stir in the wine (if using) and season to taste with the salt and black pepper. Spoon the mixture into a 2 l (3^1/$_2$ pt) baking dish or soufflé dish.

To make the crust: Preheat the oven to 220°C/425°F/gas 7. In a small bowl, combine the flour, baking powder and salt. Cut in the oil or margarine with a fork or pastry blender until coarse crumbs form. Mix in the water, a tablespoon at a time, until a dough forms.

Transfer to a lightly floured surface and roll to 5 mm (^{1}/$_4$ in) thickness. Carefully place the rolled dough over the baking dish. Trim the edges and flute or press with the tines of a fork. Cut several steam vents in the top of the crust. If desired, roll pastry scraps and cut into designs for the top of the crust.

Bake for 10 minutes. Lightly brush the top of the crust with the milk and sprinkle with the Parmesan. Bake for 5 to 10 minutes longer, or until the crust is lightly browned. Cool on a rack for 5 minutes before serving.

Makes 4 servings

Per serving: 450 calories/1881 kJ, 10 g protein, 58 g carbohydrate (of which sugars 10 g), 11 g fat, 6 g dietary fibre, 673 mg sodium

Garden Burgers with Mustard Sauce

Vegetables, grains and reduced-fat cheeses make these meat-free burgers moist, delicious and low in fat. Serve them on wholemeal or multigrain buns for extra fibre.

Garden Burgers

60 g (2 oz)	finely chopped shiitake or button mushrooms
60 g (2 oz)	finely chopped broccoli florets and stalks
30 g (1 oz)	finely chopped spring onions
2	cloves garlic, finely chopped
30 g (1 oz)	pecan pieces (optional)
½	teaspoon dried marjoram or 2 tablespoons fresh, chopped
½	teaspoon dried savory or 2 tablespoons fresh, chopped
¼	teaspoon dried thyme or 1 tablespoon fresh, chopped
50 g (1¾ oz)	instant porridge
90 g (3 oz)	cooked brown rice
60 g (2 oz)	grated half-fat Cheddar cheese
75 g (2½ oz)	reduced-fat cottage cheese
3	egg whites
¼	teaspoon ground black pepper
	Pinch of salt

Mustard Sauce

60 g (2 oz)	fat-free mayonnaise
4	teaspoons Dijon mustard
4	wholemeal or multigrain buns

To make the garden burgers: Coat a medium nonstick frying pan with cooking spray. Warm over medium heat until hot. Add the mushrooms, broccoli, spring onions, garlic, pecans (if using), marjoram, savory and thyme. Cover and cook for 5 minutes, or until the mushrooms are soft and the broccoli is crisp-tender.

Stir in the oats and rice. Cook, uncovered, for 2 to 3 minutes, stirring occasionally. Remove from the heat and cool to room temperature.

Stir in the Cheddar, cottage cheese, egg whites, pepper and salt. Mix well. Form the mixture into four 1 cm (½ in)-thick patties. (The patties will be soft, but will firm up when cooked.)

Wipe the frying pan and coat with cooking spray. Warm over medium heat until hot. Add the burgers and cook for 5 minutes on each side, or until browned.

To make the mustard sauce: In a small bowl, combine the mayonnaise and mustard. Spread on the bottoms of the buns. Top with the burgers and serve.

Makes **4** servings

Per serving: 365 calories/1526 kJ, 17 g protein, 42 g carbohydrate (of which sugars 3 g), 15 g fat (of which saturates 3 g), 5 g dietary fibre, 797 mg sodium

Grilled Peanut Butter and Banana Sandwich

It's been said that Elvis Presley regularly ate a version of this peanut butter sandwich. The bananas, which are loaded with potassium, and the wholemeal bread, which supplies fibre and other nutrients, help make this sandwich healthy.

6–8	tablespoons smooth or crunchy peanut butter
8	slices wholemeal bread
2	large ripe bananas, sliced lengthwise into a total of 16 pieces
2	tablespoons clear honey
	Butter-flavoured cooking spray

Spread about 1 tablespoon of the peanut butter on each of the bread slices. Place the banana pieces on top of the peanut butter on four of the slices and drizzle with honey. Press the remaining slices of bread on top to make four sandwiches.

Place a large, nonstick frying pan over medium-high heat. Coat the bread with cooking spray just before browning each side. Sauté (or grill) sandwiches, in batches, approximately 2 minutes per side, or until golden brown. Slice the sandwiches diagonally and serve warm.

Makes **4** servings

Per serving: 490 calories/2048 kJ, 16 g protein, 60 g carbohydrate (of which sugars 27 g), 22 g fat (of which saturates 5 g), 8 g dietary fibre, 532 mg sodium

Chunky Roasted-Vegetable Chilli

This mouthwatering yet easy-to-prepare chilli is perfect for hectic days. It's full of vitamin C, beta-carotene and fibre and is delicious served with brown rice. For an extra health boost, chop up some spinach or other greens and toss them in before serving.

685 g (1½ lb)	butternut squash, peeled, seeded and cut into 2 cm (¾ in) chunks
3	carrots, sliced
2	large peppers (red and yellow), coarsely chopped
2	courgettes, cut into 2 cm (¾ in) chunks
2	tablespoons olive oil
1½	teaspoons ground cumin
1	teaspoon salt
1	large onion, chopped
1	tablespoon finely chopped garlic
1	tablespoon chilli powder
2 x 400 g	tins chopped tomatoes in juice
2 x 400 g	tins black beans, rinsed and drained
500 ml (18 fl oz)	vegetable stock, or vegetable stock made with bouillon powder or cube
250 ml (9 fl oz)	water

Preheat the oven to 230°C/450°F/gas 8. Divide the squash, carrots, peppers, courgettes, 1 tablespoon of the oil, the cumin and ¼ teaspoon of the salt between 2 baking trays. Stir to combine. Roast for 20 minutes or until tender. Set aside.

In a casserole, heat the remaining 1 tablespoon of oil over low heat. Add the onion and sauté until softened, about 8 minutes. Add the garlic and chilli powder. Sauté for 2 minutes. Add the remaining ¾ teaspoon of salt and the tomatoes, beans, stock and water to the onions. Bring to the boil. Reduce the heat and simmer, covered, for 30 minutes.

Stir in the roasted vegetables. Bring to the boil. Cover and simmer for 15 minutes to blend the flavours.

MAKES 10 SERVINGS

Per serving: 166 calories/694 kJ, 9 g protein, 26 g carbohydrate (of which sugars 10 g), 4 g fat (of which saturates 0.5 g), 4 g dietary fibre, 352 mg sodium

FISH

Grilled Red Mullet with Gazpacho Sauce

Do you find yourself turning to the same tried-and-tested recipes when it's time to cook fish? If so, you're in for a treat with this dish, which has a tasty, orange-coloured sauce. In addition to serving the sauce with fish, try it with chicken, rice, or vegetables.

4	teaspoons olive oil
1	slice French or Italian bread, such as ciabatta, 7.5 x 5 x 1 cm (3 x 2 x ½ in) thick, toasted
3	small cloves garlic, unpeeled
115 g (4 oz)	coarsely chopped, peeled, and seeded tomatoes
115 g (4 oz)	coarsely chopped roasted red peppers or tinned peppers, drained
2	teaspoons red wine vinegar or other vinegar
	Salt
	Fresh ground black pepper
4	red mullet fillets, about 1 cm (½ in) thick and 170 g (6 oz) each, with skin
2–3	teaspoons chopped fresh basil

Preheat the grill to hot.

Heat 2 teaspoons of the oil in a small, heavy frying pan over low heat on the stove. Add the bread and garlic. Lightly brown the bread on both sides, then remove. Continue to cook the garlic, turning occasionally, for 1 to 2 minutes or until tender.

Combine the tomatoes, roasted pepper, vinegar, toasted bread broken into pieces and peeled garlic in a blender, and purée until smooth. Season.

Moisten both sides of the fillets with the remaining 2 teaspoons of oil and season with salt and pepper. Place them skin side down under the grill and cook for 4 to 5 minutes. Turn and grill 4 to 5 minutes longer, or until the skin is golden and the flesh flakes easily.

Place the fillets on plates, top with a dollop of sauce and sprinkle with the basil. Serve with the remaining sauce on the side.

MAKES 4 SERVINGS

Per serving: 220 calories/920 kJ, 31 g protein, 10 g carbohydrate (of which sugars 3 g), 6 g fat (of which saturates 1 g), 1 g dietary fibre, 290 mg sodium

Mini Salmon Cakes

Salmon is a great source of heart-healthy omega-3 fatty acids. If you know you'll be short on time, prepare and form these cakes in the morning – or even the day before. Then, all you need to do is give them a light dip in breadcrumbs before cooking. Sesame seeds could be used instead of flaxseed.

2	large eggs
4	teaspoons grated onion
1	tablespoon Dijon mustard
1	teaspoon Worcester sauce
¼	teaspoon salt
⅛	teaspoon ground black pepper
3	tablespoons finely chopped red pepper
2	teaspoons + 2 tablespoons ground flaxseed
4	teaspoons chopped fresh dill
375 g (13 oz)	cooked, coarsely flaked salmon (tinned or from 455 g/1 lb raw fillet), see note
4	teaspoons + 2 tablespoons dried breadcrumbs
	Lemon wedges

In a large bowl, stir together the eggs, onion, mustard, Worcester sauce, salt and black pepper until smooth. Stir in the pepper, 2 teaspoons of the flaxseed and the dill. Fold in the salmon and 4 teaspoons of the breadcrumbs and combine well.

Form the mixture into eight 1 cm (¹/₂ in)-thick cakes (they can be refrigerated for up to 24 hours at this point).

Mix together the remaining 2 tablespoons flaxseed and 2 tablespoons breadcrumbs on a large plate. Coat the cakes on all sides with this mixture.

Coat a large nonstick frying pan with cooking spray and set it over low heat. When it is hot, add the cakes and slowly brown them on one side for 5 to 6 minutes. Turn them over, cover, and cook until they are golden brown on the second side and hot throughout, about 5 minutes. Serve with the lemon wedges.

MAKES 4 SERVINGS

Per serving (2 cakes): 306 calories/1279 kJ, 24 g protein, 9 g carbohydrate (of which sugars 2 g), 20 g fat (of which saturates 4 g), 1 g dietary fibre, 517 mg sodium

Note: To cook salmon, grill it 10 cm (4 in) from the heat for 3 minutes per side, or until it flakes easily.

Grilled Tuna with Honey-Herb Sauce

Instead of beef steaks, cook these tuna steaks, which are a great source of heart-healthy omega-3s. Don't be scared off by the relatively large amount of oil in this recipe: since it's olive oil, it not only adds great flavour, but it also helps reduce disease-causing cholesterol and provides antioxidant protection.

15 g (½ oz)	parsley
3	tablespoons + 1 teaspoon olive oil
2	tablespoons cider vinegar
2	tablespoons fresh dill
1½	tablespoons clear honey
¼	teaspoon salt
¼	teaspoon ground black pepper
4	tuna steaks, about 2.5 cm (1 in) thick and 170 g (6 oz) each
2	teaspoons drained capers

Preheat the grill to medium-hot.

Purée the parsley, 3 tablespoons of the oil, and the vinegar, dill and honey in a blender until they form a bright green, slightly thickened sauce flecked with herbs. Season with half of the salt and half of the pepper.

Moisten both sides of the tuna steaks with the remaining 1 teaspoon of the oil and season with the remaining salt and pepper. Grill them for a total of 5 to 6 minutes, turning once, until they flake easily.

Place the tuna steaks on plates, drizzle with the sauce and sprinkle with the capers.

Makes 4 servings

Per serving: 425 calories/1776 kJ, 46 g protein, 6 g carbohydrate (of which sugars 5 g), 24 g fat (of which saturates 3 g), 0 g dietary fibre, 623 mg sodium

Poached Salmon
with Toasted Breadcrumbs and Basil

Salmon is a true treasure from the sea when you consider the high levels of omega-3 fatty acids it contains. These acids are not only good for your heart but also have a protective effect against cancer. Because the salmon in this dish is poached at a gentle simmer, it remains tender and succulent.

1	thin slice lemon
1	bay leaf
2	teaspoons olive oil
30 g (1 oz)	dried breadcrumbs
1	tablespoon chopped pine nuts or other nuts
1	clove garlic, finely chopped
1	tablespoon drained, chopped sun-dried tomatoes
2	tablespoons grated Parmesan cheese
	Salt
	Freshly ground black pepper
2	tablespoons chopped fresh basil
4	salmon fillets, about 1 cm (½ in) thick and 115 g (4 oz) each, with skin

Put 1 l (1³/₄ pt) of hot water and the lemon slice and bay leaf in a 23 or 25 cm (9 or 10 in) frying pan. Place the pan over low heat to simmer.

Warm the oil in a smaller frying pan on low heat. Stir in the breadcrumbs and nuts and cook, stirring, for about 2 minutes or until lightly toasted.

Add the garlic to the crumb mixture and cook, stirring, for 30 to 60 seconds longer or until the garlic is fragrant. Turn off the heat and stir in the tomatoes and cheese. Season with salt and pepper to taste, then stir in the basil. Set aside.

Place the fillets skin side up in the simmering water, adding more hot water if needed to just cover. Cook for 10 minutes or until the fish flakes easily. Transfer to a serving dish and remove the skin by peeling it off from one end to the other. Discard the skin and the bay leaf.

Turn the fillets over, set on plates and spoon the breadcrumb mixture on top.

MAKES 4 SERVINGS

Per serving: *338 calories/1413 kJ, 26 g protein, 5 g carbohydrate (of which sugars 0.5 g), 23 g fat (of which saturates 5 g), 0 g dietary fibre, 441 mg sodium*

Lemon Sole Veracruz

This delicious dish requires just 15 minutes to prepare, yet it's pretty enough to serve to guests. The bright red hue of the tomatoes is a sign that you're getting vitamin C and lycopene, important elements in an immune-enhancing diet.

4	lemon sole fillets (about 115 g/4 oz each)
	Juice of 1 lime
1	teaspoon dried oregano or 1 tablespoon chopped fresh
2	teaspoons olive oil
1	onion, chopped
1	clove garlic, finely chopped
400 g	tin chopped tomatoes with chilli
12	pimento-stuffed olives, coarsely chopped
2	tablespoons chopped fresh parsley

Preheat the oven to 180°C/350°F/gas 4. Coat a 20 x 20 cm (8 x 8 in) baking dish with cooking spray. Place the fillets in the prepared dish. Sprinkle with the lime juice and oregano. Set aside.

Warm the oil in a medium frying pan set over medium heat. Add the onion and garlic. Cook, stirring occasionally, for 5 to 6 minutes or until soft. Add the tomatoes, olives and parsley. Cook, stirring occasionally, for 5 minutes or until thickened. Spoon over the fillets. Cover tightly with foil.

Bake for 18 to 20 minutes, or until the fish flakes easily.

Makes 4 servings

Per serving: 144 calories/602 kJ, 21 g protein, 6 g carbohydrate (of which sugars 5 g), 4 g fat (of which saturates 0.5 g), 2 g dietary fibre, 290 mg sodium

PASTA

Linguine with Mushrooms and Peppers

White button mushrooms are a good source of niacin, a B vitamin that plays a role in the conversion of sugars into energy in your body. Shiitake mushrooms are at the top of the list of foods with anti-cancer properties.

2	teaspoons olive oil
1	sweet onion, sliced and separated into rings
1	bay leaf
60 g (2 oz)	fresh button mushrooms, sliced
60 g (2 oz)	fresh shiitake mushrooms, sliced
2	red, yellow, or green peppers, cut into thin strips
2	cloves garlic, finely chopped
½	teaspoon dried thyme or 1 tablespoon fresh, chopped
½	teaspoon dried oregano or 1 tablespoon fresh, chopped
1	teaspoon dried basil or 1 tablespoon fresh, chopped
3	tablespoons flat leaf parsley, chopped
150 ml (¼ pt)	vegetable stock or defatted chicken stock, or stock made with bouillon powder or cube
230 g (8 oz)	linguine or spaghetti
2	tablespoons grated Parmesan cheese (optional)

In a large nonstick frying pan over medium-low heat, warm the oil. Add the onion and bay leaf and sauté for about 5 minutes.

Add the button mushrooms, shiitake mushrooms, peppers and garlic, and sauté for 4 minutes or until the mushrooms begin to release their liquid. Add the thyme, oregano, basil, parsley and stock. Increase the heat to medium and simmer uncovered for 5 to 7 minutes, or until the peppers are soft and the stock has reduced slightly.

Meanwhile, in a large pan of boiling water, cook the linguine according to the package directions. Drain. Place in a serving bowl and toss with the mushroom mixture.

Remove and discard the bay leaf. Sprinkle with the Parmesan (if using).

MAKES 4 SERVINGS

Per serving: 293 calories/1225 kJ, 12 g protein, 51 g carbohydrate (of which sugars 9 g), 6 g fat (of which saturates 2 g), 5 g dietary fibre, 270 mg sodium

Pasta Primavera

A tasty mixture of half-fat crème fraîche, low-fat natural yoghurt and grated Parmesan cheese replaces the high-fat cream in this slimmed-down version of an Italian classic. Even better, this dish is packed with nutritious vegetables such as carrots, courgettes and mangetouts.

340 g (12 oz)	penne
2	teaspoons olive oil
1	small onion, thinly sliced and separated into rings
2	cloves garlic, finely chopped
150 g (5½ oz)	carrots, thinly sliced
150 g (5½ oz)	courgettes, thinly sliced
150 g (5½ oz)	mangetouts
1	medium tomato, chopped
150 g (5½ oz)	frozen peas, thawed
125 ml (4 fl oz)	low-fat natural yoghurt
125 ml (4 fl oz)	half-fat crème fraîche
2	tablespoons grated Parmesan cheese
½	teaspoon dried basil or 1 tablespoon fresh, chopped
¼	teaspoon ground black pepper

In a large pot of boiling water, cook the penne according to the package directions.

Meanwhile, in a large nonstick frying pan over medium heat, warm the oil. Add the onions and garlic. Cook and stir for 2 minutes. Add the carrots and cook, stirring frequently, for 3 minutes. Add the courgettes, mangetouts, tomato and peas and cook, stirring frequently, for 4 to 6 minutes or until the vegetables are tender.

Reduce the heat to low. Remove the frying pan from the heat and stir in the yoghurt, crème fraîche, Parmesan, basil and pepper. Return the pan to the heat and cook over very low heat for 1 to 2 minutes, or until warmed through. Do not boil.

Drain the pasta and place in a large serving bowl. Add the sauce and toss to mix well.

MAKES 4 SERVINGS

Per serving: *492 calories/2056 kJ, 21 g protein, 80 g carbohydrate (of which sugars 13 g), 12 g fat (of which saturates 6 g), 8 g dietary fibre, 178 mg sodium*

Creamy Caprese Pasta

This pasta dish from the island of Capri tastes like pesto, but it's creamier. Calcium-rich yoghurt is the secret and one of the reasons why this recipe is good for healthy bones.

455 g (1 lb)	dry wholewheat pasta shapes
1 x 200 g	pot fat-free natural yoghurt
1	tablespoon + 1 teaspoon extra-virgin olive oil
½	teaspoon salt
1	large clove garlic
30 g (1 oz)	fresh basil leaves plus additional for garnish
2	large, ripe tomatoes, chopped
1	teaspoon balsamic or red wine vinegar
170 g (6 oz)	low-fat mozzarella cheese, cubed

Prepare the pasta according to the package directions, eliminating any suggested salt or oil.

While the pasta is boiling, place the yoghurt, oil, salt and garlic in a blender. Purée until smooth. Add the basil and purée until completely blended.

Place the tomatoes in a small mixing bowl. Toss with the vinegar and add the cheese.

Drain the pasta and place it in a large mixing bowl. Immediately pour the basil sauce over the hot pasta. Toss until the mixture is coated. Serve topped with the tomato-mozzarella mixture. Garnish with additional fresh basil.

MAKES 5 SERVINGS

Per serving: 432 calories/1806 kJ, 17 g protein, 74 g carbohydrate (of which sugars 6 g), 10 g fat (of which saturates 4 g), 5 g dietary fibre, 626 mg sodium

Fiesta Pasta Salad

This colourful salad is the perfect dish to bring to a summer picnic or a party. It takes just 15 minutes to prepare, and you're likely to have most of the ingredients in your store cupboard. Furthermore, one serving contains just 5 grams of fat and 7 grams of fibre.

150 ml (¼ pt)	vegetable juice cocktail
2	tablespoons lime juice
½–1	teaspoon hot-pepper sauce
2	cloves garlic, finely chopped
½	teaspoon sugar
¼	teaspoon ground cumin
¼	teaspoon salt
230 g (8 oz)	pasta shapes, cooked and drained
90 g (3 oz)	sliced, smoked ham, cut into 2.5 cm (1 in) strips
400 g	tin red kidney beans, rinsed and drained
230 g (8 oz)	sweetcorn kernels, tinned and drained or frozen and thawed
115 g (4 oz)	grated low-fat Cheddar cheese
3	plum tomatoes, chopped
3	spring onions, sliced
60 g (2 oz)	sliced pitted black olives

In a large bowl, combine the vegetable juice, lime juice, ½ teaspoon of the hot-pepper sauce and the garlic, sugar, cumin and salt. Whisk to mix. Add the pasta, ham, beans, corn, Cheddar, tomatoes, spring onions and olives. Toss to mix. Taste and add up to ½ teaspoon more hot-pepper sauce, if desired.

Makes 8 servings

Per serving: 249 calories/1041 kJ, 15 g protein, 40 g carbohydrate (of which sugars 7 g), 5 g fat (of which saturates 2 g), 7 g dietary fibre, 787 mg sodium

Penne with Broccoli and Peppers

There's no need for a rich cream and butter sauce when you're pairing your pasta with crisp, colourful vegetables such as broccoli and pepper. To save time and washing up, you can cook the broccoli in the same pan as the penne. Simply add it for the last 5 minutes of the pasta's cooking time.

230 g (8 oz)	penne
250 g (9 oz)	broccoli florets
1	tablespoon olive oil
1	red or yellow pepper, cut into thin strips
3	large cloves garlic, slivered
125 ml (4 fl oz)	vegetable or defatted chicken stock, or stock made with bouillon powder or cube
1¼	teaspoons Dijon mustard
½	teaspoon salt (optional)
⅛	teaspoon ground black pepper
2	teaspoons balsamic vinegar
2	tablespoons grated Parmesan cheese (optional)

In a large pan of boiling water, cook the penne according to the package directions. Drain. Transfer to a serving bowl and keep warm.

Meanwhile, in a medium saucepan, cook the broccoli in a small amount of boiling water for 5 minutes, or until bright green and just tender. Drain.

In a large nonstick frying pan over medium heat, warm the oil. Add the red or yellow peppers and sauté for 2 minutes. Add the garlic and sauté for 2 minutes.

Stir in the stock and broccoli and cook for 3 minutes. Stir in the mustard, salt (if using), and black pepper.

Toss the penne with the vegetables. Drizzle with the vinegar and toss again. Sprinkle with the Parmesan (if using).

MAKES 4 SERVINGS

***Per serving:** 303 calories/1266 kJ, 14 g protein, 48 g carbohydrate (of which sugars 5 g), 7 g fat (of which saturates 2 g), 3 g dietary fibre, 626 mg sodium*

MEAT MAIN COURSES

All-American Meat Loaf

Meat loaf as part of a healthy diet? It's true – with a recipe like this one! The secret is using the leanest possible minced beef in combination with rice and healthy vegetables such as cabbage, carrots and green peppers.

145 g (5 oz)	shredded cabbage
115 g (4 oz)	chopped onions
75 g (2½ oz)	grated carrots
60 g (2 oz)	chopped green peppers
2	cloves garlic, finely chopped
200 g (7 oz)	cooked brown rice
1	teaspoon dried basil or 2 tablespoons fresh, chopped
½	teaspoon dried savory or 1 tablespoon fresh, chopped
¼	teaspoon dried thyme or 1 tablespoon fresh, chopped
455 g (1 lb)	extra-lean minced beef
3	egg whites, lightly beaten
¾	teaspoon salt
¼	teaspoon ground black pepper
	Horseradish sauce

Preheat the oven to 180°C/350°F/gas 4. Coat a 1-kg (2-lb) nonstick loaf tin with cooking spray.

Coat a large nonstick frying pan with cooking spray and warm over medium heat. Add the cabbage, onions, carrots, green peppers and garlic. Cover and cook, stirring occasionally, for 8 to 10 minutes or until the carrots are tender. Stir in the rice, basil, savory and thyme. Let stand for 5 to 10 minutes, or until cool.

Add the beef, egg whites, salt and pepper. Mix with your hands to combine. Pack the mixture into the prepared loaf tin.

Bake for about 1 hour, or until a thermometer inserted in the centre registers 82°C (160°F) and the meat is no longer pink. Remove from the oven and set aside to cool for 5 minutes. Turn out of the tin onto a serving plate and slice. Serve with the horseradish sauce.

Makes 6 servings

Per serving: 168 calories/702 kJ, 19 g protein, 15 g carbohydrate (of which sugars 3 g), 4 g fat (of which saturates 2 g), 2 g dietary fibre, 349 mg sodium

Lamb Curry with Rice

As long as you choose a lean cut such as loin or fillet and remove all visible fat, lamb can be low in fat and calories. This spicy dish is a very good source of riboflavin, vitamin B_{12}, potassium, vitamin C and thiamin.

1	medium aubergine, thinly sliced
1	onion, chopped
1	teaspoon finely chopped garlic
250 ml (9 fl oz)	defatted chicken stock, or stock made with bouillon powder or cube
455 g (1 lb)	boneless lamb, trimmed of fat and cut into 1 cm (½ in) cubes
400 g tin	chopped tomatoes (with juice)
1	tablespoon curry powder, strength according to taste
1	teaspoon ground black pepper
½	teaspoon ground coriander
340 g (12 oz)	hot cooked rice
125 ml (4 fl oz)	low-fat natural yoghurt
15 g (½ oz)	finely chopped fresh coriander

In a large nonstick frying pan over medium-high heat, cook the aubergine, onion, garlic and 80 ml (3 fl oz) of the stock for 5 minutes. Add the lamb, tomatoes (with juice), curry powder, pepper, coriander and remaining stock. Bring to the boil.

Reduce the heat to medium. Cook, stirring occasionally, for 30 minutes or until the lamb is no longer pink when tested with a sharp knife. Serve over the rice, topped with the yoghurt and chopped coriander.

MAKES 4 SERVINGS

Per serving: 373 calories/1559 kJ, 31 g protein, 37 g carbohydrate (of which sugars 8 g), 12 g fat (of which saturates 5 g), 4 g dietary fibre, 371 mg sodium

Asian Green Beans with Beef

If you're trying to cut back on the amount of meat that your family eats, this is the perfect dish. Though each serving contains just 90 g (3 oz) of beef, you'll be more than satisfied because you'll be filling up on healthy brown rice and green beans. This stir-fry works best with young, tender beans. If your beans are less than fresh, blanch or steam them to tenderise before stir-frying.

1	tablespoon cornflour
½	teaspoon ground ginger
2	tablespoons soy sauce
6	cloves garlic, finely chopped
340 g (12 oz)	rump or sirloin steak, cut into thin strips
1	tablespoon corn or groundnut oil
455 g (1 lb)	fresh green beans, cut into 5 cm (2 in) lengths
250 ml (9 fl oz)	hot water
2	tablespoons smooth peanut butter
	Juice of ½ lime
2	tablespoons chopped fresh coriander
640 g (1 lb 6 oz)	hot cooked brown rice

In a medium bowl, mix the cornflour, ginger, 1 tablespoon of the soy sauce and half of the garlic. Add the steak and stir to coat. Set aside to marinate.

Heat 1 teaspoon of the oil in a large nonstick frying pan over medium heat. Add the beans and stir-fry for 3 minutes, or until the beans are slightly browned. Add the remaining garlic and stir-fry for 1 minute. Transfer the beans to a bowl.

Mix together the water, the peanut butter and the remaining 1 tablespoon of soy sauce. Set aside.

In the same pan, heat the remaining 2 teaspoons of oil over medium-high heat. Add the steak, a little at a time, stirring constantly. Stir-fry for 3 minutes or until the steak is browned. Stir in the beans and the peanut butter mixture. Cook, stirring often, for 1 minute or until the mixture is heated through and the sauce is slightly thickened. Stir in the lime juice. Remove from the heat and sprinkle with the coriander. Serve over the rice.

Makes 4 servings

Per serving: 479 calories/2002 kJ, 27 g protein, 61 g carbohydrate (of which sugars 5 g), 16 g fat (of which saturates 4 g), 5 g dietary fibre, 528 mg sodium

DESARTS

DESSERTS

Peanut Butter–Chocolate Mousse

Excite your tastebuds with this decadent dessert created by Louis Lanza, executive chef and co-owner of Josie's Restaurant and Juice Bar in New York City. The soya protein in tofu and monounsaturated fat in peanut butter make it heart-healthy as well.

340 g (12 oz)	silken tofu
170 g (6 oz)	maple syrup
45 g (1½ oz)	cocoa powder
1½	teaspoons vanilla extract
75 g (2½ oz)	smooth peanut butter
	Pinch of salt
2	tablespoons vanilla soya milk

Place the tofu, syrup, cocoa powder, vanilla, peanut butter and salt into a food processor, slowly drizzling in the soya milk. Blend until smooth.

Spoon into 5 serving dishes and refrigerate. Chill for 1 to 2 hours before serving.

MAKES 5 SERVINGS

Per serving: 277 calories/1158 kJ, 11 g protein, 31 g carbohydrate (of which sugars 28 g), 13 g fat (of which saturates 3 g), 1 g dietary fibre, 392 mg sodium

Pink Cantaloupe Ice

This refreshing dessert – perfect for hot summer days – is a very good source of vitamins A and C. Out of season, try different combinations of fruit.

455 g (1 lb)	cubed ripe cantaloupe melon
90 g (3 oz)	fresh strawberries
75 g (2½ oz)	sugar
4	tablespoons water
1	tablespoon glucose syrup
2	tablespoons orange juice
½	teaspoon grated orange zest (optional)

Spread the melon and strawberries in a single layer in a baking dish. Cover and freeze overnight.

In a small saucepan, mix the sugar, water and glucose syrup. Cover and bring to the boil over medium-high heat. Uncover and simmer for 3 to 4 minutes. Allow to cool, then pour into a jug and stir in the orange juice and orange zest (if using). Chill 30 minutes or overnight.

Combine the frozen fruit and the cold syrup in a food processor. Pulse until the mixture is smooth, stopping often to scrape down the sides. Serve immediately or transfer to a freezer container, cover, and freeze for up to 1 week.

Makes 6 servings

Per serving: 80 calories/334 kJ, 1 g protein, 20 g carbohydrate (of which sugars 19 g), 0.5 g fat (of which saturates 0 g), 1 g dietary fibre, 12 mg sodium

Pumpkin Pudding

Pumpkin is very important when it comes to nutrition: it contains phytosterols, which help to block bad cholesterol; it's high in zinc, an important cancer-preventing mineral; and it contains beta-carotene, an infection fighter. You won't be thinking about any of that, though, when you taste this rich and decadent pudding.

1.2 l (2 pt)	**vanilla soya milk**
30 g (1 oz)	**arrowroot**
750 g (1lb 10 oz)	**tinned pumpkin or pumpkin pie filling or same weight fresh pumpkin, lightly cooked**
250 g (9 oz)	**maple syrup**
1	**teaspoon ground cinnamon**
½	**teaspoon ground allspice**
⅛	**teaspoon salt**
1	**teaspoon vanilla extract**

Preheat the oven to 180°C/350°F/gas 4. In a large bowl, mix the milk, arrowroot, pumpkin, maple syrup, cinnamon, allspice, salt and vanilla until well-combined. Pour into a 23 x 33 cm (9 x 13 in) baking dish.

Place the baking dish into a large roasting tin. Add 2.5 cm (1 in) of hot water to the roasting tin.

Bake for about 1 hour and 15 minutes. The pudding will appear soft. Remove the baking dish from the water-filled tin. Cool at room temperature. Serve at room temperature or chilled.

MAKES 8 SERVINGS

Per serving: 178 calories/744 kJ, 8 g protein, 32 g carbohydrate (of which sugars 31 g), 3 g fat (of which saturates 0.5 g), 1 g dietary fibre, 225 mg sodium

Plum-Blueberry Clafoutis

This scrumptious dessert proves that even sweet treats can help you give your body the nutrients it needs. Furthermore, whereas many desserts have 500 calories or even more per serving, this clafoutis has only 194 calories per serving.

8	plums, quartered
300 g (10½ oz)	fresh or frozen blueberries
145 g (5 oz)	sugar
2	tablespoons + 115 g (4 oz) plain flour
¾	teaspoon baking powder
⅛	teaspoon salt
125 ml (4 fl oz)	buttermilk
1	egg white, lightly beaten
1½	tablespoons vegetable oil

Preheat the oven to 190°C/375°F/gas 5. Coat a 20 x 20 cm (8 x 8 in) baking dish with cooking spray.

In a large bowl, combine the plums, the blueberries, 115 g (4 oz) of the sugar and 2 tablespoons of the flour. Pour into the prepared baking dish.

In a medium bowl, combine 3 teaspoons of the remaining sugar, the baking powder, the salt and the remaining 115 g (4 oz) flour.

In a small bowl, combine the buttermilk, egg white and oil. Pour into the bowl with the flour mixture. Stir until a thick batter forms. Drop the batter in tablespoonfuls on top of the fruit. Sprinkle with the remaining sugar.

Bake for 35 to 40 minutes, or until the top is golden and bubbly. Remove to a rack to cool. Serve warm or at room temperature.

MAKES 8 SERVINGS

Per serving: *194 calories/810 kJ, 4 g protein, 40 g carbohydrate (of which sugars 23 g), 4 g fat (of which saturates 1 g), 4 g dietary fibre, 117 mg sodium*

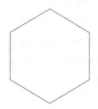

SUPER-IMMUNITY INGREDIENTS

MOST OF THE INGREDIENTS THAT FOSTER A FIRST-CLASS IMMUNE system can be found in any supermarket. Copy this list and take it with you every time you go shopping. Forage in the fresh produce area first.

Select several items from each of the categories below. Even though broccoli and carrots are excellent immune system boosters, eating just those two vegetables can get boring. Each week, try a new food and tick it off on this list.

Work your way around the shop. Detour from the list, of course, to pick up tins of tomatoes and a variety of tinned beans, a box of brown rice, a bottle of olive oil, some frozen vegetables and a package or two of frozen berry fruits.

Research shows that more variety in your diet means a healthier immune system and less disease. A study of more than 42,000 women screened for breast cancer found that there were fewer deaths from all causes among women who ate the greatest variety of foods than among those who ate the least variety.

In most of the categories below, we've listed plenty of examples to show the vast array of different flavours. Most members of each food family possess similar nutritional properties.

- Cruciferous vegetables: broccoli, brussels sprouts, cabbage, cauliflower, kohlrabi, mustard greens, pak choi, radishes, rutabagas, savoy cabbage, spring greens, turnips, watercress

- Onion family: chives, garlic, leeks, onions (red and yellow onions have more phytochemicals; white have the least), shallots, spring onions

- Dark green leafy vegetables: fresh and cooked spinach, kale, Swiss chard

- Fresh salad greens: chervil, coriander, dandelion leaves, escarole, frisée, lamb's lettuce, lettuce of all kinds, green and red, radicchio, rocket, ruby Swiss chard, parsley (curly leaf and flat-leaf), sorrel

- Carotenoid-rich fruits and vegetables: apricots, broccoli, carrots, deep orange or red citrus fruits, pumpkins, squashes of all kinds, sweet potatoes, spinach

- Peppers: peppers of all colours, chilli peppers

- Tomatoes and tomato products: ketchup, tomatoes, tomato sauce, tomato purée, tomato soup, tomatoes of all kinds

- Mushrooms: enoki, maitake, red reishi, shiitake, zhu ling

- Other vegetables: asparagus, beetroot, courgettes, green beans of all kinds, peas, okra, parsnips, potatoes, sweetcorn

- Non-citrus fruits: apples, cherries, figs, fruit juices, grapes, peaches, pears, plums

- Citrus fruits: clementines, grapefruit (both pink and white), kumquats, lemons, limes, oranges, orange or grapefruit or other citrus juices, pomelos, satsumas, tangerines, ugli fruit

- Tropical fruit: avocados, bananas, guavas, kiwi fruit, mangoes, papayas, passion fruit, pineapple, star fruit

- Melons: cantaloupes, Charentais, honeydews, watermelons

- Berries: blackberries, blueberries, cranberries, cranberry juice, elderberries, gooseberries, loganberries, mulberries, raspberries, strawberries

- Pulses: canned beans of all sorts are available; try adzuki beans, black beans, black-eyed peas, broad beans, butter beans, cannellini beans, chickpeas, flageolets, haricot beans, kidney beans, lentils, soya beans, split peas

• Baked or grilled fish and shellfish: mackerel, steamed lobster, oysters, rainbow trout, fresh or tinned salmon (not smoked), sardines, squid, fresh tuna, tuna packed in water

• Turkey or chicken, baked or stewed

• Lean meat

• Eggs

• Yoghurt and vitamin D–fortified dairy products such as skimmed and semi-skimmed milk

• Wholemeal products and other whole-grain products; barley, bulgur wheat, millet, oats, oat bran, quinoa, brown rice, wheat germ, cracked wheat, buckwheat and kasha; also try dark breads such as whole wheat, rye, or pumpernickel

• Cornbread, polenta, tortillas

• High-fibre cereals, such as bran flakes or muesli; porridge

• Nuts: almonds, Brazil nuts, chestnuts, hazelnuts, peanuts, walnuts, nut butters such as peanut butter

• Seeds: poppy, pumpkin, sesame, sunflower

• Ground flaxseed

• Grape juice, red wine

• Teas: black tea, green tea, and a type of black tea/green tea mix called semifermented oolong tea

• Spices and condiments: basil, cumin, garlic, ginger, nutmeg, black pepper, saffron, turmeric, wasabi (Japanese horseradish)

• Olive oil, especially extra-virgin

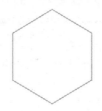

IMMUNE-BUSTING FOODS TO AVOID

W‌HEN YOU'RE RUSHED TO PREPARE DINNER FOR YOUR HUNGRY family or you're out with your friends having a good time, it's difficult to make tasty *and* healthy choices for immune power. This list is a way to start. From the left–hand column, select a few items that you eat often. This week, try the option in the right-hand column for those items. Your immunity diamond will gleam brighter.

WHEN YOU'RE SHOPPING AND COOKING . . .

INSTEAD OF:	CHOOSE:
Any old ready-to-eat-cereal	A cereal that supplies at least 7 g of fibre per serving
Bread made with white flour	Bread with wholemeal flour. If you don't like wholemeal bread, drizzle honey over toast, or spread with peanut butter.
Cream crackers	Whole-grain crispbreads such as rye crispbread, wholemeal crackers and popcorn.

WHEN YOU'RE SHOPPING AND COOKING . . . (CONT.)

INSTEAD OF:	CHOOSE:
Iceberg lettuce	Cos lettuce, escarole, endive, fresh spinach, watercress
Items with partially hydrogenated oil or hydrogenated oil	Your own home-baked biscuits, cakes and pies. And when you do buy shop-bought goodies, read the labels to find ingredients that are not hydrogenated.
Low-fat or fat-free foods	Foods with fewer calories overall. Check the label because sugars are often added to make up for lost flavour in low- or no-fat foods.
Quick/instant pasta or rice	Bulgur (cracked, partly cooked wheat kernels that are mixes in a packet ready in 15minutes). You can also try wheat berries (whole wheat kernels), kasha (whole buckwheat), Kashi (a mix of whole grains), or quinoa (a high-protein South American grain).
White rice	Brown rice or wild rice. If the package just says 'rice' or even 'enriched rice', it's naked rice that has lost its nice coat of bran and its precious rice germ. If you think it takes too long to cook brown rice, cook a big batch on Tuesday and put half of it in the fridge for dinner on Thursday.
White flour, white pasta, white bread	Products whose labels contain the magic word *whole* as in *wholemeal* or *whole grain*. 'Wheat flour' doesn't cut it. That's just white wheat flour. Same goes for pasta: find wholewheat pasta. Many supermarkets carry one or two kinds of wholewheat pasta or you could try buckwheat noodles for a change.
Wrinkling your nose at vegetables and passing them by	A little butter, olive oil, balsamic vinegar, lemon or lime or sugar added to vegetables. Or mix a vegetable you love with one you like less. Do whatever it takes to eat them, except deep-frying.
Avoiding breakfast	Cool juice or fresh fruit to surprise your stomach, and crisp, cold cereal with semi-skimmed milk. No time? Pop a slice of wholemeal bread in the toaster. Pour juice into a glass – that's all you need for a serving. As soon as your toast pops up, you can be out of the door. Also try peanut butter or a fruit spread on your toast, or a handful of pretzels, a smoothie made with several different kinds of fruit or a yoghurt.

INSTEAD OF:	CHOOSE:
Fast food hamburgers (made from meat from dozens of cows)	A piece of beef that the butcher will mince for you – or buy a mincer and mince it yourself. Freeze meat for future use.
Mayonnaise or butter on your sandwich	Mustard or barbecue sauce to moisten your bread and spice up the sandwich. Or use a trans-free margarine,one which actually lowers cholesterol.
Using sunflower, safflower, corn and soya bean oils exclusively, which means that you're getting an imbalance of omega-6 fatty acids to omega-3 fatty acids	Two servings of freshwater fish a week. Also, avoid processed foods. Cut down on all fats, and switch to olive oil and rapeseed oil whenever possible.
A nightcap	A cup of soothing herb tea

WHEN YOU'RE DINING OUT, OR AT THE BAR . . .

INSTEAD OF:	CHOOSE:
A fat, juicy steak	A 3- or 4-ounce portion of beef that has less fat, such as rump or sirloin. Trim off any fat. Or order pork tenderloin or leg of lamb. A 3-ounce serving of meat is about as big as a computer mouse or a pack of cards. A hundred years ago, people got half of their protein from plants. Now, we get only 30 per cent from plants. Buck the trend and choose more pulses and grains to supply your protein needs.
Double cheese on your pizza	The vegetarian pizza or a pizza marinara
Refried beans in that wonderful little Mexican restaurant	Another dish. Skip refried beans when dining out; enjoy them at home, made from tinned refried beans in an oil that is not hydrogenated or partially hydrogenated. Some brands of refried beans are fat-free.
Your favourite greasy spoon's special (often a special Immune Buster!)	Stock-based soups; a small hamburger; a large salad with dressing on the side; a turkey, chicken, roast beef, or ham sandwich on wholemeal bread with lettuce and tomato
Being a member of the Clean Plate Club	To divide your portion before you dig in if you are served a very large portion. Take the other half home for a meal the next day.

WHEN YOU'RE DINING OUT, OR AT THE BAR . . .(CONT.)

INSTEAD OF:	CHOOSE:
Crisps	Peanuts. They do, of course, have lots of calories, but they also have healthy monounsaturated fatty acids. Just be sure to eat a handful rather than an entire bowlful.
That second, third or fourth twist, or a drink, or 'one last drink'	A non-alcoholic beer, a mineral water with a glass of juice on the rocks

ADDITIONAL RESOURCES: AGENCIES, ASSOCIATIONS, ORGANISATIONS AND THEIR WEBSITES

THE FOLLOWING IS A LIST OF SOME ORGANISATIONS AND THEIR websites, which will give you more information about a specific immune-related condition or an immune-boosting technique. Some of these organisations may be able to put you in touch with a support group for individuals who have an immune-related condition, and their family and friends.

Acupuncture

British Acupuncture Council
Park House
206–208 Latimer Road
London W10 6RE
Tel: 020 8964 0222
www.acupuncture.org.uk

Australian Acupuncture and Chinese Medicine Association
PO Box 5142 West End
QLD 4101
www.acupuncture.org.au

Allergies and Asthma

Anaphylaxis Campaign
PO Box 149
Fleet
Hampshire
Tel: 01252 542029
www.anaphylaxis.org.uk

British Allergy Foundation
30 Bellgrove Road
Welling
Kent DA16 3PY
Tel: 020 8303 8525
www.allergyfoundation.com

Australian Society of Clinical Immunology and Allergy
PO Box 450

Balgowah
NSW 2093
Tel: 8900 6402
www.allergy.org.au

National Asthma Campaign
Providence House
Providence Place
London N1 0NT
Tel: 020 7226 2260
www.asthma.org.uk

National Asthma Campaign, Australia
Level 1, 1 Palmerston Crescent
South Melbourne
VIC 3205
Tel: 03 9214 1476
www.nationalasthma.org.au

Arthritis

Arthritis Research Campaign
Copeman House
St Mary's Court
St Mary's Gate
Chesterfield
Derbyshire S41 7TD
Tel: 01246 558033
www.arc.org.uk

Arthritis Foundation Australia
GPO Box 121
Sydney
NSW 2001

Tel: 02 9552 6058
www.arthritisfoundation.com.au

Autoimmune Diseases

Lupus UK
1 Eastern Road
Romford
Essex RM1 3NH
Tel: 01708 731251
www.uklupus.co.uk

Lupus Australia
PO Box 974
Kenmore
QLD 4069
Tel: 07 3878 9553
www.lupus.com.au

Multiple Sclerosis Society
25 Effie Road
London SW6 1EE
Tel: 020 7610 7171
www.mssociety.org.uk

MS Society of Australia
Suite 503, Level 5
157 Walker Street
Sydney
NSW 2060
Tel: 02 9955 0700
www.msaustralia.org.au

Raynaud's and Scleroderma Association
112 Crewe Road

Alsager
Cheshire ST7 2JA
Tel: 01270 872776
www.raynauds.demon.co.uk

Scleroderma Australia
St Vincent's Hospital
2nd Floor, Daly Wing West
41 Victoria Parade
Fitzroy
VIC 3065
Tel: 03 9288 3651
www.scloz.org

British Sjögren's Syndrome Association
Unit 1
Manor Workshops
West End
Nailsea
Bristol BS19 2DD
Tel: 01275 854215
www.ourworld.compuserve.com/home-pages/bssassociation

National Association for Colitis and Crohn's Disease
4 Beaumont House
Sutton Road
St Albans
Herts AL1 5HH
Tel: 01727 844296
www.nacc.org.uk

Australian Crohn's and Colitis Association
13/96 Manchester Road
PO Box 201

Mooroolbank
VIC 3138
Tel: 03 9726 9008
www.acca.org.au

Thyroid UK
32 Darcy Road
St Ostyth
Clacton-on-Sea
Essex CO16 8QF
www.thyroiduk.org

Thyroid Australia Ltd
PO Box 2575
Fitzroy Delivery Centre
VIC 3065
www.thyroid.org.au

Cancer

Macmillan Cancer Relief
15-19 Britten Street
London SW3 3TZ
Tel: 020 7351 7811
www.macmillan.org.uk

Cancer Research Campaign
10 Cambridge Terrace
London NW1 4JL
Tel: 020 7224 1333
www.crc.org.uk

The Cancer Council Australia
GPO Box 4708
Sydney
NSW 2001

Tel: 02 9380 9022
www.cancer.org.au

Diabetes

British Diabetic Association
10 Queen Anne Street
London W1M 0BD
Tel: 020 7323 1531
www.diabetes.org.uk

Diabetes Australia
218 Northbourne Avenue
Braddon
ACT 2600
Tel: 02 6230 1155
www.diabetesaustralia.com.au

Herbal Medicine

National Institute of Medical
Herbalists
56 Longbrook Street
Exeter EX4 6AH
Tel: 01392 426022
www.nimh.org.uk

National Herbalists Association of
Australia
Suite 305
PO Box 61
BST House
Broadway
NSW 2007
Tel: 02 9211 6472
www.nhaa.org.au

HIV/AIDS

Terence Higgins Trust
52-54 Grays Inn Road
London WC1X 8JU
Tel: 020 7831 0330
www.tht.org.uk

Australian Federation of AIDS
Organizations
PO Box 876
Darlinghurst
NSW 1300
www.afao.org.au

Holistic Medicine

British Complementary Medicine
Association
249 Fosse Road
Leicester LE3 1AE
www.bcma.co.uk

Institute for Complementary
Medicine
PO Box 194
London SE16 1QZ
www.icmedicine.co.uk

Australian Complementary
Health Association
247 Flinders Lane
Melbourne
VIC 3000
Tel: 03 9650 5327
www.diversity.org.au

Homeopathy

British Homeopathic Association
27a Devonshire Street
London W1N 1RJ
Tel: 020 7935 2163
www.trusthomeopathy.org

Society of Homeopaths
2 Artizan Road
Northampton NN1 4HU
Tel: 01604 621400
www.homeopathy-soh.org

Australian Homeopathic Association
PO Box 396
Drummoyne
NSW 2047
www.homeopathyoz.org

Massage

British Massage Therapy Council
Greenbank House
65a Adelphi Street
Preston PR1 7BH
Tel: 01772 881063
www.bmtc.co.uk

Massage Association of Australia
PO Box 501
Canberra
ACT 3124
Tel: 03 9885 7631
www.maa.or.au

ME and Fibromyalgia

ME Association
4 Top Angel
Buckingham Industrial Park
Buckingham MK18 1TH
Tel: 01280 816115
www.meassociation.org.uk

National ME/CFS Association of
Australia
23 Livingstone Close
Burwood
VIC 3125
Tel: 03 9888 8991
www.mecfs.org.au

Fibromyalgia Association UK
PO Box 206
Stourbridge DY9 8LY
Tel: 0870 220 1232
www.ukfibromyalgia.com

Music Therapy

Association of Professional Music
Therapists
26 Hamlyn Road
Glastonbury
BA6 8HT
Tel: 01458 834919
www.apmt.org.uk

Australian Music Therapy
Association Inc.
PO Box 79
Turramurra
NSW 2074
Tel: 02 9449 5279
www.austmta.org.au

Radon Testing

UK Department of the
Environment, Food and
Rural Affairs
www.defra.gov.uk

Australian Department of Health
and Ageing
www.health.gov.au

Sexually Transmitted Diseases

UK Health Education Authority
www.playingsafely.co.uk

Australian Department of Health
www.health.gov.au

Sleep

British Snoring and Sleep Apnoea
Association
1 Duncroft Close
Reigate
Surrey RH2 9DE
Tel: 01249 701010
www.britishsnoring.demon.co.uk

Australian Sleep Association
GPO Box 295
Sydney
NSW 1043
www.sleepaus.on.net

Water Treatment

UK Department of the Environment, Food and Rural Affairs
www.defra.gov.uk

Water Services Association of
Australia
www.wsaa.asn.au

Yoga

The British Wheel of Yoga
1 Hamilton Place
Boston Road
Sleaford NG34 7ES
Tel: 01529 306851
www.bwy.org.uk

Australian Institute of Yoga
7/71 Ormond Road
Elwood
VIC 3184
Tel: 03 9525 6951
www.hotkey.net.au

SAFE USE GUIDELINES FOR SUPPLEMENTS, ESSENTIAL OILS AND HERBS

RESEARCHERS AND SPECIALISTS IN NATURAL MEDICINE CAUTION that you should use any supplement responsibly. Foremost, if you are under a doctor's care for any health condition or are taking any medication, do not take any supplement without informing your doctor. Certain natural substances can change the way your body absorbs and processes certain medications. Also, if you are pregnant, do not self-treat with any natural remedy without the consent of your doctor or midwife. The same goes for breastfeeding mothers and women trying to conceive.

Every product has the potential to cause adverse reactions. Below are precautions for the supplements mentioned in this book that may be more likely than others to cause adverse reactions in some people. Do not exceed the recommended dosages – more is *not* better.

By familiarising yourself with this list, you can enjoy the world of natural healing and use this book with confidence.

Supplements

Reports of adverse effects from supplements are rare, especially when compared with prescription drugs, and some supplement manufacturers provide information on labels about reasonably safe recommended dosages for healthy individuals. Be aware that the potency and dosing strategy can vary significantly among products.

You should note, however, that little scientific research exists to assess the safety or long-term effects of many emerging supplements, and some supplements can complicate existing conditions or cause allergic reactions in some people. For these reasons, you should always check with your doctor before taking any supplement.

We recommend that you take supplements with food for best absorption and to avoid stomach irritation, unless otherwise directed. Never take them as a substitute for a healthy diet, since they do not provide all the nutritional benefits of whole foods.

If you are pregnant, breastfeeding or attempting to conceive, do not supplement without the supervision of a doctor.

SUPPLEMENT	SAFE USE GUIDELINES AND POSSIBLE SIDE EFFECTS
Acidophilus	If you have any serious gastrointestinal problems that require medical attention, check with your doctor before supplementing. Amounts exceeding 10 billion viable *Lactobacillus acidophilus* organisms daily may cause mild gastrointestinal distress. If you are taking antibiotics, take them at least 2 hours before supplementing.
Co-enzyme Q$_{10}$	Discuss supplementation with your doctor if you are taking the blood thinner warfarin (Marevan). On rare occasions, CoQ$_{10}$ may reduce warfarin's effectiveness. Supplementation should be observed by a knowledgeable naturopathic or medical doctor if taken for more than 20 days at levels of 120 mg a day or higher. Side effects are rare but may include heartburn, nausea, or stomach ache, which can be prevented by consuming the supplement with a meal.
Curcumin	May cause heartburn in some people

SUPPLEMENT	SAFE USE GUIDELINES AND POSSIBLE SIDE EFFECTS
Fish oil (omega-3 fatty acids, omega-6 fatty acids, eicosapentaenoic acid [EPA], and docosahexaenoic acid [DHA])	Do not take if any of the following apply to you: a bleeding disorder, uncontrolled high blood pressure, anticoagulants (blood thinners) or regular aspirin use, allergy to any kind of fish. People with diabetes should not take fish oil because of its high fat content. Increases bleeding time, possibly resulting in nosebleeds and easy bruising, and may cause upset stomach. Take fish oil, not fish-liver oil, because fish-liver oil is high in vitamins A and D – toxic in high amounts.
Glucosamine	May cause upset stomach, heartburn, or diarrhoea
Glutamine	If you have problems with your kidneys or liver, check with your doctor before supplementing.
Omega-3 fatty acids	In some people, doses as low as 2 g may reduce blood clotting ability, resulting in bleeding or, in extreme instances, leading to haemorrhages.
Propolis, bee	Do not take if you have asthma; contains allergens that can worsen asthma. May also cause a rash when handled
Quercetin (bioflavonoid)	Doses above 100 mg may dilate blood vessels and cause blood thinning in some people. Should be avoided by individuals who are at risk for low blood pressure or who have problems with blood clotting

Essential Oils

Essential oils are inhaled or applied topically to the skin. With few exceptions, they are never taken internally.

Of the most common essential oils, lavender, tea tree, lemon, sandalwood and rose can be used undiluted. The rest should be diluted in a carrier base, which can be an oil (such as almond), a cream or a gel, before being applied to the skin.

Many essential oils may cause irritation or allergic reactions in people with sensitive skin. Before applying any new oil to your skin, always carry out a patch test. Put a few drops of the essential oil, mixed with the carrier, on the back of your wrist and wait for an hour or more. If irritation or redness occurs, wash the area with cold water. In the future, use half the amount of essential oil or avoid it altogether.

Do not use essential oils at home for serious medical problems. During pregnancy, do not use essential oils unless they're approved by your doctor.

Some essential oils (such as lavender and Roman camomile) can safely be used in a vaporiser for the benefit of children and even babies. Do not add to bathwater or use directly on a child's skin.

Store essential oils in dark bottles, away from light and heat and out of the reach of children and pets.

ESSENTIAL OIL	SAFE USE GUIDELINES AND POSSIBLE SIDE EFFECTS
Basil *(Ocimum basilicum)*	Do not use while breastfeeding or over extended periods of time. Do not use more than 3 drops in the bath.
Cajeput *(Melaleuca cajeputi)*	Do not use more than 3 drops in the bath.
Clary sage *(Salvia sclarea)*	Do not use when drinking alcohol because it can cause lethargy and exaggerate drunkenness.
Eucalyptus *(Eucalyptus globulus)*	Do not use for more than 2 weeks without the guidance of a qualified practitioner. Do not use more than 3 drops in the bath. Do not use at the same time as homeopathic remedies.
Hyssop *(Hyssopus officinalis)*	Do not use for more than 2 weeks without the guidance of a qualified practitioner because of toxicity levels. Do not use if you have hypertension. Do not use if you have epilepsy, due to the powerful action on the nervous system.
Lavender (true) *(Lavandula angustifolia)*	Safe. Can be used undiluted, but keep it away from your eyes.

Herbs

While herbs are generally safe and cause few, if any, side effects, you should use them responsibly. Foremost, if you are under a doctor's care for any health condition or are taking any medication, don't take any herb without informing your doctor. Certain natural substances can change the way your body absorbs and processes certain medications. Also, if you are pregnant, do not self-treat with any herb without the consent of your doctor or midwife. The same applies to breastfeeding mothers and women trying to conceive.

Every product has the potential to cause adverse reactions. Below are precautions for the herbs mentioned in this book that may be more likely than others to cause adverse reactions in some people. Though such occurrences are rare, you should be aware of what they are and discontinue use of the herb if you experience an unusual reaction. Also, do not exceed the recommended dosages: more is *not* better.

HERB	SAFE USE GUIDELINES AND POSSIBLE SIDE EFFECTS
Aloe *(Aloe vera)*	May delay wound healing; do not use gel externally on any surgical incision. Do not ingest the dried leaf gel, as it is a habit-forming laxative.
Birch tea *(Betula spp.)*	Do not take birch bark if you need to avoid aspirin because its active ingredient, salicin, is related to aspirin.
Borage seed oil *(Borago officinalis)*	Safe. For external use only. Long-term use is not recommended.
California poppy *(Eschscholzia californica)*	Do not use with antidepressant MAO-inhibitor drugs such as phenelzine (Nardil) and tranylcypromine (Parnate) unless under medical supervision.
Camomile *(Matricaria recutita)*	Very rarely can cause an allergic reaction when ingested. People allergic to closely related plants such as ragweed, asters and chrysanthemums should drink the tea with caution.
Chasteberry (also known as vitex) *(Vitex agnus-castus)*	May counteract the effectiveness of birth control pills.
Echinacea *(Echinacea, various spp.)*	Do not use if allergic to closely related plants such ragweed, asters and chrysanthemums. Do not use if you have tuberculosis or an autoimmune condition such as lupus or multiple sclerosis because echinacea stimulates the immune system.
Elderberry extract *(Sambucus canadensis)*	Seeds, bark, leaves and unripe fruit can cause vomiting or severe diarrhoea.
(S. nigra)	Unripe fruit may cause vomiting.
Flaxseed *(Linum usitatissimum)*	Do not take if you have a bowel obstruction. Take with at least 240 ml (8 fl oz) of water. *(Note:* This precaution pertains to flaxseed only. Flaxseed oil is considered safe.)
Garlic *(Allium sativum)*	Do not use supplements if you're on anticoagulants or before undergoing surgery because garlic thins the blood and may increase bleeding. Do not use if you're taking drugs to lower your blood sugar.

HERB	SAFE USE GUIDELINES AND POSSIBLE SIDE EFFECTS
Ginger *(Zingiber officinale)*	May increase bile secretion. If you have gallstones, do not use therapeutic amounts of the dried root or powder without guidance from a healthcare practitioner.
Ginkgo *(Ginkgo biloba)*	Do not use with antidepressant MAO-inhibitor drugs such as phenelzine (Nardil) or tranylcypromine (Parnate); with aspirin or other nonsteroidal anti-inflammatory medications; or with blood-thinning medications such as warfarin (Marevan). Can cause dermatitis, diarrhoea and vomiting in doses higher than 240 mg of concentrated extract.
Ginseng, American *(Panax quinquefolius)* **and Korean** *(P. ginseng)*	May cause irritability if taken with caffeine or other stimulants. Do not take if you have high blood pressure.
Ginseng, Siberian *(Eleutherococcus senitcosus)*	Safe. This is not a true ginseng.
Goldenseal *(Hydrastis canadensis)*	Do not use if you have high blood pressure.
Hawthorn *(Crataegus oxycantha;* *C. laevigata;* *C. monogyna)*	If you have a cardiovascular condition, do not take hawthorn regularly for more than a few weeks without medical supervision. You may require lower doses of other medications, such as high blood pressure drugs. If you have low blood pressure caused by heart valve problems, do not use without medical supervision.
Hops *(Humulus lupulus)*	Do not take if prone to depression. Rarely, it can cause skin rash, so handle fresh or dried hops carefully.
Jewelweed *(Impatiens capensis)*	Do not use internally without the guidance of a qualified practitioner.
Licorice root *(Glycyrrhiza glabra)*	Do not use if you have diabetes, high blood pressure, liver or kidney disorders or low potassium levels. Do not use daily for more than 4 to 6 weeks because overuse can lead to water retention, high blood pressure caused by potassium loss, or impaired heart and kidney function.
Lomatium *(Lomatium dissectum)*	May cause skin rashes when used internally.
Nettle *(Urtica dioica)*	If you have allergies, your symptoms may worsen, so take only one dose a day for the first few days.
Parsley tea *(Petroselinum crispum)*	Do not use if you have kidney disease, because it increases urine flow when used in therapeutic amounts. Safe as a garnish or ingredient in food.

HERB	SAFE USE GUIDELINES AND POSSIBLE SIDE EFFECTS
Reishi mushroom *(Ganoderma lucidum)*	Rarely, can cause dry mouth or stomach upset when used for more than 3 months.
St. John's wort *(Hypericum perforatum)*	Do not use with antidepressants or other prescription medicine without medical approval. May cause photosensitivity. Avoid overexposure to direct sunlight.
Saw palmetto *(Serenoa repens)*	Consult your doctor for proper diagnosis and monitoring before using to treat an enlarged prostate.
Turmeric *(Curcuma domestica)*	Do not use as a home remedy if you have high stomach acid or ulcers, gallstones or bile duct obstruction.
Valerian *(Valeriana officinalis)*	Do not use with sleep-enhancing or mood-regulating medications because it may intensify their effects. May cause heart palpitations and nervousness in sensitive individuals. If such stimulant action occurs, discontinue use.
Yarrow *(Achillea millefolium)*	Rarely, handling flowers can cause skin rash.

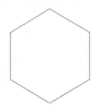

INDEX

*Page references in **bold** type indicate illustrations. <u>Underlined</u> references indicate boxed text.*

E

Conversion Chart

These equivalents have been slightly rounded to make measuring easier.

VOLUME MEASUREMENTS		WEIGHT MEASUREMENTS		LENGTH MEASUREMENTS	
Metric	*Imperial*	*Metric*	*Imperial*	*Metric*	*Imperial*
1 ml	¼ tsp	30 g	1 oz	0.6 cm	¼ in
2 ml	½ tsp	60 g	2 oz	1.25 cm	½ in
5 ml	1 tsp	115 g	4 oz (¼ lb)	2.5 cm	1 in
15 ml	1 tbsp	145 g	5 oz (⅓ lb)	5 cm	2 in
30 ml	1 fl oz	170 g	6 oz	11 cm	4 in
60 ml	2 fl oz	200 g	7 oz	15 cm	6 in
80 ml	3 fl oz	230 g	8 oz (½ lb)	20 cm	8 in
120 ml	4 fl oz	285 g	10 oz	25 cm	10 in
160 ml	5 fl oz	340 g	12 oz (¾ lb)	30 cm	12 in (1 ft)
180 ml	6 fl oz	400 g	14 oz		
240 ml	8 fl oz	455 g	16 oz (1 lb)		
		1 kg	2.2 lb		

PAN SIZES

Metric	*Imperial*
20 x 4 cm sandwich or cake tin	8 in cake tin
23 x 3.5 cm sandwich or cake tin	9 in cake tin
28 x 18 cm baking tin	11 x 7 in baking tin
32.5 x 23 cm baking tin	13 x 9 in baking tin
38 x 25.5 cm baking tin (Swiss roll tin)	15 x 10 in baking tin
1.5 litre baking dish	1½ quart baking dish
2 litre baking dish	2 qt baking dish
30 x 19cm baking dish	2 qt rectangular baking dish
22 x 4 or 23 x 4 cm pie plate	9 in pie plate
18 or 20 cm springform or loose-bottom cake tin	7 or 8 in springform tin
23 x 13 cm or 2 lb narrow loaf tin or pâté tin	9 x 5 in loaf tin

TEMPERATURES

Centigrade	*Fahrenheit*	*Gas*
60°	140°F	–
70°	160°F	–
80°	180°F	–
105°	225°F	¼
120°	250°F	½
135°	275°F	1
150°	300°F	2
160°	325°F	3
180°	350°F	4
190°	375°F	5
200°	400°F	6
220°	425°F	7
230°	450°F	8
245°	465°F	9
260°	500°F	–

OTHER RODALE BOOKS
AVAILABLE FROM PAN MACMILLAN

1-4050-0667-6	The Green Pharmacy	*Dr James A. Duke*	£14.99
1-4050-0674-9	The Hormone Connection	*Gail Maleskey & Mary Kittel*	£15.99
1-4050-2101-2	8 Minutes in the Morning	*Jorge Cruise*	£12.99
1-4050-0672-2	Pilates for Every Body	*Denise Austin*	£12.99
1-4050-0665-X	Get A Real Food Life	*Janine Whiteson*	£12.99
1-4050-3286-3	Stay Fertile Longer	*Mary Kittel*	£12.99
1-4050-0666-8	Banish Your Belly, Butt & Thighs Forever!	*The Editors of* Prevention *Health Books for Women*	£10.99
1-4050-2097-0	6 Questions that Can Change Your Life	*Dr Joseph Nowinski*	£8.99

All Pan Macmillan titles can be ordered from our website, *www.panmacmillan.com,*
or from your local bookshop and are also available by post from:

Bookpost, PO Box 29, Douglas, Isle of Man IM99 1BQ
Credit cards accepted. For details:
Telephone: 01624 836000
Fax: 01624 670923
E-mail: bookshop@enterprise.net
www.bookpost.co.uk

Free postage and packing in the United Kingdom

Prices shown above were correct at time of going to press.
Pan Macmillan reserve the right to show new retail prices on covers which may differ from
those previously advertised in the text or elsewhere.

For information about buying *Rodale* titles in **Australia**, contact Pan Macmillan Australia.
Tel: 1300 135 113; fax: 1300 135 103; e-mail: *customer.service@macmillan.com.au*;
or visit: *www.panmacmillan.com.au*

For information about buying *Rodale* titles in **New Zealand**, contact Macmillan Publishers
New Zealand Limited. Tel: (09) 414 0356; fax: (09) 414 0352; e-mail: *lyn@macmillan.co.nz*;
or visit: *www.macmillan.co.nz*